UNDERSTANDING AND MANAGING FLUENCY DISORDERS

This accessible book provides an overview of fluency disorders. Written by a team of speech-language pathology researchers and practitioners in India, it examines the concepts of fluency and disfluency with illustrative examples in English and Indian languages.

Understanding and Managing Fluency Disorders gives an overview of current research and evidence-based practice in the context of a theoretical background. Clinical aspects of each fluency disorder are described, and the book outlines assessment protocols and intervention methods. Maruthy and Kelkar address key concepts related to different fluency disorders, including cluttering and acquired neurogenic stuttering. One of the highlights of the book is the chapter dedicated to typical disfluency, which could be of immense use to beginning clinicians who wish to increase the specificity and accuracy of their assessment. Other salient features include case vignettes, activity examples, easy steps to carry out intervention approaches and the added advantage of an ICF perspective, making this a practitioner's guide to management of fluency disorders.

Offering a comprehensive overview of theoretical and clinical aspects of stuttering, cluttering and fluency disorders, this volume will be highly relevant reading for students of fluency disorders and speech and language therapy. It will also provide clinicians and trainees working in the field with up-to-date theoretical and clinical information about assessment and intervention.

Santosh Maruthy, Ph.D., is Professor of Speech Sciences in the Department of Speech-Language Sciences at the All India Institute of Speech and Hearing, Mysore, India. His research focuses on the mechanisms underlying stuttering as well as bilingualism and stuttering, speech science, speech perception and voice disorders in professional voice users.

Pallavi Kelkar, Ph.D., is Associate Professor at the School of Audiology and Speech-Language Pathology, Bharati Vidyapeeth (Deemed to be University), Pune, India. She is also the international representative for India at the International Cluttering Association. Her current body of work includes clinical practice, research and community work in the area of stuttering, cluttering and professional voice.

Understanding and Managing Fluency Disorders

From Theory to Practice

**Edited by Santosh Maruthy
and Pallavi Kelkar**

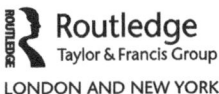
Routledge
Taylor & Francis Group

LONDON AND NEW YORK

Cover image: © Andriy Onufriyenko/Getty Images

First published 2023
by Routledge
4 Park Square, Milton Park, Abingdon, Oxon OX14 4RN

and by Routledge
605 Third Avenue, New York, NY 10158

Routledge is an imprint of the Taylor & Francis Group, an informa business

© 2023 selection and editorial matter, Santosh Maruthy and Pallavi Kelkar; individual chapters, the contributors

The right of Santosh Maruthy and Pallavi Kelkar to be identified as the authors of the editorial material, and of the authors for their individual chapters, has been asserted in accordance with sections 77 and 78 of the Copyright, Designs and Patents Act 1988.

All rights reserved. No part of this book may be reprinted or reproduced or utilised in any form or by any electronic, mechanical, or other means, now known or hereafter invented, including photocopying and recording, or in any information storage or retrieval system, without permission in writing from the publishers.

Trademark notice: Product or corporate names may be trademarks or registered trademarks, and are used only for identification and explanation without intent to infringe.

British Library Cataloguing-in-Publication Data
A catalogue record for this book is available from the British Library

ISBN: 978-1-032-43514-5 (hbk)
ISBN: 978-1-032-43512-1 (pbk)
ISBN: 978-1-003-36767-3 (ebk)

DOI: 10.4324/9781003367673

Typeset in Bembo
by Apex CoVantage, LLC

Contents

Contributors

Amudhu Sankar, Ph.D., is Assistant Professor at Sri Ramachandra Faculty of Audiology and Speech-Language Pathology, SRIHER (DU), Chennai, India. Her areas of work include stuttering and childhood language disorders. She is a Hanen certified speech-language pathologist. Her current research focus is on development of applications for guiding parents of children with stuttering.

Anjana B. Ram, Ph.D., is Assistant Professor in Speech Pathology, Department of Speech-Language Pathology, All India Institute of Speech and Hearing, Mysore. Her areas of interest include stuttering in children, adolescents and adults. Her clinical, research and academic work are in the fields of stuttering, motor speech disorders and autism.

Chanchal Chaudhary is Assistant Professor at the Department of Audiology and Speech-Language Pathology, Kasturba Medical College, Mangalore. She is currently pursuing her Ph.D. in fluency disorders. Her research involves understanding mechanisms underlying stuttering, speech motor learning in stuttering and evidence-based practice in stuttering management.

Divya Seth, Ph.D., is Assistant Professor of Speech-Language Pathology in the Department of Audiology and Speech-Language Pathology at the Kasturba Medical College, Mangalore, India. Her current research focuses on mechanisms underlying stuttering and the intervention of stuttering. Her research interests also include speech science and speech sound disorders.

Gagan Bajaj, Ph.D., is Associate Professor at Kasturba Medical College, Mangalore, Manipal Academy of Higher Education, Karnataka, India. He is passionate about exploring the heterogenous nature of fluency disorders, studying age-linked cognitive communicative changes and applying principles of ICF to communication disorders.

Maya Sanghi served as Assistant Professor at the Audiology and Speech Therapy School, T.N. Medical College, Mumbai, India till 2010 and was an international representative (India) at the International Cluttering Association till 2017. Her present work includes management of individuals with neuro-communication disorders, voice and fluency disorders.

Pallavi Kelkar, Ph.D., is Associate Professor at the School of Audiology and Speech–Language Pathology, Bharati Vidyapeeth (Deemed to be University), Pune, India. She is currently the international representative for India at the International Cluttering Association. Her current body of work includes clinical practice, research and community work in the area of stuttering, cluttering and professional voice.

Santosh Maruthy, Ph.D., is Professor of Speech Sciences in the Department of Speech–Language Sciences at the All India Institute of Speech and Hearing, Mysore, India. His research focuses on the mechanisms underlying stuttering as well as bilingualism and stuttering, speech science, speech perception and voice disorders in professional voice users.

Rakesh Chowkalli Veerabhadrappa, Ph.D., is Assistant Professor in Speech–Language Pathology at Manipal University. He received the prestigious Travers Reid award at the 2021 Oxford Dysfluency Conference, UK. His research focuses on mechanisms underlying stuttering, treatment and emotional issues in stuttering.

Foreword

It gives us immense pleasure and satisfaction to finally be able to put out a go-to book for students and practitioners interested in fluency disorders. *Understanding and Managing Fluency Disorders* is an amalgamation of the experience, expertise and hard work of many academicians, all of them from different parts of India.

For the uninitiated, India is a country synonymous with diversity. Diversity in terms of geographical landscape, languages, religions and cultures is inseparable from the Indian sociocultural fabric. In the present day and age, as technology and accessibility makes the world shrink, students across the globe must keep themselves abreast of how different facets of a disorder vary across countries and cultures. Putting out a book from India to the rest of the world, then, was something we foresaw as a necessity for broadening readers' perspectives on fluency and its disorders.

You will find in this book, numerous examples of this diversity through examples and case vignettes. The case vignettes will also reflect two other features prominently seen among the Indian population. Firstly, the fact that bilingualism or multilingualism is a rule rather than an exception. Secondly, the culture here is predominantly collectivistic or group oriented. While collectivism, on one hand, brings with it strong family support, on the other hand, it also adds to barriers faced by patients in the form of societal pressure to conform or blend in.

Speaking of barriers, another salient feature of this book is the inclusion of an ICF perspective. All the authors of this book have found assessment, intervention and documentation along the lines of the ICF to be extremely useful. This, in our opinion, would aid beginning clinicians of fluency in understanding the multifactorial mosaic that is a fluency disorder. It would help them look at the people behind the disfluencies.

This last task is, in fact, practically very feasible for students in India. With a population which is the second largest in the world, students get abundant exposure to the entire continuum of fluency to disfluency. However, the sheer numbers of cases seen on a daily basis make systematic documentation a difficult task. This comes in the way of gaining a broader insight into the people they see through assessment. To increase the ease and time efficiency of record keeping, therefore, we bring to the readers a detailed protocol for documenting assessment-related information. We have also included a complete impact assessment tool, the ISACS, which is the only tool that can assess impact of stuttering and/or cluttering from two perspectives – that of the person with disfluencies and that of their significant other. It has the added advantage of an indigenous normative, so culture specific impact assessment is finally possible. The systematic record-keeping protocol as well as the ISACS can be found in the Appendices.

We would like to take this opportunity to thank the publishers for giving wings to our ideas and our respective institutes for encouraging us in this endeavour. We thank all the contributing authors for giving us their time, efforts and cooperation in putting this book together. We extend our heartfelt gratitude to those who gave prompt and valuable feedback when we consulted them about some aspect of the book. Most importantly, we can't but thank all the people who visited our clinics and took us a step closer to understanding fluency better. Finally, a special thank you to our parents, in-laws, spouses and above all, our kids, for that little nudge of motivation when meeting deadlines seemed impossible, for their patience and understanding when we spent long hours poring over the manuscript and for smiles at the end of long days that energized us to keep going till the end!

We hope that our efforts translate to positive educational outcomes for students of fluency and consequently for persons with fluency disorders.

Santosh Maruthy, Ph.D.
Pallavi Kelkar, Ph.D.

1 Introduction to fluency and its development

Santosh Maruthy

Introduction

Speech is produced with simultaneous and successive programming of muscular movements. The different dimensions of speech include voice, articulation, fluency and prosody. This chapter mainly aims to define and elaborate on the concept of fluency, different components of speech fluency and prosody. Development of fluency and factors affecting it are also discussed.

What is fluency?

The word "fluency" is derived from Latin word *fluere*, which means "to flow". Based on this root word, anything that involves a smooth flow can be considered as fluent. In the domain of language, fluency may be interchangeably used with proficiency. A person is considered as fluent if he or she is able to speak either the first language (L1) or the second language (L2) rapidly and continuously without any difficulty. Fluency in the written modality could be defined as being able to read or write in a particular language in a smooth, uninterrupted manner. In order to be fluent in a language, then, an individual must gain fluency in each linguistic component; in other words, syntactic fluency, semantic fluency, phonologic fluency and pragmatic fluency. A person is thought to be *phonologically* fluent if they are able to construct long and complicated strings of phonological sequences without any difficulty; *syntactically* fluent if they are able construct highly complex sentences; *semantically* fluent if they possess an ability to access a large vocabulary; and *pragmatically* fluent if they are skilled at speaking at a variety of speaking situations.

Dimensions of fluency

In speech communication, fluency may be defined as effortless continuous speech uttered at a rapid rate (Starkweather, 1987). This definition highlights that fluent speech needs to be uttered continuously, at a rapid rate with a minimal amount of effort. Hence, fluency is a multidimensional behaviour, its domains being continuity, rate and effort. Starkweather (1987) also added speech rhythm as the fourth domain. Each of these dimensions of fluency are discussed briefly below.

DOI: 10.4324/9781003367673-1

Continuity

Continuity refers to smooth flow of speech. It reflects how speech flows from one sound to another in a word, from one word to another in a phrase and from one phrase to another in a sentence. Although ideally fluent speech needs to be devoid of any interruptions, conversational or spontaneous speech is sometimes interrupted by different sets of behaviours, which may break the smooth flow of speech. One kind of speech interruptions that are seen in typically speaking individuals are called as *dis*fluencies. Examples of these behaviours are pauses (filled and unfilled), revisions, parenthetical remarks, multisyllabic word repetitions, etc. The second type of speech interruptions that are majorly seen in individuals who have fluency disorders are referred to in many textbooks as *dys*fluencies. These refer to abnormal motoric breakdowns in speech. For example, repeating a sound or syllable multiple times, prolonging a sound (voiced or voiceless) or uttering a broken word. Individuals with fluency disorders may have *dis*fluencies, that is, the stoppages that are usually seen in typical speakers, along with *dys*fluencies. Some textbooks, on the other hand, use the word "disfluencies" to refer to stoppages of any kind. We would be using the uniform term "disfluencies" in the present text. Further classification of these disfluencies into typical and atypical ones will be discussed in Chapters 2 and 3. A detailed account of different types of disfluencies which are characteristic of typically speaking individuals and persons with fluency disorders is given below.

Pauses

The continuity of fluent speech is often interrupted by filled or unfilled pauses. In case of filled pauses, the utterances used to fill the pause are meaningless or neutral utterances such as "um, uh, am, ah, eh, er, I mean, you know", etc. Unfilled pauses are silences which are longer than 250 milliseconds (Goldman-Eisler, 1958). Clarke (1971) classified these pauses as conventional pauses and idiosyncratic pauses. Conventional pauses are those which a fluent or proficient speaker uses to signal something that is important. For example, if the speaker wants the listener to know that he is coming on *Wednesday* and not on *Monday*, he may pause just before the word Wednesday and Monday. Idiosyncratic pauses are those pauses that are used by less proficient or uncertain speakers who may not be sure of word choice, meaning or the syntax. Conventional pauses help listeners to comprehend a message better. In contrast, idiosyncratic pauses often increase listeners' processing load and could be a barrier to comprehension of messages. Pauses in general occur more often before words that are grammatically loaded, such as nouns, verbs, adjectives and adverbs compared to words which are less grammatically loaded, such as articles, prepositions and conjunctions. Pauses are seen more often in conventional spontaneous speech or conversational speech tasks than during loud reading. Further, pauses are more synchronized with breathing in reading tasks than during conversational tasks. The available evidence also suggests that pauses occur more frequently before words with high uncertainty (Cook, 1971), words which are longer and phonetically complex (Cook et al., 1974), and at the beginning of the clauses rather than within clauses (Boomer, 1970). Frequency and duration of pauses can be documented for both filled and unfilled pauses.

Repetitions

Like pauses, repetitions also interrupt the continuity and forward flow of fluent speech. As its name implies, a repetition involves repeated production of an utterance. A person might repeat a sound, syllable, word or phrase. For example, "p p pen" would be sound repetition, "ca ca camp", a syllable repetition, "ball ball ball", a word repetition, and "I want I want I want coffee", a phrase repetition. Sound and syllable repetitions can be combined under the blanket term "part-word repetitions". Word repetitions can involve monosyllabic words, such as "I I I want coffee" or multisyllabic words, such as "Mohan Mohan Mohan, can you come here?" Frequency of repetitions in speech can be calculated in terms of a percentage. This is done by counting all the repeated syllables/words, dividing the number by the total number of syllables/words and then multiplying the resultant number by 100. For instance, if there are 25 part-word repetitions in a total of 300 words, then $(25/300)^*100 = 8.33\%$. Some researchers also note the total number of repeated units (Ambrose & Yairi, 1999). For instance, the sentence "m m m my name is Jagadeesh" has three repeated units.

False starts/revisions, parenthetical remarks and interjections

When a speaker interrupts the forward flow of speech and restarts or changes the utterance they had originally planned to speak, the result is a false start or a revision (e.g. "This is a blue – a purple bag"). The modification may be in terms of replacing the word with an entire new word as in the previous example or insertion of a word in a word sequence (e.g. "This is a bag – blue bag"). Changes in the grammatical structure of the sentence are also called revisions (e.g. "I will – I shall do it"). False starts or revisions can thus serve as self-repair strategies as well. Parenthetical remarks are words or phrases that are meaningful in nature but not appropriate for the sentence (e.g. "I mean, like, you know, well"). Interjections are the addition of extraneous sounds that are meaningless in nature (e.g. "uh, um"). It may be recalled that these examples (of interjections and parenthetical remarks) were also given while mentioning filled pauses. Interjections and parenthetical remarks are thus, often used to fill pauses when the speaker may not want to remain silent for a long time between two words. These utterances may be repeated by the speaker several times. Similar to repetitions, the frequency of false starts, parenthetical remarks and interjections can also be calculated as a percentage.

Broken words or blocks and prolongations

The next two chapters would get the reader familiarized with stuttering, one of the various fluency disorders. In persons who stutter (PWS), apart from the above-mentioned disfluencies, another common type of speech discontinuity or disfluency is broken words or blocks. Broken words are within-word disfluencies characterized by a break in the smooth flow of speech. These breaks are accompanied by fixed articulatory postures and often a stoppage in the outflow of air that is customary while speaking (e.g. "I am g . . . oing"). In this example, during the production of the /g/ sound the articulator is fixed, which is accompanied by a discontinuity in the flow of air.

Prolongations, in contrast, are characterized by an undue persistence of a speech sound. Only continuants such as vowels, nasals and fricatives are prolonged. During a prolongation of speech sounds, although the articulator is fixed, there will be continuous flow of air or voicing. If there is a flow of air accompanied by voicing, the prolongation is said to be "voiced". A prolongation which involves only the flow of air, but no voicing is a "voiceless" prolongation. Both the frequency and duration of broken words and prolongations can be calculated. For example, if the person who stutters prolongs utterances for 500 milliseconds to 4 seconds, you can calculate the average duration of the prolongation by adding durations of all prolonged instances in the speech sample and then dividing the sum by the number of instances prolonged. The frequency of prolongations and blocks can be calculated in a manner similar to pauses, repetitions, etc.

Rate of speech

Rate of speech or speech rate is the second dimension of fluency. It refers to the speed with which one can speak. Speech rate could be influenced by mood, environment, linguistic structure, a person's age, culture, speed of articulatory movement and co-articulation. As per the definition of fluency (Starkweather, 1987), fluent speech is uttered at a rapid rate. However, speech rate varies continuously based on the situation. Speech rate may be measured in syllables per second, syllables per minute or words per minute. It can be calculated using the formula:

$$\frac{Total\ number\ of\ words\ or\ syllables\ read\ (excluding\ disfluent\ utterances)}{Total\ time\ taken\ to\ read\ the\ passage}$$

Adult speakers whose native language is English, on an average, speak at a rate of 5 to 6 syllables per second (Walker & Black, 1950). If documented in words per minute, normal rates of speech vary between 80–180 words per minute. The upper range of rate can vary between 250 to 280 words per minute if speech is intelligible. Another pertinent measurement in fluency literature and clinical practice is articulation rate (AR). AR is the total number of utterances produced (after removing unfilled pauses and disfluencies) within the time taken only for articulation (devoid of any silences) (Costa et al., 2016, p. 43)

It is given by the formula:

$$\frac{Total\ number\ of\ syllables\ (without\ pauses\ and\ disfluent\ utterances)\ read}{Total\ time\ taken\ to\ read\ the\ passage\ (without\ unfilled\ pauses)}$$

Effort

The third dimension of fluency, effort, could imply muscular or mental effort. Muscular effort refers to the amount of energy spent in the movement of different muscles involved in speech production (respiratory, laryngeal or articulatory). Mental effort refers to the effort involved during the planning of the speech utterances. Fluent speech is considered to be effortless speech, requiring little thought and muscular effort (Starkweather, 1987). Muscular effort may be documented indirectly by measuring action potentials from muscles involved in speech production. However, mental effort is difficult to document. Indirect measures such as reaction time (RT) have been used in some studies to document mental effort.

Rhythm

Rhythm is defined as a pattern of movement that occurs with temporal regularity. Speech might not have as regular a rhythm as music, though it is certainly rhythmic in nature. Rhythm enables speakers to divide an utterance into phrases while speaking and provides them some respite from continuous production of utterances. From the point of view of the listener, rhythm is an essential component to facilitate speech intelligibility. Languages characteristically differ with regard to rhythm. There are three types of languages based on the rhythm: Stress-timed languages (English, French), syllable-timed languages (Hindi, Telugu) and mora-timed languages (Japanese) (Pike, 1945).

The concept of a mora

To understand this better, the beginning student of fluency needs to know concepts such as syllables and mora. In simple terms, a word is divided into syllables, and syllables are further divisible into mora. For example, the word "cut" is comprised of only one syllable. This syllable has a CVC structure (consonant-vowel-consonant). Each of these components of the syllable is assigned a moraic value. Mora is the unit of syllable weight. The assignment of moraic values to syllables must follow certain predefined rules. For instance, prevocalic consonants do not carry any moraic value. A short or lax vowel has a weight of one mora. Post-vocalic consonants have one mora of weight. Therefore, the weight of the syllable (which, in this case, is also a word) is two moras. Now, imagine if the /t/ at the end did not exist. In that case, this utterance would not mean anything in English. It follows then, that in the English language, an utterance must have at least two moras of weight for it to be meaningful.

Stress-timed languages are those in which stress occurs at regular intervals. Languages in which each syllable takes an equal interval of time to be produced are called syllable-timed languages. Analogous to this, languages in which each mora is produced at the same time interval as the previous and the next are called mora-timed languages.

The metric used for quantification of rhythm in different languages is called the pairwise variability index (PVI). PVI documents rhythm by measuring the variability in successive vocalic and intervocalic intervals (Low, 2006). Normalized pairwise variability index (nPVI) is calculated for vocalic intervals and raw pairwise variability index is calculated for the intervocalic intervals (rPVI). In stress-timed languages both nPVI and rPVI values will be higher. In syllable-timed languages nPVI values will be lower; however, rPVI values will be higher. In mora-timed languages both nPVI and rPVI values will be low. There are no absolute cutoff values for different languages as PVI values will vary depending on the frequency of occurrences of consonants and vowels. Researchers have used PVI measures and classified languages into different categories. Stress-timed languages include English, Dutch, and German. Syllable-timed languages include French and Spanish; and mora-timed languages include Japanese (Grabe & Low, 2002). Savithri et al. (2007) compared Indo-Aryan and Dravidian languages and suggested Assamese, Punjabi, Kannada and Telugu to be mora-timed and Bengali, Malayalam, Tamil and Kashmiri to be syllable-timed languages. Data on PVI values of 60 typically developing Kannada-speaking children suggested that 3–4-year-old children had syllable-timed rhythm, 8–9-year-old and 11–12-year-old children had mora-timed rhythm (Savithri et al., 2010). rPVI values reduced from the younger to the older age group, while no such trend was seen in nPVI values.

The superimposition of a rhythm pattern of a native language on the second language, then, produces what is commonly called a native accent. Therefore, to learn a language in its entirety, a language learner must observe and listen not only to the phonemes (segmentals) of that language, but also to the suprasegmental or prosodic features such as rhythm. As their name suggests, suprasegmental aspects of speech are the nuances that are superimposed on speech utterances. They add to the perceived fluency and meaning of utterances and make speech sound typical to a language or culture. Some other suprasegmental features are discussed in detail below.

Prosody

As mentioned above, prosody adds to language fluency through knowledge of its suprasegmental features and to speech fluency through production of the desired rhythm, and consequently, accent. From the perspective of a student of fluency, therefore, speech that lacks prosody can sound disfluent. One of the aspects of prosody, rhythm, was already discussed under the section on dimensions of fluency. We elaborate on some other prosodic features below.

Stress

Stress can be defined from a listener's as well as from a speaker's perspective. From a listener's perspective, stress can be defined as change in the perceived loudness of a syllable/word in an utterance. For instance, stressed syllables are perceived louder than unstressed syllables. From a speaker's perspective, during the production of stressed syllables, there is greater muscular effort compared to unstressed syllables.

During speech perception, stress helps the listener in the segmentation of a continuous stream of acoustic events into separate units for further processing. At the *syntactical level*, it helps differentiate between sentence types by marking the beginning or end of a phrase. At the *lexical level* it helps identify a verb from a noun (e.g. pre*sent*, which is a verb versus *pres*ent, a noun). At the *pragmatic* level, stress helps clarify the content to the listener (e.g. Are you from Pune? No, I'm from *Kerala*).

In line with its functions, stress can be classified as phonemic stress/word-level stress, morphological stress and sentence-level stress. *In phonemic stress or word-level stress*, the minimum size of the unit of stress placement is the syllable. However, one can identify a syllable as stressed or unstressed only in contrast to another syllable. It follows then that stress on monosyllabic words can be distinguished only in the context of a larger utterance, at least two syllables long. Hence, to identify whether there is stress on a particular syllable or not, at least two syllables are needed. At the word level, if the placement of the stress is not governed by either the lexical, syntactical or the morphological rules of the languages, such stress is termed as free stress. In contrast, some languages involve fixed placement of stress (bound stress) on a certain syllable in a word. In these languages, if the stress placement does not occur on that particular syllable, it could result in a change in the meaning of the word, or the word may become a non-meaningful word. For instance, in the Czech language, speakers stress the first syllable; in Polish, there is stress placement on the penultimate syllable; and in French, the last syllable is stressed. Perceptually one can do four kinds of stress analysis. First, stress is used in place of an unstressed syllable/ word; second, unstressed syllable/word is used in place of a stressed syllable/word; third, there is equal stress on all syllables; and fourth, there is no stress on any syllable.

Stress can also function at the sentence level. In such cases, the meanings of words do not change, but their relative importance in the sentence does. There are three types of sentence-level stress. The first, *primary stress (non-emphatic)*, involves placement of stress on certain syllables or words in the sentence based on the rules of the language. For example, English being a stress-timed language will have stress occurring at regular intervals. The second, *emphatic stress*, refers to stress placement on a particular syllable or word in order to highlight it or lay emphasis on it (e.g. I came by *bus* today). The third type of sentence stress is *contrastive stress*, in which stress on a particular syllable or word occurs in a sequence of phrases or sentences with similar constituents barring one contrasting word or morpheme. Hence, by placing stress on a particular syllable/word, two contrasting elements in successive sentences or phrases can be differentiated (e.g. That book is *blue*, not *yellow*).

Different authors have put forth different cues for perception of stress in different languages. According to Trager and Smith (1951), stress is perceived through changes in loudness. According to Fant (1958) lengthening of syllables is the most obvious physical correlate of stress. Bolinger (1958) considers stress as accent. Thus, for Bolinger (1958), the primary cue of stress is pitch prominence. Lieberman (1960) considers stress as rhythm. It appears that the perceptual cue of stress differs from one language to another. In languages where vowel durations are distinct, an increased vowel duration may be a prominent cue. In languages where vowel duration distinctions are not distinct, pitch or loudness prominence may serve as a cue to

Table 1.1 Review of literature on cues to stress perception

Author	Language	Cues
Fry (1955)	English	Duration, intensity
Fant (1958)	Swedish	Duration
Bolinger (1958)	English	Frequency, duration
Rigault (1962)	French	Frequency, duration
Morton and Jassem (1965)	English	Frequency
Westin et al. (1966)	Swedish	Frequency
Lehiste (1968)	Estonian	Duration
Jassem et al. (1968)	Polish	Frequency
Rehder (1968)	Serbo-Croatian	Frequency
Bertinetto (1980)	Italian	Duration
Balasubramanian (1980)	Tamil	Duration
Savithri (1987, 1999)	Kannada	Duration
Rajupratap (1991)	Kannada	Duration

perception of stress. In general, across different languages, major cues for stress perception include increased durations of vowels, increased pitch and increased loudness. Table 1.1 presents a brief review of findings reported in these studies.

Overall, the findings reveal that acoustically, fundamental frequency, amplitude, phoneme duration and the frequency of the second formant of a phoneme can be measured and compared with the adjacent phoneme to determine which of the two has greater stress placement.

Intonation

Intonation is defined as the fundamental frequency (pitch) variations in phrases, clauses, or sentences in a temporal dimension. Tone refers to the pitch variation at word level. Based on the tonal characteristics or tonality, languages across the world are classified as tone languages, stress accent languages and pitch accent languages. Identification of intonation of a language can be carried out using subjective and/ or objective methods. Irrespective of the method used, the layout of the intonation contour/curve operates within a baseline and top line. These lines represent the pitch levels within which there are pitch excursions constituting the intonation contour as shown in Figure 1.1. The variations in the pitch curve are determined by a combination of various factors, such as the phonetic, phonological and grammatical constituents of an utterance; the attitude of the speaker; the placement of accented syllables in the utterance, etc.

The intonational features of European languages are well reported in literature. In comparison, the information available on intonation in Indian languages is limited. It is observed but not proven that some Indian languages, which have a common origin, for example, Dravidian languages, share some features of intonation, rendering support to a universal theory of intonation. Usually, any language exhibits idiosyncratic features unique to that language. Intonation, in addition, also varies across the dialects of a given language. Thus, analysis of intonation of a language could be

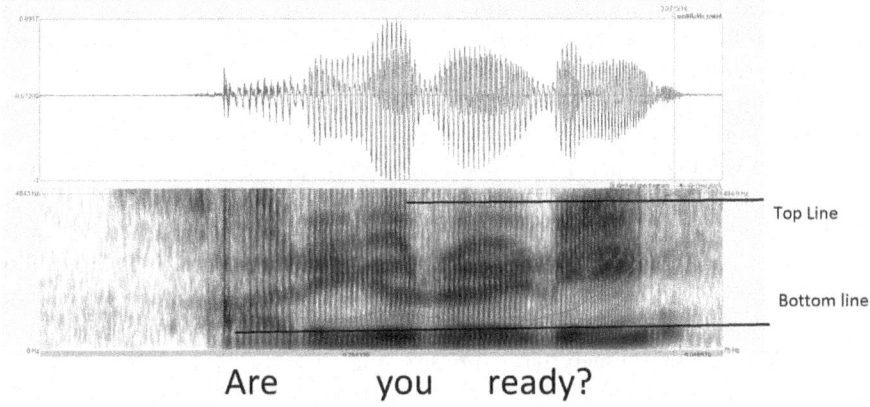

Figure 1.1 An example of an intonational contour

a challenging and complex task. The availability of various instruments for analysis of intonation in the present day makes this task relatively easier. Nonetheless, a lot about the relationship between the intonation curve and the underlying linguistic or segmental constituents is not yet completely understood. Hence a combination of subjective and objective analyses is often recommended as ideal for understanding the intonation patterns of a language.

Why study prosody?

Prosody is an integral aspect of speech fluency. In addition, it also gives a listener cues about the speaker's intent, state of mind and background. For speech output to be fluent, the speaker must possess fluency in the different domains of language and a well-coordinated speech mechanism. However, despite these being present, a listener might not perceive a speaker as fluent if the speaker does not use suprasegmentals appropriate to that language. Such speech would sound unnatural. Students of fluency must therefore be aware of the various aspects of prosody, their variations across languages and their uses and applications. The study of prosody enables the fluency therapist to work towards speech that is continuous as well as natural sounding.

Speech naturalness

Speech naturalness refers to the social acceptance of speech. The need to include speech naturalness as one of the domains of fluency arises from the documented outcomes of some stuttering treatment approaches. Intervention techniques such as prolonged speech therapy and syllable-timed speech have been successful in treating stuttering as will be described in Chapter 6 of this book. However, in individuals who used these therapy approaches, the post-therapeutic speech was found to be unnatural (Onslow, 1996). Martin et al. (1984) developed a standardized speech naturalness rating scale. It is a 9-point scale in which highly unnatural speech is represented at one end with a value of 1, and highly natural sounding speech is represented at the other end with a value of 9. This scale has since been used by many researchers to document changes in speech naturalness in those who stutter. However, a few researchers argued that speech naturalness is a multifaceted variable which imbibes several sub-components, such as stress, intonation, rhythm, articulation and breathing patterns or breath groups. Disruption in any of these variables might affect speech naturalness (Franken et al., 1995). To account for these other variables, Franken et al. (1995) developed a speech quality instrument, which included a speech naturalness scale. This instrument comprised of 14 adjectival pairs descriptive of a person's speech, namely low pitch-high pitch, slow-quick, slovenly-polished, flat-expressive, shrill-deep, soft-loud, monotonous-melodious, tense-relaxed, weak accentuation-strong accent, unpleasant-pleasant, slurred-precise, fluent-halting, weak-powerful and unnatural-natural. The clinician rated each of these 14 pairs on a 7-point bipolar scale in order to give a holistic description of the perceived speech output.

A substantial amount of research has been conducted to investigate speech naturalness in adults who stutter post-treatment (Harrison et al., 1998; Ingham et al., 1989; Ingham & Packman, 1978; Kalinowski et al., 1994; Metz et al., 1990; O'Brian et al., 2003). However, limited literature is available on speech naturalness in children who stutter (Druce et al., 1997; Onslow et al., 1990), especially in the context of pre-therapy and post-therapy comparisons.

In the Indian context, Subramanian (1997) and Kanchan (1997) investigated speech naturalness rating of 40 adults who stutter who underwent non-programmed prolonged speech treatment. Both these studies used binary scales instead of the traditional 9-point scale (Martin et al., 1984) used by previous researchers. These scales incorporated several parameters that are believed to contribute to speech naturalness. Subramanian's (1997) scale included attributes such as confidence, command over language, clarity, speed, continuity, stuttering and an overall rating of speech naturalness. Kanchan's (1997) scale included rate, continuity, effort, stress, intonation, rhythm, articulation, breathing pattern and an overall rating of speech naturalness. Each of these parameters is based on a set criteria where the speech is rated on a binary scale as natural or unnatural. Their results showed a significant increase in mean naturalness scores post-treatment.

Development of fluency

Children's speech is less fluent compared to adults. With an increase in age, children achieve better proficiency in language and speech motor abilities and become increasingly fluent. Understanding the development of speech fluency in typically developing children helps clinicians and parents in differentiating typical disfluencies from disfluencies indicative of stuttering. Most studies elaborating on the development of fluency have investigated fluency development in the English language. However, a few attempts have also been made in other languages. Some studies have tried to compare the nature of disfluencies between children who stutter and children who do not stutter (elaborated in Chapter 2) in an attempt to understand similarities and differences in the two kinds of disfluencies. In other words, these studies have attempted to answer the question as to whether stuttering and typical disfluency lie on the same continuum and vary only in terms of the frequency of disfluencies or whether they are separate disorders.

One of earliest studies to investigate the development of fluency was done by Kowal et al. (1975) who studied the development of disfluencies in 168 typically developing children from kindergarten to the 12th grade. They reported that at a younger age (kindergarten children) a large proportion of the total number of disfluencies were part-word repetitions. Unfilled and filled pauses were noticed more in younger children, and as they grew older, they used more sophisticated types of disfluencies such as parenthetical remarks. However, the overall frequency of disfluencies changed very minimally from kindergarten to the 12th grade. Yairi (1981) studied 33 children, 18 girls and 15 boys ranging in age from 24 and 33 months. Data collected from the children included spontaneous speech samples. The collected speech samples were transcribed, and different types of disfluencies were identified. Results suggested that the frequency of total number of disfluencies varied across the participants. Part-word repetitions, single-syllable word repetitions, interjections and revisions were the major types of disfluencies observed. Further, the number of repetition units were two in a majority of the children. In a subsequent study, Yairi (1982) divided the children into two groups. Subgroup I consisted of 13 younger children in the age range of 24 to 26 months. Subgroup II comprised of older children (10 boys and 10 girls) in the age range of 29 to 33 months. Results showed that although there was an overall decrease in the frequency of disfluencies, the results varied between both subgroups. In children who were in subgroup I, disfluencies increased as age progressed. In contrast, children who were in subgroup II showed a decline in disfluencies during the eight-month period. The author concluded that 2-year-old children should not be treated as a homogenous group in studies of disfluency.

Wexler (1982) studied disfluency characteristics in 36 typically developing males aged 2, 4 and 6 years (12 in each age group). They identified the total frequency of various disfluency types, cluster disfluencies and oscillations (the number of repetitions per instance of disfluency). In a cluster disfluency, there may be more than one type of disfluency in the same disfluent episode. These might be on the same syllable or different syllables in the word. Revisions and incomplete phrases were the most commonly occurring type of disfluencies followed by phrase repetitions and word repetitions. Part-word repetitions were the least occurring types of disfluency types. Furthermore, they compared disfluency types across the different age groups. Results indicated that overall, part-word repetitions and phrase repetitions occurred with a greater frequency in 2-year-old children than 4 or 6-year-old children. Although the frequency of cluster disfluencies and oscillations decreased with age, the results were not statistically significant. DeJoy and Gregory (1985) studied 60 typically developing males aged 3.5 and 5 years of age and found that repetitions, incomplete phrases and disrhythmic phonations declined significantly across younger to older children. Part-word repetitions and disrhythmic phonations significantly discriminated between older and younger children. However, no significant change in the frequency of interjections and ungrammatical pauses indicates that these disfluencies might be seen in the speech of typical adults as well. Brutten and Miller (1988) studied the nature of disfluencies in African-American first grade children. Their results suggested that among the different types of disfluencies, interjections occurred most frequently, and broken words were the least frequently occurring types of disfluencies. Among the different types of repetitions, the frequency of whole-word repetitions was higher compared to the frequency of part-word and phrase repetitions.

In the Indian context, a few unpublished master's theses (Indu, 1990; Nagapoornima, 1990; Rajendraswamy, 1991; Yamini, 1990) involved the study of the development of fluency in different age groups in children who spoke Kannada, a south Indian Dravidian language. This was based on disfluency data of 12 children in the age groups of 3 to 4 years (Nagapoornima, 1990), 4 to 5 years (Indu, 1990), 5 to 6 years (Yamini, 1990) and 6 to 7 years (Rajendraswamy, 1991). The material used for these studies was in the form of simple cartoons and pictures depicting stories of the Panchatantra. A total disfluency of greater than 25% to 30% was considered to be abnormal. This percentage cutoff value was high because unlike other studies where several iterations of sound/syllable are considered as one instance of repetition, the authors in the present study calculated each iteration as one repetition. Rathika et al. (2012) analyzed disfluencies in 48 typically developing 4- to 8-year-old Tamil speaking children. The analysis of disfluencies across age groups suggested that pauses were the most frequently occurring type of disfluencies. Among repetitions, whole-word repetitions followed by part-word repetitions were more frequently observed, compared to the other repetition types. The frequency of disfluencies ranged from 17% to 30%.

Anjana (2015) studied the development of disfluencies in typically developing 2 to 6-year-old Kannada-speaking children. Frequency, duration and types of disfluencies as well as number of units of repetitions were studied. The age range was divided into four subgroups: 2 to 3 years, 3.1 to 4 years, 4.1 to 5 years, 5.1 to 6 years with 30 children (15 boys and 15 girls) in each group. Recordings of conversational speech and picture description tasks were obtained and analyzed. Median percentage of total disfluencies varied between 2.21% to 3.38% across the age range. Number of repetition units varied between 1 to 4.

Variables affecting the development of fluency

As seen from the above studies on the development of fluency, the process of fluency development may be affected by several variables internal and external to a child. Of these, the variables which have been predominantly studied are discussed below.

Intrinsic variables

Age

Several studies (DeJoy & Gregory, 1985; Haynes & Hood, 1977; Wexler, 1982) reported a decrease in the frequency of disfluencies of typically speaking children with an increase in age (4 to 8 years). Haynes and Hood (1977) reported interjections to significantly increase between ages 4 and 8. Word repetitions, however, exhibited a noticeable downward shift. DeJoy and Gregory (1985) reported that with an increase in age, the frequency of different types of disfluencies (word, part-word and phrase repetitions, incomplete phrases and disrhythmic phonations) decreased. However, Ambrose and Yairi (1999) did not find any significant difference in the number of disfluencies across age in children from 2 to 5 years of age. Even so, part-word repetitions and single-syllable word repetitions reduced and were replaced with other types of disfluencies. Also, repetition units were highest in 3-year-olds but decreased later.

Gender

Multiple studies have reported that sex did not have any significant effect on the frequency of disfluencies (Ambrose & Yairi, 1999; Haynes & Hood, 1977; Johnson et al., 1959; Kools & Berryman, 1971; Ratusnik et al., 1979). However, there is general perception that fluency in females is slightly better than males, although both are within the normal range. A recent meta-analysis by Hirnstein et al. (2022) shed more light on this topic and revealed that females were found to perform better than males in phonemic fluency, but there was no significant difference in semantic fluency across gender.

Extrinsic variables

Bilingualism

In the only available published literature on effect of bilingualism on the frequency of disfluencies, Eggers et al. (2020) studied frequency and types of typical disfluencies and disfluencies indicative of stuttering in typically developing bilingual Yiddish-Dutch speaking children. Yiddish was the dominant language of these children, and Dutch was the non-dominant language. The frequency of both typical and atypical disfluencies was significantly higher in the non-dominant language compared to the dominant language.

Speech and language input

It may be surmised based on the concepts of language fluency and speech fluency introduced in this chapter that the nature of speech and language input given by parents might affect a child's fluency. However, based on a review by Bancroft (2011), the findings related to this variable are presently inconclusive.

The degree to which each of the above variables or their combinations affect fluency development is unique to each individual. Broadly speaking, though, studies on development of fluency show that disfluencies show an increasing trend as children grow and peak around four years of age. Research findings also show that children use an immature pattern of disfluencies (consisting of repetitions and pauses) during their early years of life. These patterns develop into more mature and sophisticated use of disfluencies (such as false starts) as these children develop. The occurrence of normal disfluencies and its increase occurs with concurrent development of syntactically longer and complex sentences used by children during the developmental period. However, as the nature of fluency development might vary across languages and cultures, normative data specific to different countries through large scale studies could help clinicians achieve a more complete understanding of fluency and facilitate more accurate diagnoses of atypical from typical fluency.

Points to remember

- Fluency is a multidimensional behaviour, with the key components being continuity, rate, effort, rhythm and speech naturalness.
- Continuity refers to smooth flow of speech from one sound to another.
- Speech rate varies based on several factors; it is therefore difficult to comment on average rate of speech for a particular individual.
- It is possible to document muscular effort directly, but not mental effort.
- Commonly occurring disfluencies in typical children are whole-word repetitions, interjections, parenthetical remarks and filled and unfilled pauses.
- The frequency and types of disfluencies change with age.

Answer the following questions

1. Define fluency. What are the components of fluency?
2. What are the different discontinuities that can affect the smooth flow of speech?
3. How do we measure rate of speech?
4. Describe the development of fluency with supportive evidence.

2 Typical disfluency

Chanchal Chaudhary

Introduction

Fluent speech is speech that is free from interruptions or hesitations, with continuity, rate, rhythm, and effort as its characteristic features (Starkweather, 1987). Expecting a hundred percent fluency, however, is unrealistic. Children and adults have occasional disruptions in their speech, referred to as "disfluencies" (Guo et al., 2008; Yairi, 1981). Disfluencies are a part of the normal developmental process, and children usually present with these between ages 3 and 4 (Feldman & Messick, 2009). Some children may experience little or no disfluencies during this period. In contrast, others may show a marked degree of disfluency in their speech.

In children, these disfluencies might be considered a red flag by speech-language pathologists (SLPs) and parents. This is because the time window during which they occur concurs with the age of diagnosis of stuttering. Most children who stutter are identified between ages 2 and 4 (Yairi & Ambrose, 2013). It is, therefore, important to identify normally disfluent speech in children and differentiate it from a childhood-onset fluency disorder (Ram & Savithri, 2007).

Several terminologies have been interchangeably used to define disfluencies and can potentially confuse a new student of speech-language pathology. Some authors use the term disfluency for any interruption in speech (in normal or stuttered speech) (Guitar, 2019; Yairi & Seery, 2014); others specifically mention the term "normal disfluency", "typical disfluency" or "normal non-fluency" (Dalton & Hardcastle, 1989). The term "dysfluent" has also been used by some authors to imply stuttering (Yairi & Seery, 2014; Savithri, 2019). Dysfluency, according to them, signifies an abnormality in fluency (Wingate, 1984) while disfluency refers to normal non-fluency. In this book, we have used the term "disfluency" to refer to interruptions in speech of any kind, "stuttering-like disfluencies" (SLDs) to refer to interruptions that indicate stuttering, and "typical disfluencies" for those seen in typically developing children as part of the normal developmental process or in adults who do not have stuttering.

A historical perspective

Research for identification of characteristics of typical disfluencies and differentiation of these from early stuttering have been an area of research for decades. The

DOI: 10.4324/9781003367673-2

earliest of these attempts was made by Johnson and his colleagues (1959) at the Iowa State University. They compared the speech of 89 children who stuttered (CWS) in the age range of 2.5 to 8 years and an equal number of age and gender matched children with no stuttering (CWNS). Their results suggested that non-fluencies occur in children's speech, and there is no demarcation between normal and abnormal degrees of non-fluency (Johnson et al., 1959). They highlighted similarities between normal disfluencies and stuttering in both groups stating that stuttering develops due to a misdiagnosis of normal disfluencies by an overly concerned parent or caregiver (Guitar, 2019) and a limited understanding of the nature of disfluencies. Along these lines, Bloodstein (1970) proposed a continuity hypothesis, in which he described normal disfluency and stuttering as part of a continuum. He specified that all young children experience communicative pressure during speech, leading to minor disruptions. When these communicative pressures are excessive, these minor disruptions could develop into episodes of stuttering. As per Johnson et al. (1959) and Bloodstein (1969), there were no marked differences between normal and abnormal behaviours, and the characteristics of these two groups were overlapping in nature. Both these views hinted at an interactive nature of normal disfluencies and stuttering.

The view was later replaced by one that perceived normal disfluencies and stuttering to have a dichotomous nature rather than an interactive one. The new perspective of dichotomy was supported by a number of researchers who provided evidence of differences in the type and amount of disfluencies exhibited by children who do and do not stutter (Conture, 1990a; Ambrose & Yairi, 1999; Meyers, 1986; Yairi & Lewis, 1984). Terminologies such as within and between word disfluencies, SLDs and ODs, more usual and more unusual disfluencies (Teesson et al., 2003), were used to differentiate CWS and CWNS (Table 2.1).

Yairi and Lewis (1984) studied ten 2-year-old and ten 3-year-old CWS (five boys and five girls) and ten matched CWNS. Their results suggested that the overall frequency of disfluencies in CWS was three and a half times more than CWNS. Furthermore, their results also highlighted that 2- and 3-year-old CWS exhibited interjections, revisions and single unit part-word repetitions. CWS repeated part words two or more times per moment of stuttering, whereas CWNS rarely repeated a segment more than once.

Meyers (1986) studied disfluencies in 24 young children who do and do not stutter (4 to 5 years old). Twelve of these were CWS and 12 were CWNS. CWS had a higher percentage of stuttering behaviour (M = 13.5%, SD = 6.4%) than CWNS (M = 0.2%, SD = 0.4%). Furthermore, CWS had significantly more part-word repetitions, prolongations, and tense pauses compared to CWNS. The most common type of SLD for CWS was part-word repetitions. CWNS had a few part-word repetitions and no prolongations, tense pauses, or broken words. CWNS had significantly more whole-word repetitions and revisions than CWS. However, CWS and CWNS did not differ with regard to other types of typical disfluency (i.e., phrase repetitions, incomplete phrases, and interjections).

Table 2.1 Different terminologies used for typical disfluencies and those seen in stuttering

Author and year	Disfluency description/categorization
Lidcombe behavioural data language (Teesson et al., 2003)	Repeated movements: Syllable repetition, incomplete syllable repetition, multisyllabic unit repetition Fixed Postures: With audible airflow, without audible airflow Superfluous behaviours: Verbal, non-verbal
Ambrose and Yairi (1999)	Stuttering-like disfluencies (SLDs): Part-word repetitions, monosyllabic word repetitions, dysrhythmic phonation Other disfluencies (ODs): Interjections, phrase repetitions, revisions/ incomplete phrases were categorized as other disfluencies
Conture (1990a)	Within-word disfluencies: Monosyllabic whole-word repetitions, sound/syllable repetitions, audible prolongations, inaudible prolongations Between word disfluencies: Phrase repetitions, polysyllabic whole-word repetitions, interjections, revisions
Campbell and Hill (1987)	Less typical disfluencies: Monosyllabic word repetitions (three or more repetitions), part-word/syllable repetitions (three or more repetitions), sound prolongations, prolongation, blocks More typical disfluencies: Hesitations, interjection, revision, phrase repetition, monosyllabic word repetition (two or less, no tension), part-word repetitions (two or less, no tension)

Zebrowski (1991) studied ten CWS and ten CWNS (mean age 4 years). The total frequency of disfluency in CWS was significantly higher (13%) than CWNS (5%). Further, there was no significant difference between the two groups in either the average duration of sound/syllable repetitions and sound prolongations or the average number of repeated units.

Ambrose and Yairi (1999) recorded speech samples from 90 CWS in the age range of 2 to 5 years and from 54 age matched CWNS. They used a six-category classification system for the identification of disfluencies. These included (1) part-word repetitions, (2) single-syllable word repetitions, (3) disrhythmic phonation (comprising of prolongations, blocks and broken words), (4) interjections, (5) revision or abandoned utterances and (6) multisyllable or phrase repetitions. The first three types were combined under the umbrella term of SLDs, and the next three categories were grouped as other disfluencies (OD). For part-word and single-syllable word repetitions, if a segment was repeated more than the required times, it was computed as repetition units (RU). The authors found the main difference between the groups in terms of number of SLDs. Among CWS, SLDs constituted 66% of the total disfluency, whereas for CWNS it was 34%. Other disfluencies constituted 34% of the total disfluency for the CWS group and 76% for the CWNS group. In the CWS group, part-word repetitions were the major type of disfluency, whereas in the CWNS group interjections and revisions contributed majorly to the disfluency count. Furthermore, part-word repetitions tended to significantly decrease with age. Other disfluencies tended to increase with age, but these did not reach statistical significance.

Ambrose and Yairi (1999) developed a weighted measure for SLD which was the weighted sum of part and one syllable word repetitions and disrhythmic phonation per 100 syllables. They described its computation as follows:

> Weighed SLD measure: It is calculated by adding together part- and single-syllable word repetitions per 100 syllables (pw + ss) and multiplying by the mean number of repetition units (ru). This yields the mean number per 100 syllables of extra productions of sounds, syllables, or single-syllable words. This accounts for the frequency and extent of repetitions. To account for the presence and duration of disrhythmic phonation (dp), its frequency is weighted and then added to the number above. These scores also allow for assessing severity: 4.00–9.99, mild; 10.00–29.99, moderate; 30 and above, severe.
>
> (p. 902)

Combining the two formulae given above for repetitions and dysrhythmic phonations, the overall weighted SLD measure can be computed using the following formula:

$$\frac{\left(Repetitive\ disfluencies \times Mean\ number\ of\ repetition\ units\right) + \left(Disrhythmic\ phonations \times 2\right)}{100}$$

Using this measure, with a cutoff of 4, all children were correctly assigned to their respective fluency groups. In other words, weighted SLD scores were found to be continuous across age groups and were below 4.00 for all the CWNS and above 4.00 for the CWS group. Pellowski and Conture (2002) studied disfluencies in 72 children (3 to 4 years of age) of which 36 were CWS and the remaining 36 were age and gender matched CWNS. They measured SLD, OD, total disfluencies (TD) and the number of repetition units (RU). They also calculated the weighted SLD measure as described by Ambrose and Yairi (1999). Results showed a statistically significant difference between the groups for SLDs and total disfluencies. Eighty-one percent and 42% of the total disfluencies comprised of SLDs in the CWS and CWNS groups respectively. Fifty-eight percent of the total disfluencies in CWNS, and 19 % in the CWS group were ODs. The mean weighted SLD measure was 20.1 in CWS and 1.2 in CWNS. A weighted SLD value of 4 and unweighted SLD of 3, thus, correctly classified 97% of the children as CWS or typically disfluent children.

Natke et al. (2006) studied the speech disfluencies of German-speaking pre-school CWS and age and gender matched CWNS. Speech samples were both audio and video recorded. SLDs and ODs were identified. The number of iterations for repeated units were then counted separately. Results showed that CWS and CWNS differed significantly at a very early age, and all disfluency types classified as SLD were produced significantly more often by CWS than by CWNS.

Boey et al. (2007) compared Dutch speaking children who stutter (n= 693) with a group of typically developing children (n=79). Their findings suggested that the frequency of SLD in the stuttering group (M= 15.71) was significantly higher than in the control group (M= 0.42). Further, duration of SLD was longer for CWS than

CWNS; and physical tension during SLD was estimated as higher for stuttering than non-stuttering children. Valente and Jesus (2011) studied SLDs in eight monolingual Portuguese school age CWS (mean age 10 years) and an equal number of typically disfluent children. They found that SLDs were more frequent in CWS than in typically disfluent children. Further, the mean number of RUs for the group with stuttering was higher than for the normal group in congruence with studies by Ambrose and Yairi (1999). The dichotomy perspective is therefore prevalent even in current clinical practices for assessment and diagnosis of typical disfluency.

Probable causes of disfluent speech

Fluent speech involves uninterrupted flow through speech segments and continuous flow of information (Jayaram & Savithri, 1993). Some children undergo a phase of disfluency during their development process. These disfluencies peak between the ages of 2.5 and 4 years (Culatta & Leeper, 1989). Children undergo a rapid development process during these early years of life. A plausible reason for this period of disfluency during the early years of life could be the complex nature of the interaction between developmental processes that co-occur at this age (Zebrowski & Kelly, 2002). When placed on a speech planning system, heavier demands could also increase disfluencies (Bortfeld et al., 2001). The following section describes some factors that can cause a surge of disfluencies in children.

Development of language

Most of children's phonological and syntactic developments occur between 2 and 4 years of age. With an increase in their phonetic inventory during this age (Rosal et al., 2013), children also develop phonological processes to approximate adult productions. Along with developments in phonology, children begin developing sentences that contain mainly content words around 2 years of age. These sentences then take the form of complex sentence structures with evidence of complete syntactic structures of language (Dalton & Hardcastle, 1989; Maner et al., 2000). Instances of increased disfluencies in producing linguistically complex sentences (Guitar, 2019) and the occurrence of disfluencies in children on function words and longer sentences (Brown, 1945), supports that the development of these complex process can interfere with the fluency of speech.

Speech motor skills

Disfluencies in children coincides with the learning of articulatory skills. Children require speech motor skills and articulatory processes to develop simultaneously to be linguistically proficient. Fluent productions require precise coordination between oral-motor movements. The articulatory speed markedly increases in a non-monotonic way from one year to adulthood (Nip et al., 2009). This immature control over the speech motor system may affect a child's ability to speak fluently (Guitar, 2019; Maner et al., 2000).

Demands exceeding capacities

Some researchers reported that typical disfluencies could also occur due to children's demands exceeding their capacities (Starkweather & Gottwald, 1990). Complex language production demands that require coordination between speech structures and linguistic planning and processing, along with environmental stressors (such as parents' expectation of fluent speech) might cause the child to experience excessive disfluencies (Bloodstein, 2006).

Psychological stressors

Some authors also highlight the role of psychological stressors that elicit emotions such as sadness or excitement, in the occurrence of disfluencies in children (Guitar, 2019).

Characteristics of typical disfluency

Typical disfluencies and stuttering show quantitative and qualitative differences (Myers & Wall, 1981; Lickley, 2017). Quantitative differences include number of disfluencies, duration of disfluencies and the relative proportion of different types of disfluencies. Qualitative differences encompass associated behaviours, such as abnormal laryngeal tension and inappropriate articulatory gestures. The speech and non-speech behaviours that characterize typical disfluencies are described below.

Core behaviours

We will now discuss some of the visible and observable features of typical disfluency below in terms of their types, frequency and duration.

Types of disfluencies

It may be recalled that the kind of interruptions seen in a child exhibiting typical disfluency are different from those exhibited by CWS. The classifications of disfluencies into dichotomous categories have generated easy to distinguish evidence into identifying the nature of disfluencies in CWS and CWNS. Several authors have categorized the two types of disfluencies in slightly different ways. Some popular classifications are displayed in Table 2.1.

Among the different terminologies given in Table 2.1, SLD is the most commonly used term for speech interruptions seen in stuttering. Disfluencies not typical of stuttering, on the other hand, are labelled as non-stuttering-like disfluencies (NSLD), normal disfluencies or typical disfluencies. Some examples of NSLD can be seen in Table 2.2. These disfluencies are also seen in typically speaking adults as a result of increases in cognitive, linguistic or emotional load while speaking (Roberts et al., 2009).

RELATIVE PROPORTION OF TYPICAL DISFLUENCIES AND SLDs

It is essential to understand that CWS and CWNS produce all the disfluencies (both SLDs and ODs) listed above. However, there is a marked difference in the frequency

Table 2.2 Disfluencies of typical speakers

S. No.	Description of the disfluency with examples	Specific label given to the disfluency
1.	Single-syllable repetitions not accompanied by struggle (e.g. M-Mummy, come here fast)	One repetition of the syllable followed by successful production
2.	An entire word is repeated – (e.g.- call-call-call Mummy)	Whole-word repetition (WWR) Also, part-word repetitions and single repetitions of syllables
3.	An entire phrase is repeated (e.g. Can you please -can you please -can you please)	Phrase repetition
4.	Addition of extra sounds or words to fill in the gaps of silence so as to escape a disfluency (e.g.- um, er, uh, you know, I mean)	Interjections
5.	Trying to edit an initial attempt to formulate a phrase or sentence (e.g. You can give – I mean – you can opine on this issue. Or I was going to call – I mean – I asked about you.)	Revisions (phrase or sentence)

of disfluencies. CWS produce more SLDs as compared to CWNS (Savithri, 2019). Some studies have reported that CWS produce twice the number of SLDs than CWNS (Zebrowski & Kelly, 2002). The frequency of part-word repetitions, monosyllabic word repetitions, and disrhythmic phonation is much higher (approximately eight times) in CWS compared to CWNS (Yairi & Ambrose, 1992). CWNS show a meagre percentage of repetitions, and disrhythmic phonations are rarely observed. They also show more interjections and revisions.

AMOUNT OF DISFLUENCY

The total percentage of disfluencies in CWS is much higher than CWNS (Natke et al., 2006; Tumanova et al., 2014). Some studies reveal that a child with NNF would exhibit 3% disfluencies or less (Tumanova et al., 2014), while some assert a relatively lax criterion of 10% disfluencies (Johnson et al., 1959; Yairi & Ambrose, 1992) to differentially diagnose normal non-fluency from stuttering. According to Guitar (2013), when measured using syllables, we can expect only about six disfluencies per 100 syllables in a child with typical disfluencies. It is also important to note that the range of disfluencies in typically developing children is vast, with some children exhibiting as low as one or two disfluencies per hundred syllables, to some being normally disfluent to a greater extent (Yairi, 1981).

NUMBER OF UNITS OF REPETITION AND DURATION OF DISFLUENCIES

Another parameter that differentiates typical disfluency and stuttering is the number of units of repetition (Ambrose & Yairi, 1999; Johnson et al., 1959; Pellowski & Conture,

2002; Zebrowski, 1991). Normal disfluencies constitute only one or two units of repetitions (Guitar, 2019). In contrast to normal disfluencies, a hallmark feature of stuttering is extra units of iterations on all repetitions (Ambrose & Yairi, 1999; Johnson et al., 1959). The duration of normal disfluencies is relatively shorter than those seen in stuttering (Lickley, 2017). However, no precise differentiation is present to use this measure as a significant feature to differentiate CWS and CWNS (Zebrowski & Kelly, 2002).

DEVELOPMENTAL TREND/CHANGE IN DISFLUENCY TYPE

Disfluencies in typically developing children follow a developmental trend (Kowal et al., 1975; Yairi, 1981; Savithri, 2019). Findings from literature show that children begin to use an immature pattern of disfluencies (consisting of repetitions and pauses) during their early years of life. These patterns develop into more mature and sophisticated forms of disfluencies (such as false starts)[1] around 4 years of age (Kowal et al., 1975; Yairi, 1981; Savithri, 2019). The occurrence of normal disfluencies and its increase occurs with concurrent development of syntactically longer and complex sentences used by children during this age. The studies pertaining to this section have been discussed in detail in Chapter 1.

Associated behaviour

Associated behaviours, known as "secondary behaviours" in CWS are generally thought to occur due to an escape from stuttering, which later becomes integrated into stuttering behaviours (Yairi & Seery, 2014). These will be explained in detail in the Chapter 3. In typically developing children, disfluencies occur as a part of their normal developmental process, and these children rarely show any signs of concern towards their disfluencies. As a result, no associated behaviours are seen in children who exhibit typical disfluencies.

Assessment

In our routine clinical practice, we get many concerned parents who bring in their children for assessments when they notice disfluencies in their child's speech. Our primary goal during assessment is to establish whether the child shows typical disfluencies or is at the onset of stuttering. Along with this differentiation, it is also the examiner's responsibility to assess whether the child is at risk for developing stuttering in future.

The assessment process is an amalgamation of a parental interview, direct observation by the clinician, and assessing risks for the development of stuttering (Figure 2.1). Information obtained in the parental interview needs to be corroborated by direct observation and assessment by the clinician. The two processes, the parent interview and direct observation are not necessarily sequential, but in fact, overlapping. For instance, the clinician might check for behaviour reported by parents during in–clinic assessment and also seek clarifications for behaviour observed in the session, through questions posed to parents. The outcomes of both of these procedures then feed information for risk assessment.

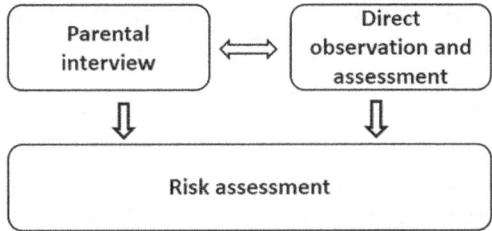

Figure 2.1 Assessment of typical disfluencies

Parental interview

Time spent on parental interviews for gathering information about the child's disfluencies is time well spent (Conture, 2001). Parental reports can help determine characteristics that differentiate typical disfluencies from stuttering. Parents spend the most time with children and can be a great source to provide detailed descriptions of their child's disfluencies. The speech-language pathologist can obtain significant details pertaining to a child's speech by asking open-ended questions to parents as these would allow them to describe the condition using their own words (Guitar, 2019). Along with routine case history questions that are asked in conducting a speech and language evaluation, the following questions must be included in the parental interview of a child with disfluencies:

Questions pertaining to type and amount of disfluencies

 i. What did you notice in your child's speech that raised your concern?
 ii. When did you first notice these disfluencies? What was the child doing at that time?
iii. What type of disfluencies do you notice in your child's speech? Can you demonstrate these disfluencies?

The questions mentioned above are crucial in identifying whether the child exhibits characteristics of typically disfluent speech (as described in the previous section) or disfluencies indicating the onset of stuttering (see Chapter 3). Answers to questions (i) and (iii), specifically, could elicit responses that could help determine the nature of disfluencies (Table 2.2). In response to these questions, the parents might describe the type of disfluency that the child exhibited, such as whether the child repeated "*I wa. . .wa . . . wa . . . want a toy*" or "*I want . . . want a toy*". This information can help classify the child's disfluencies as SLDs or ODs. Information indicative of rapid repetitions, long pauses can also hint towards SLDs rather than typical disfluencies (Yairi, Ambrose, Paden, et al., 1996).

Questions pertaining to frequency and consistency of disfluencies

 i. Do these disfluencies occur frequently or rarely?
ii. Do these disfluencies vary on a day-to-day basis?

Responses that indicate a lack of variation on a daily basis and a high frequency of occurrence could hint at onset and persistence of stuttering (Van Riper, 1971).

Questions pertaining to the child's and the caregiver's reaction to disfluencies

i. Does the child react in any way to the occurrence of these disfluencies?
ii. What do you do when your child experiences a disfluency?
iii. What do you think caused this problem?

As mentioned in the section on associated behaviours, children who are normally disfluent do not have any concerns about their disfluencies; however, children at the onset of stuttering might be aware and show some signs of frustration or muscular tension (Yairi & Seery, 2014). Question (iii) could help the clinician determine whether parents have any incorrect beliefs or negative attitudes related to the child's disfluencies. This information does not directly help in the diagnostic process but is useful for making decisions about concerns that need to be addressed during management and counselling.

Direct observations and assessments

If a clinician is thoroughly familiar with the characteristics of typically disfluent children with reference to the type of disfluencies, number of disfluencies, units of occurrence of disfluencies, and associated behaviours, a clinical judgement can be made about the child's speech based largely upon the results from parental interviews and observation of the child's speech. Recording interactions with a child will help facilitate accurate assessment and diagnosis and also aid outcome measurement on follow-up visits. It is advisable to video record samples as they help capture essential features of speech such as secondary behaviours, that can help differentiate normal disfluencies from stuttering. At least two speech samples, a conversation, and a narration of a minimum of 300 syllables, are necessary to examine a child's speech performance across speaking tasks (Leadholm & Miller, 1994; Yaruss, 1997a; Roberts et al., 2009; Conture, 2001). Conversational samples could be recorded during a parent-child conversation and/or a clinician-child conversation. Narrative speech samples elicit longer utterances in young children (Byrd, McGill, et al., 2015). If eliciting a long enough speech sample proves to be a challenge, as it often does in the case of children, a story retelling task can serve as an excellent method for obtaining speech samples. The clinician first looks at a story and describes it; the child then retells the story after the clinician. After narrating the first story in this manner, children often tell another story without any model (Byrd, McGill, et al., 2015). In addition to this, the following analyses are important to differentially diagnose typical disfluency from stuttering and to detect or rule out the presence of concomitant disorders.

Disfluency analysis

Speech samples should be recorded, transcribed, and analyzed for calculating the number of disfluencies. Children begin to use multisyllabic utterances as they grow up. Stuttering can occur on more than one syllable in a multisyllabic word. As a majority of Indian languages (such as Kannada and Hindi) are rich in multisyllabic words, calculating disfluencies per 100 syllables attempted is recommended (Andrews & Ingham, 1971; Guitar, 2019). Other than the frequency of disfluencies, analysis should also quantify the type and duration of disfluencies, units of repetitions, and the presence or absence of associated behaviours, such as secondary movements, tension or struggle, and the severity of disfluencies should be noted (Guitar, 2019; Yairi & Seery, 2014; Yaruss, 1997a).

Language evaluation

Language skills should be screened informally if parents report any concerns related to language difficulties in the child or if the clinician feels that the child is showing some sign of language difficulty. In some children, disfluencies can occur as a result of difficulties faced in the production of complex language structures (Guitar, 2019) or when children start speaking multi-word utterances (Packman & Kuhn, 2009). Hence, administering a language test to screen for language abilities adds information about the child's language abilities and helps identify whether the child is exhibiting any subtle signs of language deficits.

Risk assessment

A clinician should look for factors that might put a child at risk of developing stuttering. These help the clinician get a clearer picture of the diagnosis of typical disfluencies in a child. Some of these include:

Excessive disfluencies

As seen in the subsection on characteristics of typical disfluency, the frequency of typical disfluencies varies between 3 to 10 per 100 syllables spoken. There might also be a few children who show frequencies higher than these values (Ambrose & Yairi, 1999). Children at the onset of stuttering show a higher number of disfluencies in their speech. Regardless of the type of disfluencies, highly disfluent children will have difficulty with oral communication (Zebrowski & Kelly, 2002). These children will experience failure to attempt fluent speech and may receive negative evaluations of their speech.

Reactions to disfluencies

Children who are typically disfluent, rarely show any signs of concern towards their speech. However, very young children at the onset of stuttering show concerns towards their speech. If a typically disfluent child appears to show high levels of concern towards their speech, counselling parents to watch out for the development of any negative feelings and attitudes is essential.

Positive family history of stuttering

Many children who stutter have a family member with a history of stuttering. Children who show typical disfluencies with a positive family history should be observed for the development of stuttering behaviours.

Language difficulties

Although some studies show no differences between language skills in CWS and CWNS (Nippold et al., 1991; Bajaj, 2007), others have reported slight difficulties in syntactic and phonological abilities of CWS (Anderson & Conture, 2000; Ntourou et al., 2011).

At the end of our assessment, we are likely to be able to classify the child as fitting into one of the three diagnoses shown below:

Table 2.3 Probable diagnostic labels post-assessment

Typically disfluent child with no additional concerns	Typically disfluent child at risk for stuttering	A child exhibiting the onset of stuttering

The process of assessment and diagnosis can be understood better from the case examples below.

Case example 1

Child MK, a 3-year-old, was brought to an outpatient SLP clinic with a complaint of difficulty in speaking. The child was accompanied by his parents, who were somewhat concerned about the change in his speech. They reported observing this change in the last two weeks. As per their report, he often repeated some sounds in words but primarily repeated phrases while speaking. They added that he was unaware of this change in his speech and continued talking with ease, even with repetitions.

Analysis of speech samples showed whole-word easy repetitions with no tension or struggle associated with speaking. The parents did not report any positive family history of stuttering. A complete assessment revealed that the child was experiencing normal disfluencies in his speech. The parents were counselled regarding the current status and sent back.

Case example 2

Child AP's mother contacted our SLP clinic through tele-mode. She expressed concern over her 5-year-old son's disfluencies that she had observed in the past two months. She reported that AP mainly had repetitions in his speech, with some struggle associated with speaking. She reported increased disruptions in his speech during moments of excitement; however, units of repetition were always around two or three. She also reported that family members often interrupt him during moments of disfluency and instruct him to breathe and speak slowly.

In AP's speech analysis, we found that the disfluency type and number of disfluencies correlated with normal disfluencies. Although the child was aware of these disruptions in his speech, he was not negatively affected by them. He was diagnosed as a typically disfluent child. However, parents were counselled regarding some environmental modifications conducive to fluency. They were also asked to return to the clinic for a follow-up in three months.

Case example 3

Child NM, 4.5 years old, was referred for a speech evaluation by his pediatrician. The child reportedly had excessive disruptions in his speech. He had also started avoiding speaking situations at home and most other social situations. His speech had approximately eight to nine units of repetition, and he often prolonged the initial sounds of a word. His efforts to speak were also associated with struggle to get the words across.

NM's speech samples were analyzed and assessed for disfluencies. His speech was associated with a lot of struggle and tension. Analysis revealed a presence of stuttering-like disfluencies (SLDs) along with typical disfluencies. The proportion of SLDs was around 5%. On examining the case history and verifying the type and number of disfluencies, the child was diagnosed as exhibiting an onset of stuttering. Parents were explained the diagnosis and treatment plan.

The above case examples illustrate the importance of putting together information from the case history, parental interview, clinical observation and risk assessment to arrive at a diagnosis and intervention plan. This might sound slightly complicated to beginning clinicians. We have, therefore, summarized the contrasting features between typical disfluency and stuttering in Table 2.4 below.

Management of typical disfluency

It is clear so far from the present chapter that many children experience a period of disfluency, which is a part of their normal development process. Some children can have excessive disfluency, though, and others might experience disfluency only to a mild degree. Once we establish after thorough assessment that the characteristics exhibited by the child resemble those seen in typically disfluent children and not stuttering, we can establish whether some clinical intervention is warranted or not.

Table 2.4 Typical disfluencies versus stuttering: Differential Diagnosis

Characteristic Feature	Typical disfluency	Stuttering
Frequency (Guitar, 2019)	Less than ten disfluencies, stuttering-like or otherwise, per hundred syllables	More than ten disfluencies per hundred syllables
Total disfluencies (stuttered and non-stuttered) (Tumanova et al., 2014)	Lower proportion of SLDs to total disfluencies, higher proportion of ODs	Higher proportion of SLDs to total disfluencies, lower proportion of ODs
Types of disfluencies (Ambrose & Yairi, 1999)	More number of interjections and revisions. Disrhythmic phonations are rare	Part-word repetitions, single-syllable word repetition, disrhythmic phonation (blocks, prolongation, broken words)
Units of repetition (Guitar, 2019; Ambrose & Yairi, 1999)	Two or less than two units of repetition. 1.10 Mean number of units per repetition	More than two units of repetition. 1.54 Mean number of units per repetition
Speed of repetition	Same as speaking rate	Faster than speaking rate
Duration	Relatively shorter in duration (e.g. just over 400 msec for filled pause)	Longer in duration (average around 1 msec, can extend up to 5 seconds or more)
Weighed SLD score (Ambrose & Yairi, 1999)	A weighted score of less than 4	A weighted score of 4 or above (regardless of the number of SLD)
Associated behaviours	Absent	Present
Awareness (Guitar, 2019; Boey et al., 2009)	Children are unaware of disfluencies	Children show some awareness of disfluencies
Reaction to disfluencies (Yairi & Seery. 2014)	No negative reactions	Negative reactions might be present
Qualitative differences (Van Riper, 1971; Myers & Wall, 1981; Jayaram & Savithri, 1993)	No vocal tension or phonatory arrests observed; disfluencies are effortless	Inappropriate articulatory gestures; laryngeal and oral tension; abrupt termination of voice and airflow

Note: *SLDs – Stuttering-like disfluencies; ODs – Other disfluencies*

Managing disfluencies in children and counselling parents of children with typical disfluency is essential. The outcomes of such intervention are prevention of the possible occurrence of excessive disfluencies or the onset of stuttering and an improvement in fluency. Both these outcomes, prevention and recovery, are discussed below in the context of two of the diagnostic labels mentioned in Table 2.3. For the first diagnostic label, the outcome that the clinician is looking for is, essentially, prevention of potential stuttering; while in the case of the second diagnosis, intervention is targeted towards recovery or a reduction in disfluency and an enhancement in fluency.

Typically disfluent child with no additional concerns: prevention

Parental counselling

A clinician must explain to the parents the current status of their child's speech. This explanation should involve describing the normal process of speech development and the factors that can affect this developmental process. The clinician must describe the results of assessment that led them to conclude that the child is exhibiting typical disfluency, such as the type and number of disfluencies obtained during the assessment, the lack of associated symptoms or struggle, etc. Such information giving is followed by counselling parents to develop positive interactive styles to facilitate fluency in the child.

INDUCING A POSITIVE INTERACTIVE ENVIRONMENT

The child's speaking environment must be modified, if required, to ensure a reduction in the emotional stress in the form of interactive and linguistic demands associated with communication.

1. Reducing rate of speech

   A reduction in speaking rate is demonstrated by the clinician, asking the parent to model an unhurried way of speaking. Rather than asking the child to slow down, modelling a slow rate encourages the child to follow suit. The child's slow rate can then be reinforced through attention and praise.

2. Increasing the length of pauses between speaking turns

   Some children might feel an additional pressure to get their words out before somebody else starts speaking. Allow for longer pauses between turns during a conversation. If there is competition (with a sibling, cousin or a friend) for speaking or a need to hold the floor, set up a practice of taking turns so that each child gets the first turn to speak on every alternate conversation, or simpler still, on every alternate day.

3. Reducing the number of questions you ask in succession

   When we usually talk to children, we sometimes might inadvertently pepper children with many questions. This might place a high demand on the child. We need to develop an alternative conversation style that involves a balance of comments and questions. Also, open-ended questions can be avoided to reduce the cognitive and linguistic demands involved in formulating a long sequence of sentences.

4. Decrease length and complexity of sentences

   Children tend to imitate the grammar and sentences used by their parents. Reducing the complexity of the language and using more straightforward sentences will help create a less demanding environment for your child.

5. Follow the child's lead in play

   During play activities, follow the child's conversation. This would reduce the number of verbal instructions and questions during play. Maintain good eye contact and praises throughout the conversation (during both fluent and non-fluent productions).

All the above modifications are directed towards making communication a pleasurable experience for the child.

The instructions given above must be supplemented with an information brochure to ensure that parents retain and implement what has been recommended in the session. Clinicians can also provide brochures on normal speech and language development and instruct parents to monitor any delays or deviance. Parents can also be provided with links to information available on the internet (e.g. https://eyaslanding.com) if they have access to it. A follow-up must be scheduled to ensure that the child will be monitored for changes in fluency, if any.

Once the parents have understood the current status of the child's speech and instructions provided to reduce the communicative stress, they can be asked to monitor the child's speech at home. A follow-up can be scheduled either via telephone calls or clinic visits and should continue for three to six months. During the last follow-up, clinicians can conduct a re-evaluation to examine current disfluency levels.

Typically disfluent child at risk for stuttering: recovery

Parental counselling

Although children in this diagnostic category are normally disfluent, we identify specific concerns that might increase the child's disfluencies and put him at risk of stuttering. Parents, in this case, must be explained what constitutes "risk factors". After addressing parental concerns, the clinician must encourage frequent follow-up sessions to monitor change (Shenker & Santayana, 2018). Curlee (1990) recommended enrolling the child for fluency enhancing sessions (a total of four sessions, two per week, and one hour in length). In the author's own opinion, the frequency and total number of follow-up sessions need not be a blanket rule, but should, in fact, be decided based on the presenting features shown by each individual child in combination with the environmental variables that could alleviate or exacerbate these presenting features. Irrespective of the session frequency or modality (in person or online), parents must involve themselves in these sessions, observe the activities conducted by the clinician, and most importantly, observe clinician-child interactions. In addition to these sessions, parents are encouraged to model positive interactive styles (mentioned in the context of the first diagnostic category) at home. The instructions given to parents of a child who is at risk for stuttering, however, would include certain additions.

In addition to the instructions given to parents whose child is not at an apparent risk for stuttering, parents of a child who might be at risk for stuttering must also note days when the child is excessively disfluent. More of non-speech activities such as arts and crafts or activities that require a closed set response mode (e.g. making a choice between two food items) can be engaged in. Exhibit speech, or situations where the child is asked to tell their name, say a poem or tell a story to someone (say, for instance, a guest or an acquaintance) must be avoided. This especially occurs in collectivistic cultures where a joint family system and social visits are highly prevalent. A disciplinary reaction to incorrect behaviour (e.g. breaking a vase) can involve speaking calmly and giving a timeout rather than a loud verbal reprimand or a demand for a response, during the process of which the child might speak disfluently.

MONITORING DISFLUENCIES

Typically disfluent children with some additional concerns such as a high number of disfluencies, a positive family history of stuttering, or atypical speech and language development must be monitored because they might be at a risk of developing stuttering. Parents of these children can be asked to identify environments and situations that cause an increase in a child's disfluencies and maintain a diary for their child's speech behaviours. To this diary, parents can add any questions or comments that they might have regarding their child's speech. Along with this, a daily disfluency tracking form can be shared with parents in which they can rate their child's disfluency on a Likert scale (0=no disfluency; 1=very little disfluency, 2= very severe disfluencies). A review of entries made in the diary and clarification of queries, if any, can be done at every clinic visit. It goes without saying that implementation and follow-up must be maintained in these children as well.

Although typical disfluencies may be experienced by children and adults alike, in children, occurrence of these disfluencies can be a cause of alarm and concern for parents. An observant clinician, however, can help ease the worries experienced by parents of children with typical disfluency. Careful assessment, an accurate diagnosis, and intervention comprising of the right kind of counselling and guidance can go a long way in alleviating any potential distress that might be faced by the child as well as the family.

Summary points to remember

- Disfluencies are a part of the normal developmental process, and children usually present with these between the ages 3 and 4. Some children may experience little or no disfluencies during this period, while others may show an increase in disfluencies in their speech.
- It is essential to thoroughly assess a child presenting with disfluencies as the age at which children exhibit typical disfluencies in their speech coincides with the age of onset of stuttering.
- The assessment process is an amalgamation of a parental interview, direct observation by the clinician, and assessing risks for the development of stuttering.
- Historically, typical disfluencies and SLDs were considered to be a part of a continuum. However, many authors differentiated between these in terms of type of

disfluencies, number of disfluencies, number of units of repetitions and relative proportion of typical and SLDs in one's speech.
• Managing disfluencies in children and counselling parents of children with typical disfluency is essential. The outcomes of such intervention are prevention of the possible occurrence of excessive disfluencies or the onset of stuttering and an improvement in fluency.

Study questions

1. What causes an increase in disfluencies in typically developing children?
2. Differentiate stuttering-like disfluencies (SLDs) from other disfluencies (ODs).
3. Describe the process of recording and analysis of speech samples in the assessment of typical disfluencies.
4. Mention any five characteristics of typically disfluent speech.
5. Describe positive interactive styles to enhance fluency/preventive counselling for typically disfluent children who are not at an apparent risk for stuttering.

Note

1 False starts: Grammatical correction of a word or a syllable.

3 Stuttering and other fluency disorders: an overview

Maya Sanghi and Pallavi Kelkar

Disorders of fluency

A *disorder* is an illness that disrupts normal physical or mental function (Merriam-Webster, 2022). Trying to understand disorders in a little more detail, they are physical or mental conditions that disturb regular functioning or interfere with day-to-day activities. Such difficulties in functioning might not be faced in every situation with the same severity. Every individual's experience with the same disorder would, therefore, vary. Finally, as a disorder can best be understood against the background of normalcy, we urge the reader to refer to Chapter 2 of this book for a better understanding of normal non-fluency.

An individual is said to have a *fluency disorder* when they are unable to express themselves using speech that flows continuously with ease; and they experience this difficulty consistently and frequently across various speaking situations. The phrase "flows continuously with ease" implies that the speaker does not experience an excess effort and/or interruptions in the articulation of speech sounds while expressing their thoughts to a listener.

Individuals with a fluency disorder can broadly be classified into three types:-

1. Developmental Stuttering[1]
2. Acquired Stuttering, further classified as:
   a. Neurogenic Stuttering
   b. Psychogenic Stuttering
3. Cluttering

Van Riper (1982) proposed a third type of acquired stuttering known as occult stuttering (OS). The cause of this type of stuttering is neither neurogenic nor psychological in its origin. According to Van Riper (1982), OS could be developmental stuttering that went undetected in early childhood or was in a state of remission and made a comeback in later stages of life. The term "occult stuttering" is hardly ever used in clinics as most clinicians are unaware of this possible subtype of stuttering.

Diagnosing the type of fluency disorder an individual is experiencing enables the speech–language pathologist (SLP) to focus on an appropriate management strategy.

DOI: 10.4324/9781003367673-3

Therefore, it is important that the SLP understands the characteristic features of each type of fluency disorder. This chapter elaborates on developmental and psychogenic stuttering. Neurogenic stuttering and cluttering have been discussed in detail in Chapters 8 and 9 of this book.

Developmental stuttering

The most commonly encountered among all the subtypes of fluency disorders, developmental stuttering has been an enigma and continues to be one till date. Efforts to unravel this condition in its totality have been ongoing for several decades, although the answers with reference to its etiology and management are not complete till date. The age of technology and neuroimaging has added interesting dimensions and insights to this disorder, but we are still a long way away from understanding it in its entirety.

Historically, knowledge about stuttering dates back to ancient times. Descriptions are available from the Egyptian era as long as 2000 BC, the Old Testament passages of the Bible, and ancient Sanskrit literature. Excerpts from the Old Testament show that Moses stuttered. Greek Orator Demosthenes, a contemporary of Aristotle, asked individuals with stuttering to speak with pebbles in their mouth in order to correct their speech. In the beginning of the 19th century, a French otologist and physician, Jean Marc Gaspard Itard (1774–1838), suggested that weakness in the muscles of the larynx was a possible cause for the development of stuttering. As a cure, he invented a small, forked gold plate to be kept under the tongue. In the Indian context, ancient Sanskrit texts (Vedic period 2000–2500 BC to 700–750 BC) on Ayurveda refer to stuttering using the term *Vakesangha*. The cause of stuttering was attributed to attenuation of functioning of the central and sympathetic nervous system. It is also suggested that *Devadharu*, honey, or seeds of brinjal ground into a paste were very good cures for stuttering. There have also been claims that oil of *Ajeyas* could cure stuttering. There is, however, no scientific evidence for any of these practices. The systematic study on stuttering started only in the beginning of the 20th century (1920s), with the early work done by Travis and his coworkers (Travis et al., 1934). Brown (1937, 1938) published a series of systematic studies on the effect of different linguistic factors on the loci of stuttering. Johnson and his colleagues (Johnson et al., 1959; Johnson & Knott, 1937) published extensively on the characteristics of stuttering, the cause of stuttering, and the management of stuttering. The growth in the field since then has produced an enormous amount of evidence on different aspects of stuttering.

Defining stuttering

Traditionally, stuttering[2] has been viewed as a disorder in which the rhythm or fluency of speech is impaired by interruptions or blockages (Bloodstein, 1995). However, defining stuttering in a few words has been a challenge due to its multidimensional and complex nature. Literature holds innumerable definitions and explanations of stuttering. A few of them are discussed below.

We begin with definitions based on speech behaviours in stuttering. The tenth revision of the International statistical Classification of Diseases and health related problems or the ICD-10 by the World Health Organization (WHO, 2016) defines stuttering as

> Speech that is characterized by frequent repetition or prolongation of sounds or syllables or words, or by frequent hesitations or pauses that disrupt the rhythmic flow of speech. It should be classified as a disorder only if its severity is such as to markedly disturb the fluency of speech.
>
> (F 98.5, p. 345)

One of the recent explanations by Guitar (2013) that succinctly captures the predominant features of stuttering states that

> Stuttering is characterised by an abnormally[3] high frequency and/or duration of stoppages in the forward flow of speech. These stoppages usually take the form of (a) repetitions of sound, syllables, or one syllable words, (b) prolongations of sounds, or (c) "blocks" of air flow and/or voicing in speech.
>
> (p. 7)

Some definitions give a broader perspective by including speech behaviours as well as other accompanying features. According to Van Riper and Erickson (1996), "Stuttering occurs when the forward flow of speech is interrupted abnormally by repetitions or prolongations of a sound syllable, syllable or articulatory posture or by avoidance or struggle behaviours" (p. 249). They have also described the various aspects of this condition as:

> Stuttering shows breaks in the usual time sequence of utterances. The usual flow is interrupted. There are conspicuous oscillations and fixations, repetitions and prolongations of sounds and syllables. There are gaps of silence that call attention to themselves. If you ask a question, the answer may not be forthcoming at the proper time. Some sounds are held too long. Odd contortions and struggles occur that interfere with communication. And the person who stutters may show marked signs of fear or embarrassment.
>
> (p. 119).

One of the most exhaustive descriptions has been put forth by Wingate (1964b) in what was one of the earliest attempts to define stuttering. As per this definition, the term "stuttering" means:

> I. (a) Disruption in the fluency of verbal expression, which is (b) characterized by involuntary, audible or silent, repetitions or prolongations in the utterance of short speech elements, namely: sounds, syllables, and words of one syllable. These disruptions (c) usually occur frequently or are marked in character and (d) are not readily controllable. II. Sometimes the disruptions

are (e) accompanied by accessory activities involving the speech apparatus, related or unrelated body structures, or stereotyped speech utterances. These activities give the appearance of being speech-related struggle. III. Also, there are not infrequently (f) indications or report of the presence of an emotional state, ranging from a general condition of "excitement" or "tension" to more specific emotions of a negative nature such as fear, embarrassment, irritation, or the like. (g) The immediate source of stuttering is some incoordination expressed in the peripheral speech mechanism; the ultimate cause is presently unknown and may be complex or compound.

(Wingate, 1964b, p. 488)

A shortcoming of the above definitions, however, is the exclusion of the challenges experienced by individuals with stuttering. These, together with the key features of stuttering, can be summarized using the International Classification of Functioning, Disability, and Health (ICF; WHO, 2001). Yaruss and Quesal (2004) conceptualized an ICF-based model of stuttering which encompasses impairment of speech functions as well as the limitations experienced in terms of participation in society when the individual feels unable to execute his speech performance to societal expectations (Yairi & Seery, 2014). ICF-based descriptions of stuttering acknowledge the immense diversity among any two individuals who stutter. In fact, the same individual's experience of stuttering may vary from day to day and across people and situations. Coping mechanisms vary and so do each individual's unique ways of avoiding and escaping from speaking situations. Despite this diversity, one does find some common elements seen in every person who stutters[4] (PWS):

1. **Speech behaviours:** Frequent interruptions in speech which are atypical in duration and disrupt the ability to communicate with ease.
2. **Accompanying non-speech behaviours:** Avoidance and struggle behaviours which result from the individual's attempt to hide his speech problem,
3. **Internal aspects:** Negative feelings and attitudes resulting from failure to maintain a smooth flow of speech to communicate.
4. **Accompanying physiological changes:** The physiological changes often experienced during moments of stuttering

Speech behaviours

As mentioned in the first two chapters of this book, interruptions in speech are seen in any individual; no one is absolutely fluent in every speaking situation. However, the nature of speech behaviours observed in a PWS is different from those seen in typical speakers. The surface features heard and seen by listeners are known as *core behaviours* of stuttering (Van Riper, 1982). Table 3.1 displays the types and examples of stuttering-like disfluencies. These types of behaviours (within-word disfluencies) are seen more frequently in PWS. Some of these examples are in Indian languages

Table 3.1 Stuttering–like disfluencies

S. No.	Description of the disfluency with examples	Specific label given to the disfluency
1.	Either a syllable is repeated, or a sound is repeated (e.g. m-m-m my, ke-ke-kettle; /pa-pa-pa-pa-paani pi lo/)(Hindi: Drink water).	Part-word repetitions sound repetition or syllable repetition
2.	The movement of the articulators stops and the sound is stretched in an atypical way – Bo . . . y; /ga . . . di/ (Hindi: car)	Sound prolongation
3.	Abrupt cessation of voice and movement of articulators simultaneously for a conspicuous duration of time (e.g. /ai mala p – ani de/ Marathi: Mommy, give me water)	Blockage or block

and are therefore displayed phonetically for readers to understand. The meanings of the utterances are given in brackets.

REPETITION

When speech output consists of frequent repetition of sounds or syllables, part-words, or mono-syllabic whole words accompanied by increased effort or spoken in an arrhythmic manner, the listener gets an impression of atypical speech. In developmental stuttering, it has been observed that these repetitions are almost always seen in the initial segments of speech and not in the medial or final positions of words.

Teesson et al. (2003) described a behavioural taxonomy to classify observable behaviours in PWS. Also known as Lidcombe Behavioral Data Language, this taxonomy was developed to train parents to identify stuttering-like disfluencies in their children as part of the Lidcombe programme for stuttering intervention (see Chapter 6). It further classifies repetitions into three types: Syllable repetitions ("my-my-my name . . . ", "I-I-I wil l. . . "), incomplete syllable repetitions, ("m-m-m-my name . . . ", "uh-uh-uh-I will . . . ") and multisyllable unit repetitions (I will-I will-I will go . . . "). It must, however, be noted that multisyllable unit repetitions are not strictly stuttering-like disfluencies. Repetitions are more frequently seen in children who stutter. Initially they begin as easy, slow, evenly repetitions, but with advanced age they become more effortful, fast and irregular in nature.

PROLONGATION

Some PWS speak words with inappropriate stretching out of the vowel of a syllable. Most often experienced on initial segments of words, these can be seen in almost all sounds (continuants) with the exception of plosive consonants. Teesson et al. (2003) refer to these as fixed postures with audible airflow either in the form of a sound or frication. Prolongations occur when there is fixation of the articulator but continuation of airflow or voicing. Prolongations could be voiced or voiceless prolongations depending on the type of speech sounds.

BLOCKAGE, BLOCKS OR BROKEN WORDS

Also known as "hard attack", this is an explosive type of initiation of speech seen only on stop plosive consonants. The stop phase of the consonant is prolonged followed by excessive aspiration of the plosive phase (Bloodstein, 1995). Guitar (2013) aptly describes this speech behaviour as

> Blocks occur when a person inappropriately stops the flow of air or voice and often the movement of articulators as well. Blocks may involve any level of the speech production mechanism – respiratory, laryngeal, or articulatory. There is some evidence and much theorizing that inappropriate muscle activity at the laryngeal level characterizes most blocks.
>
> (p. 23)

The Lidcombe Behavioral Data Language taxonomy (Teesson et al., 2003) describes these as fixed postures with inaudible airflow.

SILENT PAUSE

This type of speech interruption is described as an "inappropriate pause" or "tense pause". This implies that the person's speech stops abruptly at an inappropriate juncture, disrupting the smooth flow of communication.

The above types of disfluencies can be seen individually or in combination or in isolation or in clusters in different individuals who stutter (Bona, 2019). Clustering of disfluencies refers to the phenomenon of two or more disfluencies occurring on one word. These might even be adjacent to one another. They might be a combination of two or more stuttering-like disfluencies or a combination of stuttering-like and typical disfluencies (Bona, 2019; Mahesh & Raju, 2020). Further, durations of the above-mentioned disfluency types have also been documented in many studies. The mean duration of disfluencies (mean duration of part-word repetitions, prolongations) may be less than a second (Kelly & Conture, 1992) to almost five seconds (Johnson & Colley, 1945).

Accompanying behaviours

These are also known as secondary behaviours, associated symptoms (Van Riper, 1982; Yairi & Seery, 2023), accessory features (Wingate, 1964b) or superfluous behaviours (Teesson et al., 2003). Individuals experiencing speech interruptions often try to hide, avoid or terminate them. In an attempt to do so, they subconsciously use additional behaviours unrelated to the speech mechanism, such as clenching fists or a backward jerk of the head. This makes stuttered speech appear atypical and, at times, unpleasant. Secondary behaviours are unique to every individual and might be related to the face, voice or the extremities. The ones related to the voice can also be termed verbal superfluous behaviours (Teesson et al., 2003) or interjections (Johnson et al., 1959). An "uh", "um", "I mean", etc., might be inserted repeatedly when it is redundant to the meaning of the utterance. Behaviours related to the face, breath-stream or extremities are called non-verbal superfluous behaviours (Teesson et al., 2003). The long, not exhaustive list of such behaviours might include eye blinking, facial grimaces, flaring the nostrils, head movements, tongue protrusion, jaw jerks, gasping, exhaling explosively, finger snapping, clenching a fist, moving an arm in many different ways, stamping the feet, foot tapping, or coin jingling.

Each behaviour facilitates an escape from the speech interruption the PWS is about to experience or is already in and might result in a feeling of relief. With the passage of time, however, the behaviour loses its effectiveness. This leads to the person picking up another behaviour in addition to the earlier one. Some PWS might display three to four such behaviours before they escape a block. The resultant speech seems unnatural or distracting to listeners, consequently making the PWS extremely self-conscious of their speech and triggering negative thoughts or avoidance behaviours.

Case example

A 30-year-old male, working at a movie theatre was taking sessions for individual as well as group therapy for his stuttering. The group was run jointly by two speech-language pathologists who had sessions every alternate week. In one of their case discussions, the two therapists started exchanging clinical notes about this person who stutters. Based on his description and session notes, they knew they were talking about the same person, though there seemed to be some discrepancy between the name on his case file and the name each of them identified him by. When they asked him for a clarification in the subsequent session, he confessed that he kept changing his name in response to being asked to give an introduction by a new person. This is an example of the degree to which word substitutions might be used by PWS to avoid or escape the negative experience of a stutter.

Internal aspects or covert aspects

These refer to feelings and attitudes a PWS develops after repeated experiences of stuttering. PWS who are able to describe their experience of stuttering express feelings of shame, frustration and embarrassment. These feelings increase their muscular tension, particularly of the speech mechanism. We have had many individuals complain of abdominal pain after speaking for some time. This tension further makes speaking difficult, and as they struggle to come up with the word, develop a fear related to speech. A feeling of loss of control over speech organs sets in. Gradually, word and sound fears develop. The conviction that they have a problem with specific sounds or words leads to the anticipation or expectancy of the blockage, which in turn makes them anxious. As a result, they develop a habit of avoiding difficult words by substituting them with their synonyms. If using another word is not possible, they may resort to using circumlocutions, describing the word at length instead of saying the exact word. For instance, "my father's aunt's son" for the word "cousin". All these experiences of frustration, shame, and anxiety makes them develop distorted attitudes towards themselves as speakers.

This can be the result of the listener's reactions to their speech or their own. Bloodstein (1987) has vividly described some of these listener reactions as "cover up smiles, look away, look up sharply with a surprise finish the word for the speaker, a few listeners say 'take it easy'" (p. 116–117). Some PWS, however, might begin to perceive unfavourable reactions from listeners such as pity, impatience, shock or amusement even though the listener might be paying sincere attention. This might be a consequence of repeated negative communicative experiences with different listeners. This once again triggers avoidance reactions, such as avoiding eye contact or avoiding the speaking situation itself. The way each individual reacts to their stuttering experiences depends on many factors, and therefore, we see innumerable variations in these reactions. The more severe the negative feelings and attitudes, the more challenges the person experiences in their ability to express in a smooth and easy manner.

The above information might give readers the impression that secondary behaviours and negative attitudes to communication go hand in hand. This might, however, not be the case for every PWS, especially children. The case vignette below clarifies that core behaviours might be accompanied by secondary behaviours, although negative thoughts and feelings may not have crystallized yet in a child who stutters.

Case example

A 2 years 8 months old boy reported to the clinic with a complaint of disfluencies. The parent seemed anxious, although she was trying her best not to express her anxiety before the child. When asked if the child ever spoke about his speech or seemed to be aware, the parent replied in the negative. She said that he was a shy and quiet child and did not initiate communication in most situations outside the home environment. Assessment revealed that the severity of stuttering was mild. However, it was observed that every time this child stuttered, he tended to cup his palm close to his mouth, as if to cover it. This makes us realize that the age of the child (in this case less than 3 years), or parental reports cannot be taken as predictors or indicators of the level of awareness in the child. It underlines the importance of video recordings during assessment, as well as keen observation on the part of the clinician.

Physiological aspects accompanying moments of stuttering

These are physiological events occurring during moments of stuttering which influence the processes of respiration, phonation and articulation. It has been observed that these events occur only during moments of stuttering and not when they are silent or when they are speaking fluently. The possibility of a psychological process being the cause of these abnormal physiologic events, therefore, cannot be eliminated. The reader must note that every PWS might have a unique combination of some of these symptoms.

RESPIRATION

Studies using pneumographic research have shown the following accompanying abnormal breathing patterns with stuttering (Bloodstein, 1995):

1. Antagonisms between abdominal and thoracic breathing
2. Irregularities of consecutive respiratory cycles
3. Prolonged expirations or inspirations
4. Complete cessation of breathing
5. Interruption of expiration by inspiration
6. Attempts to speak on intake of air

PHONATION

Electromyography and electroglottography have facilitated understanding of the laryngeal events accompanying stuttering. Silverman (1992) reported the following abnormalities at the laryngeal level:

1. Breaks in the rhythm of vocal fold vibration and a clonic fluttering of the folds
2. Vocal folds fixed in either an open or closed position
3. Excessive muscular activity
4. Simultaneous contractions of antagonistic laryngeal muscles

ARTICULATION

The movements of the articulators have been studied during stuttering. Studies have found frequent evidence of excessive muscular activity and tension, poor coordination of muscles and inappropriate bursts of activity during silence, and the occurrence of tremors in the speech muscles.

The degree of stuttering might vary from mild to severe depending on the frequency and duration of disfluencies and the noticeability of secondary behaviours that accompany these disfluencies. Some individuals with severe stuttering might even experience a disfluency on every second word to the point of making verbal communication difficult and might occasionally choose to switch over to writing as a mode of expression.

Most individuals, however, start stuttering with a mild degree of severity, although there might be exceptions to this rule (Van Riper, 1982). Some children who stutter might initially display typical disfluencies which might then progress to stuttering.

Development of stuttering

A number of theories related to the development of stuttering have been put forth by various researchers. These have been discussed in chronological order below.

Bluemel's description of primary and secondary stuttering

Bluemel (1931) defined two distinct phases of development of stuttering. The first phase, primary stuttering, comprised easy repetitions and prolongations not always accompanied by awareness of the disfluencies. The second phase, secondary stuttering, in contrast, involved a significant amount of struggle, self-consciousness, anticipation and negative feelings related to stuttering, and consequent avoidance of words and situations. Bluemel's theory over-simplified the process of development of stuttering, not accounting for differences in stuttering severity or exceptions to the sequence of progression from easy to struggle-filled disfluencies. It did not account for a phase of normal non-fluency which might sometimes precede stuttering. One of these limitations was addressed by Bloodstein's theory of development of stuttering.

Four phases of stuttering development by Bloodstein

This description was relatively more detailed than the one by Bluemel. Bloodstein's (1960, 1995) account of stuttering development entailed four phases. He studied behaviour changes in a cohort of 400 children with stuttering aged between 2–16 years. Stuttering in the first phase was episodic, or in other words, periods of stuttering were interspersed with periods of fluent speech. It coincided with situations which might excite or upset a child and consisted predominantly of repetitions of syllables or words. It could be seen on all kinds of words, unlike later stages of stuttering which might be seen more on content words. In this phase, the child did not exhibit concern about speaking or the self-concept of a person who stutters. Phase 1 was usually associated with preschoolers who stuttered.

In contrast to Phase 1, Phase 2 is associated largely with elementary school children who stutter and consists of stuttering that is chronic and increases in situations that provoke excitement or a fast rate of speech. Stuttering in this phase would occur on mainly content words. Whole-word repetitions are not commonly seen in this phase. According to Bloodstein, although a child in this phase has the self-concept of a person who stutters, he/she still does not experience a great deal of concern or self-consciousness about stuttering.

In Phase 3, stuttering is experienced largely in response to specific words, situations or people (e.g. speaking to an unfamiliar person or conversing on the telephone). As a result, the PWS experiences frustration, and consequently shows word substitutions or circumlocutions when faced with difficult words or situations. However, fear or embarrassment is not yet seen, and there is, therefore, no avoidance of speech situations. Phase 3 is associated with late childhood or early adolescence.

Phase 4, however, involves fear, embarrassment and anticipation of stuttering and a higher frequency of word substitutions and circumlocutions as compared to Phase 3. As a result, the person who stutters tends to avoid speaking situations. Bloodstein stated that although Phase 4 was associated with late adolescence or adulthood, many PWS might not reach Phase 4. Thus, some adults could also display stuttering at Phase 2 or 3.

Although this theory provided a more detailed account of stuttering development, it tended to combine the features of normal non-fluency and early stuttering in Phase 1. A limitation common to Bluemel and Bloodstein's theories was that neither of them acknowledged the inherent variation in symptom combinations across children who stutter. Further, the four phases did not account for the development of sudden onset of stuttering in 40–50 % of children who stutter (Yairi & Ambrose, 2013). In addition, these theories did not attempt to explain the processes underlying the development of stuttering. Theories by Peters and Guitar (Peters & Guitar, 1991) and Van Riper (1982) attempted to fill these gaps.

Van Riper's tracks of development of stuttering

Van Riper (1982) put forth that the development of stuttering could follow one of four continua, which he called "tracks". Table 3.2 displays details of the four tracks contrasting them along their salient features. Van Riper studied the case histories of 300 PWS (44 of which had longitudinal data on onset of stuttering) and proposed the four tracks.

As seen in Table 3.2, although all four tracks seem to describe developmental stuttering, some of them might resemble other fluency disorders. For instance, Track 2 resembles cluttering, and Track 3 seems to suggest psychogenic stuttering.

Peters and Guitar's theory of stuttering development

In one of the most detailed and analytical accounts of development of stuttering, Peters and Guitar (1991) asserted that stuttering development progressed through five phases. Further, each phase was described in detail in terms of core behaviours, secondary behaviours, feelings and attitudes and the processes underlying the phase. These have been summarized in Table 3.3.

In addition to giving an exhaustive description of the development of stuttering, this last theory also acknowledges that although most children progress through all of these stages sequentially, there might be exceptions to this rule. The theory also doubles up as a classification of severity of stuttering and helps guide diagnosis and intervention to the present day.

Table 3.2 Contrast between the four tracks of stuttering

	Track I	Track II	Track III	Track IV
Onset	2.5 to 4 years, gradual	Around 3.5 years or later, gradual	Sudden onset at any age after a shock, a frightening experience or a sudden change in their environment	Sudden onset after around 4 years of age
Nature	Cyclic with long remissions in the initial phase	Steady nature	Steady overall, with occasional remissions	Erratic but with no remissions
Speech characteristics	No articulatory errors or rate abnormalities. Initially repetitions emerge, then increase and become irregular and tense. Prolongations emerge then, followed by blocks.	Articulatory errors and fast spurts of speech present. Mostly syllable repetitions, revisions, word repetitions are present. These increase in frequency gradually. Language output seems unorganized.	No articulatory errors, slow rate of speech. Mostly prolongations which are unvoiced and laryngeal blocks are present. Primary tonic blocks with multiple occlusions of the airway are seen. Repetitions follow prolongations as the problem progresses, and they are more retrials than clonic repetitions. Each repetition begins with a slight prolongation of the first sound (tonoclonus).	No articulatory errors or rate abnormalities. Disfluencies are not typical, mostly unusual. Repetition of words that were spoken fluently at the first attempt, repeating a phrase multiple times might be seen. Sometimes there are no repetitions, but frequent gaps and pauses.
Loci	First words sentences, function words. There is no consistent pattern initially, but it becomes more consistent over time.	Throughout the sentence, more for longer, complex words, content words. No consistent pattern.	Usually at the beginning of utterances, after a pause. A consistent pattern is seen.	Mostly content words and first words of an utterance. A consistent pattern is seen. However, when they are fluent, they are extremely fluent.
Struggle	As the problem progresses, tension and struggle increase, tremors and facial contortions might accompany disfluencies.	No visible tension, tremors or struggle is seen at the outset or even as the problem progresses.	A significant amount of tension and tremors are seen. This increases as the problem progresses, with multiple attempts, gasping, etc. An intermittent vocal fry suggests a struggle for phonation.	Tension might be seen inconsistently. Occasional tremors might be observed. These don't change significantly in nature or frequency as the problem persists.

| **Feelings** | Initially there is no frustration or awareness, but as the problem persists, frustration increases and gives rise to fear and avoidance. Poor eye contact during speaking might be a sign of hesitation or embarrassment. | There is poor awareness, no frustration, and a willingness to talk. As the problem progresses, slight awareness and fear of situations might be seen. However, there is no avoidance of words or sounds. | Awareness and frustration is very high. There is a lot of hesitancy to speak, word and situation fears. Poor eye contact and avoidance is seen. Sometimes the person stops trying to speak. Some of these people might develop interiorized stuttering (elaborated on page 33). | There is a high level of awareness but no frustration or fear. The person stutters openly with good eye contact and is very willing to talk. They like to talk about the negative effects of their speech problem, but there is no evidence of stress. They often watch for listeners' reactions to their stuttering. |

Table 3.3 Phases of stuttering development according to Peters and Guitar (1991)

	Core behaviours	Secondary behaviours	Feelings and attitudes	Underlying processes
Normal disfluency Many children experience this phase characterized by some fluent and some disfluent days during the course of early language and motor development.	Interjections, revisions, part-word repetitions, single unit syllable repetitions. As the child matures beyond 3 years of age, part-word repetitions reduce and give way to word and phrase repetitions.	No secondary behaviours are seen in this phase. Occasional tense pauses might be seen in some children.	The child is unaware of the disfluencies and displays no frustration or embarrassment.	This phase usually peaks at 2 to 3.5 years of age, a period that coincides with rapid development of language and speech motor control. For production of long or complex utterances, these activities might compete with fluency for the use of cortical resources. In addition, stressors in the environment might add to the demands on the speech mechanism.
Borderline stuttering This indicates a grey area between normal disfluency and stuttering. A child might swing between normal disfluency and borderline stuttering. Some of these children recover spontaneously while some progress to further stages of stuttering.	The types of disfluencies might be the same as normal disfluency. However, the frequency might be more than 10%. Also, there might be more than single unit syllable repetitions seen.	These are rare. Disfluencies are relaxed with no evidence of tension or effort.	The child is usually unaware but might occasionally be surprised or frustrated at being unable to complete his/her utterance.	Constitutional as well as environmental variables play a role in borderline stuttering. Developmental and environmental pressures add to basic differences in cerebral organization, resulting in borderline stuttering.

Beginning stuttering When a child with borderline stuttering starts experiencing greater tension and a faster speed of repetitions, accompanied by frustration and low tolerance of stuttering, beginning stuttering emerges.	Multiple unit syllable repetitions occur at a rapid or irregular rate. Repeated syllables might be accompanied by a schwa vowel (e.g. Puh-puh-puh-please). They might also be accompanied by tenseness and a rise in pitch. Prolongations and hard blocks also appear in this phase. The child often shows groping movements of articulators in the struggle to resume speaking.	These begin as voluntary escape behaviours meant to push a word out or get out of the moment of stuttering. Head nodding, eye blinking, or adding an extra sound might result in escaping from the negative experience of stuttering. Gradually, these escape behaviours start to appear earlier and earlier and become instinctive.	There is definite awareness of stuttering and specific moments of stuttering. However, there is no fear or anticipation of it. Predominant feelings include frustration, annoyance, helplessness, and a slight amount of embarrassment. However, these are episodic and do not imply the self-concept of a defective speaker.	Classical and instrumental conditioning might be responsible for this phase. Classical conditioning: A child's inherent sensitivity to stress results in the emotion of frustration, triggering a tension response. Stuttering is another stimulus that evokes frustration. After repeated pairing, the disfluency itself would elicit increased tension and rate. Instrumental conditioning: The negative reinforcement of escape behaviours when frustration is terminated, or positive reinforcement in the form of completion of an utterance increases their frequency.
Intermediate stuttering This is usually seen in school aged children between 6–13 years, and is characterized primarily by fear of and, consequently, avoidance of stuttering.	Hard blocks predominate this phase. There are stoppages in airflow, voicing, and/or movement as the child struggles to continue speaking. Pressing the lips together or jamming the tongue against the roof of the mouth might be evidenced. The child might be unaware of these explicit behaviours but completely aware of the moment of stuttering.	In the face of frustration and helplessness in addition to being faced with a surprised or uncomfortable listener, the child might resort to escape behaviours such as the ones listed in the previous phase. In this phase, however, the escape behaviours might turn be accompanied by avoidance behaviours in anticipation of a block. Sentence starters such as 'I mean . . . ', word substitutions, circumlocutions, or avoidance of situations might be seen.	Fear and embarrassment are now accompanied by shame during moments of stuttering. Looking away from the listener, turning stiff or uneasy in an impending speaking situation might be common.	The conditioned frustration mentioned in the previous phase changes to fear, and avoidance conditioning shapes further stuttering behaviours. The escape behaviours that got reinforced in the previous phase now begin to occur earlier as the child expects stuttering and tries to avoid it. The fear and avoidance generalizes to more situations through associative learning. For example, fear of speaking to particular teachers might generalize to fear of speaking to any person in authority.

(Continued)

Table 3.3 (Continued)

	Core behaviours	Secondary behaviours	Feelings and attitudes	Underlying processes
Advanced stuttering This is seen largely in older adolescents and adults and involves stuttering becoming a part of the person's identity.	Long and tense blocks with lip, tongue or jaw tremors. Repetitions or prolongations might be seen in addition to this.	Complex escape and avoidance behaviours are seen, many of which the person might not even be aware of.	The person has the self-concept of an impaired speaker and negative thoughts and feelings related to communication pervade beyond actual moments of stuttering.	The conditioned responses, escape and avoidance behaviours become automatic over years of practice. Impatience and rejection by listeners in the immediate environment and perceptions of significant others might have a major impact on their self-concept. This in turn would further shape the perceptions of listeners, becoming a vicious cycle.

Facts about stuttering

Although the above theories help get a clear picture of the symptomatology of stuttering, understanding the phenomenon of stuttering in all its complexity would not be possible without familiarizing oneself with some of the well-researched facts about stuttering. We will therefore proceed to elaborating on the nature of stuttering by discussing various well-known facts about developmental stuttering.

Prevalence and incidence

Prevalence refers to the number of cases of a disease in a given population at a given time. Incidence, on the other hand, refers to the number of new cases that develop in a given time frame (Stoppler, 2021). In other words, prevalence figures indicate how widespread stuttering is at a given time in a given population or how many individuals currently stutter.

Prevalence of stuttering is therefore the number of individuals observed to have stuttering in a given population at a given time; and incidence of stuttering refers to the number of new individuals having stuttering at a given time in a given population. Early research on prevalence reported prevalence figures of 1% (Bloodstein, 1995). However, an extensive study by Craig et al. (2002) revealed a slightly lower lifetime prevalence of around 0.72%. Prevalence, according to Craig et al. (2002) was higher in children till about 4 years of age, following which it reduced 0.37%. Although 5% has been commonly cited as the lifetime incidence of stuttering, more recent findings indicate the possibility that it is as high as 8% or even higher (Bloodstein et al., 2021).

Age of onset

Most of the studies regarding the age at which most children begin to stutter have repeatedly found it to be in early childhood. It is commonly reported between the age range of 2 to 5 years, coinciding with the period when most children's growth is seen in the physical, linguistic, neurological and cognitive realms. Early studies reported onset of stuttering to be around 4 years of age, while recent studies report an earlier age of onset, at about 2 years 9 months (Bloodstein & Bernstein Ratner, 2008). Darmody et al. (2022) reported in their cohort of 739 PWS (age range 2–80 years) that the median age of onset was 3.0 years with a mean of 3.7 years. It appears that more than 60% of the children who stutter begin doing so prior to or at around 3 years of age, a figure that climbs to 85% by 4 years of age (Yairi & Ambrose, 2005). Some older children may begin to stutter at a later age, up to 12 years or even later, but this is found to be rare. When the onset of stuttering is at a later age, the type of disfluency may have a specific cause and is likely to be of a different type like psychogenic stuttering or neurogenic stuttering.

Gender Ratio

The ratio of stuttering males to females was found to be around 2:1 in very young preschool children (Ambrose & Yairi, 1999). An extensive review by Bloodstein (1995) concluded that the gender ratio in general is approximately 3:1 with more boys than girls exhibiting stuttering. In the previous decade, Van Borsel (2006) reiterated that stuttering was more frequently seen in males. In India, a retrospective study of 132 PWS reported a male-to-female ratio of about 3:1 (Sudhi et al., 2010). They found that that females who stutter had an earlier age of onset compared to males. Males were more likely to have moderate to severe stuttering, while females tended to have mild stuttering. Females showed a stronger genetic basis of stuttering and had more first-degree relatives who stuttered compared to males.

Most studies have consistently reported that with increasing age, there is a tendency for an increase in this gender ratio. Mansson (2000) studied children who were 3 years old and reported a gender ratio of 1.65:1 (males to females). A reassessment after two years revealed a change in the original ratio to 2.8:1. The finding was reconfirmed by Bloodstein and Bernstein Ratner (2008) in their review, which revealed an increase in the male-to-female ratio from 3:1 to 5:1 as children graduated from the third to the fifth grade. Females have a higher likelihood of spontaneous recovery than males as indicated by the male-to-female ratio in adulthood, which is 4:1. Further, more boys develop stuttering later than girls (Darmody et al., 2022). These differences in numbers of males and females who stutter suggest a strong contribution of genes to stuttering.

Heredity

In literature, there is adequate evidence to suggest that stuttering can be inherited. In other words, for many people who stutter, one or both of their parents had some predisposition to stuttering that was transmitted in their genes. Some researchers suggest that as many as 50% of those who stutter have a family history of the disorder (Riaz et al., 2005). A genetic predisposition, however, interacts with other variables in the environment, a phenomenon observed in other chronic problems such as asthma as well (Kidd, 1984, as cited in Guitar, 2013). There are three main approaches used to gather evidence about heritability and stuttering. We will briefly discuss these studies to understand this important relationship. A more detailed account of these studies can be found in Chapter 4, which talks about different theoretical perspectives on stuttering.

Family studies

Researchers study the family trees of a group of individuals (Group I) with stuttering and compare the findings of this group with the family trees of an equal number of individuals in a group (Group II) with no stuttering. The number of individuals having stuttering in the family of participant is counted. The total count in each group tells the researcher whether Group I has a larger number of relatives with stuttering as compared to Group II. Approximately 30% to 60% of PWS have some family history of stuttering. In other words, the remaining individuals who stutter could have developed stuttering through some other mechanism or predisposing factor (Yairi, Ambrose & Cox, 1996) Family aggregation studies[5] (Kidd, 1977) indicate a higher risk of chronic stuttering in males. Females, on the other hand, probably have some form of natural resistance to persistent stuttering and seem to recover spontaneously from stuttering more easily than males. Viswanath et al. (2004) asserted that stuttering follows an autosomal dominant pattern of inheritance. However, based on a review of family studies on stuttering, Frigerio-Domingues and Drayna (2017) concluded that evidence for a mode of inheritance was inconsistent. In their words, "while the evidence for heritable factors in stuttering is strong, stuttering is most likely a complex genetic trait" (p. 96).

Twin studies

Some studies investigating inheritance of stuttering compared the incidence of stuttering in identical and fraternal twins. Identical or monozygotic twins share all of their genes while only 50% genes are shared among fraternal or dizygotic twins. If both twins in a pair stutter, the pair is said to be *concordant*. If one of the twins does not stutter, however, the pair is termed *discordant*. A higher concordance rate in monozygotic twins indicates that stuttering has a strong genetic component (Frigerio-Domingues & Drayna, 2017). However, some monozygotic twin pairs are, in fact, discordant, indicating the influence of factors other than genetics as well. In the study by Howie (1981), concordance was reported in two-thirds of the group of identical twins, while one-third of the group was discordant. A single case study from India (Sanghi et al., 2009) reported stuttering in a pair of monozygotic twins who had a family history of stuttering in their father as well as the father's first cousin (maternal). However, the study also reported the presence of exacerbating factors in the children's environment. Based on their findings from a twin study, Fagnani et al. (2011) recently estimated the heritability of stuttering to be between 0.81 to 0.84.

Adoption studies

The rationale for adoption studies is that there will be evidence of the role of genetics if there is a higher incidence of stuttering among the birth parents of adopted children. In contrast, a higher incidence among the relatives of the adoptive family will support the role of environment. An adoption study by Felsenfeld and Plomin (1997) did not find evidence of incidence of stuttering being higher in children whose adoptive parents stuttered, as compared to children in the general population. They concluded that although both heredity and environment play a role in the occurrence of stuttering, the role of heredity is relatively stronger.

Linkage studies

Some studies attempted to identify the loci of genes that manifest stuttering on chromosomes. A significant finding based on studies involving consanguineous families from Pakistan concluded that the loci of such genes was on chromosomes 3, 12 and 16 (Riaz et al., 2005; Raza et al., 2010).

Bilingualism and stuttering

The earliest work on bilingualism and stuttering (Travis et al., 1937) asserted that bilingual children are at an increased risk of stuttering. This assertion was supported by several researchers whose studies demonstrated that more bilinguals than mono-linguals stutter and that the chances of recovery from stuttering are higher in chil-dren who are either monolingual or speak only one language at home, till the second language is introduced in school (Howell et al., 2009). Researchers from this school of thought recommended that exposure to a second language for educational purposes be deferred. However, this viewpoint has received several criticisms (Pack-man et al., 2009; Gahl, 2020), citing that studies along these lines probably involve misdiagnosis of stuttering in bilingual children (Byrd, 2018; Byrd, Watson, et al., 2015; Byrd, Bedore, et al., 2015) and that the benefits of bilingualism far exceed the (possible) benefits of delaying exposure to a second language (Packman et al., 2009).

Bilingual children who stutter have been known to show one of three patterns: Stuttering in only one of the two languages, stuttering about equally in both lan-guages, or stuttering to a greater extent in one of the two languages (Maruthy et al., 2015). The third pattern can have two possible variations: Stuttering to a greater extent in the first or dominant language (L1) or the second or non-dominant lan-guage (L2). Recent findings, however, lend empirical support to more disfluencies being observed in the non-dominant language (Maruthy et al., 2015; Chaudhary et al., 2021). A systematic review of language-related factors in bilinguals who stut-ter revealed that in addition to language proficiency, the nature of the language and the task can also determine the degree of disfluencies seen in either of the languages (Chaudhary et al., 2021). It is important for clinicians to stay abreast of these facts about bilingualism and stuttering in order to be able to apply them appropriately in assessment and therapy for stuttering. Improvement in one lan-guage, for instance, has been known to generalize to the second language to some extent (Priyanka & Maruthy, 2019). With an increase in the number of bilinguals the world over (Brundage et al., 2016), there is a need for continued research in this area to further strengthen the existing notions related to bilingualism and stuttering (Chaudhary et al., 2021).

Temperament, anxiety and stuttering

The relationship between temperament and stuttering is a complex one and is still in the process of being unravelled. A lot of recent literature suggests that PWS have a temperament that predisposes them to stutter (Druker et al., 2019). Some theories and models of stuttering are based on this point of view and will be discussed in the next chapter. However, some studies do not support this notion. A study by Rocha et al. (2019), for instance, demonstrated that no temperamental differences such as higher emotional reactivity exist in children who stutter aged 7–9 years as compared to their non-stuttering peers. The same study showed that temperamental differ-ences did exist in 9–12-year-old children who stutter.

Another ongoing debate is whether PWS have trait anxiety that predisposes them to stutter, whether stuttering leads to increased anxiety in those who stutter or whether stuttering and anxiety simply have a higher tendency to coexist. Many recent studies have found the concomitant presence of social anxiety disorder (SAD) in individuals who stutter (Iverach, Jones, et al., 2009; Iverach, O'Brian, et al., 2009). Treatment approaches that target communicative anxiety and negative thoughts related to speaking have been known to inadvertently reduce the frequency of stuttering behaviours (Menzies, O'Brian, et al., 2019). Overall, a larger body of literature supports the view that stuttering puts a PWS at risk for SAD or other anxiety-related symptoms (Messenger et al., 2015). Anxiety-related disorders are seen more frequently in adolescents or adults as compared to preschool and school-age children who stutter and more frequently in those with chronic stuttering, suggesting that anxiety results from an increasing impact of stuttering perceived by the PWS (Ahmed & Mohammad, 2018; Rocha et al., 2019; van der Merwe et al., 2011). In any case, dealing with communicative anxiety has to be an essential component of management of stuttering to ensure long-term well-being (Menzies, Packman, et al., 2019).

Variability and predictability

Although the symptomatology of stuttering varies to a great extent across individuals, an interesting fact about stuttering is that stuttering events can be predictable, that is, they occur in a predictable pattern. This predictability is well researched and will be discussed under the subheadings anticipation, consistency, adaptation, linguistic aspects, and conditions which reduce stuttering.

Anticipation

This simply means that the individual can predict, in advance, the words he is likely to stutter on (Johnson & Solomon, 1937, as cited in Guitar, 2019). To evaluate anticipation, the PWS is asked to read a passage silently and mark the words they think they are highly likely to stutter on. This marked passage is then kept with the therapist. The PWS is then given a fresh copy of the same passage and asked to read it aloud. In a lot of PWS, stuttering moments while reading aloud occur on a majority of the words that the PWS marks during silent reading. This probably occurs because the anxiety of anticipating the stutter leads to physical tension in an attempt to control the stutter. This ability to anticipate has been used in many therapy techniques such as "preparatory sets" which can be found in Chapter 7 of this book.

Consistency

This is the tendency of the individual to stutter on the same words repeatedly. If a PWS is asked to read the same passage five times and the therapist marks the words he stutters on in each of the readings, it is observed that most PWS tend to stutter on the same words in all the readings. Johnson and Knott (1937) were the first to publish this observation. This phenomenon is known as the *consistency effect*. The terms that are used while calculating the consistency effect are

TSW = Total number of words stuttered
Rx = the earlier reading of the five consecutive readings
Ry = the later readings of the five consecutive readings

Thus, if Ry indicates the fifth reading, then Rx could be R1, R2, R3 or R4.

Consistency effect is generally measured between the first reading R1 and the last reading R5 and is generally calculated (in percentage) by using the formula (Ham, 1999):

$$\frac{\text{Ry stutters that occurred on the same words in Rx}}{\text{TSW in Rx}} = \underline{\quad} \text{x } 100$$

Consistency has been interpreted in terms of learning theories, in that once a word has been associated with stuttering, it acquires the role of a stimulus to trigger stuttering on subsequent occasions (Johnson & Knott, 1937). Ham (1999) suggested that consistency measures can be of value to therapy planning. Individuals whose consistency percentage is well below 50% might respond better to fluency reinforcement programmes as opposed to symptom modification approaches.

Adaptation

On repeatedly reading the same passage, PWS are known to stutter progressively less frequently (Johnson & Knott, 1937). To quantify adaptation, a PWS is asked to read a passage five times, and the words stuttered on are marked (R1 to R5). The formula used to calculate adaptation is

$$\frac{(\text{TSW in Rx}) - (\text{TSW in Ry})}{\text{TSW in Rx}} = \underline{\quad} \text{x } 100 = \text{adaptation percentage for RxRy}$$

Linguistic aspects

The term loci of stuttering has been used to specify locations in the utterances where stuttering events consistently occur. Brown (1937) reported that the occurrence of the stuttering of adolescents and adults was not random. Stuttering was, in fact, associated with specific language structures. On analysis of speech samples, he observed that stuttering tended to occur on (1) content words (versus function words), including nouns, verbs, adjectives, adverbs; (2) long words (versus short words); (3) consonant-initial (versus vowel-initial) word locations; and (4) sentence-initial (versus final) locations. The more the number of factors congregated on a single word, the higher was its chance to be stuttered. These locations became known as "Brown's four factors" because they supposedly accounted for most stuttering instances (Yairi & Seery, 2014). Stuttering also has a propensity towards stressed syllables (Natke et al., 2002) or utterances with higher grammatical complexity (Blomgren & Goberman, 2007; Jayaram, 1984). However, it has been repeatedly observed that the frequency as well as the loci of stuttering show a different trend in preschool children who stutter. In preschoolers, stuttering tends to occur more frequently on pronouns and conjunctions, in contrast to content words such as nouns, adjectives, verbs, etc. (Guitar, 2019).

In a study reported from Iran, Masumi et al. (2015) found disfluencies to be more frequent for difficult syllable structures in non-word reading tasks. In India, Mahesh and Raju (2020) studied the effect of syllable complexity on the frequency and type of disfluencies in Kannada-speaking adults who stutter. Disfluencies were seen more frequently on words with consonant clusters. Also, there was a higher likelihood of cluster disfluencies being present on words with consonant clusters as compared to words without consonant clusters. The difference, however, was statistically significant only for persons with severe stuttering. Seth and Maruthy (2019) studied the effect of phonological and morphological factors on the frequency of stuttering-like disfluencies in Kannada-speaking preschool children. Words beginning with consonants were stuttered more often than words beginning with vowels; stuttering occurred more on content words compared to function words; and more often in the word-initial position.

Conditions under which stuttering decreases

An interesting observation about stuttering is that it does diminish temporarily under some specific conditions with a fair amount of consistency. Bloodstein (1995) was one of the first to study the speech of PWS in 115 conditions and reported that stuttering reduced to a great extent in many of these conditions. Some of these conditions were speaking to an animal or an infant, speaking when alone, speaking in unison with another speaker, singing, or speaking simultaneously while writing. Literature also suggests that a reduction in frequency of stuttering occurs when PWS speak under delayed auditory feedback (DAF), frequency-altered auditory feedback (FAF), masking noise, and unison or choral reading (Ingham & Packman, 1979; Kiefte & Armson, 2008; Kalinowski et al., 1993; Martin & Haroldson, 1979; Max et al., 1997; Soderberg, 1969; Stuart et al., 1996; Stuart et al., 2008). Among the several conditions mentioned above, choral reading has been found to produce the maximum effect on fluency (Andrews et al., 1983; Ingham & Packman, 1979). In a study on auditory temporal processing in 30 children with stuttering from Mumbai, India (Kekade & Valame, 2014), the performance of typically speaking children was significantly poorer on the Gap Detection Test and the Duration Pattern Test. The researchers concluded that these deficits in auditory temporal processing might place additional demands on the feedback mechanism. This is probably why DAF, or the person hearing the sound of their own voice after a lag of some milliseconds, induces fluent speech. Dechamma and Maruthy (2018) studied the effect of choral reading on 17 Kannada-speaking adults who stutter. There was significant reduction in stuttering-like disfluencies (3.38%) during choral reading task as compared to solo reading task (9.33%). Along with the reduction in the frequency of disfluencies, there was also significant reduction in the rate of speech and changes in speech rhythm.

Unfortunately, the reduction in stuttering in these conditions is experienced only while the condition is present. When removed, stuttering resumes its previous level. These fluency-inducing conditions have been incorporated in the management of stuttering, which will be discussed in Chapter 7 of this book.

The facts discussed so far pertained to factors intrinsic to an individual who stutters. As explained in the ICF model of stuttering, these factors interact with several extrinsic variables that can further increase or decrease stuttering.

Extrinsic variables that can affect stuttering

It has been commonly reported by individuals who stutter that they always experience an increase in stuttering in situations such as addressing a large audience or participating in a group discussion. *Situations of communicative pressure* tend to trigger more frequent or worse episodes of stuttering (Bloodstein & Bernstein Ratner, 2008).

Communicative content is another variable that could exacerbate stuttering. Stuttering occurs more on content that is conceptually more complex or difficult to explain. Content that conveys crucial information might increase stuttering (e.g. telling one's name). Similarly, delivery of emotionally laden content is often more difficult for PWS. Most PWS report increased stuttering when sad, angry, or excited (Bloodstein et al., 2021).

An important variable that influences stuttering is the *nature of listeners*. PWS stutter less in response to empathetic listeners; stuttering increases in response to listeners who might react negatively to their speech (Bloodstein et al., 2021; Guitar, 2013). Many PWS also report an increase in stuttering while speaking to persons in authority.

Each individual person might react differently to the above extrinsic variables. The ICF (WHO, 2001) maps most of these variables onto its component titled environmental factors (Yaruss, 2007). The presence of factors that exacerbate stuttering is considered a barrier to intervention. Helping a PWS cope with these extrinsic factors, therefore, paves the way for long-term improvement.

Spontaneous recovery

Although the term "spontaneous recovery" has been commonly used, Yairi and Seery (2023) prefer the use of the term "natural recovery" in order to give due credit to environmental factors in the recovery process. It has been observed that approximately 50% of children outgrow their stuttering over a period of time without any professional treatment. In a longitudinal study involving 84 children over a span of four years after the onset of their stuttering, Yairi and Ambrose (1999) reported that 74% of the children recovered without any treatment for their stuttering.

In a longitudinal study of 89 preschool children in the age group 23 to 65 months conducted at the University of Illinois (Yairi & Ambrose, 2005), researchers ensured that children were assessed close to onset of stuttering. In order to avoid ambiguity of interpretation of the term "recovery", the researchers employed specific inclusion criteria. These were based on parents' and therapists' ratings of stuttering severity being less than 1 on a severity rating scale, and the frequency of stuttering less than 3%, for a minimum of a year and maintained for four years. The overall natural recovery rate reported was 79%. They found that even though a reduction in stuttering might begin within a few weeks after onset, the time period needed to reach complete recovery varied. The figures indicated that a small percentage of children will need intensive therapy. The therapist therefore needs to make informed decisions regarding which child should be taken for therapy and when.

Based on their findings, Yairi and Ambrose (2005) underlined factors that indicate persistent stuttering, which are relevant to guide the beginning clinician. Some important predictors are children who begin to stutter relatively later (onset after 3.5 years); family history where stuttering persisted; girls whose stuttering has persisted for more than a year; children whose stuttering frequency and severity does not reduce for over a year after onset; children who have increased duration of stuttering moments (e.g. three or more unit repetitions and duration of prolongations not decreasing over time); children whose phonological skills are not age appropriate; children with an unstable speech motor system; and children whose mothers engage in nondirective interaction using simple language with the child. In another multicentric longitudinal study of 81 children who stuttered, Ambrose et al. (2015) found similar trends as the earlier study by Yairi and Ambrose (2005), except for age at onset and male-to-female ratio which did not differ significantly across children who recovered from stuttering and those who did not. Based on their findings, they concluded that there is a need to distinguish between persistent stuttering and recovered stuttering as subtypes of developmental stuttering.

The chances for recovery reduces as the number of years for which stuttering has persisted increases. If the child stutters longer, there are lesser chances of recovery (Ingham & Bothe, 2001) and higher chances of persistence (Conture, 1982). Between the ages of 2–16 years, the recovery rate is 76%, and the recovery after teenage year is lower (Andrews & Harris, 1964). A systematic review by Sugathan and Maruthy (2021) identified 35 studies and 44 variables from which four factors, namely phonological abilities, articulatory rate, change in the pattern of disfluency and the time since onset were identified. It must be noted, however, that there were variations in the study design of each study included in the review.

Interiorized stuttering

The discussion so far has focused on developmental stuttering, its definition, symptomatology, nature and stages of development. As mentioned earlier in this chapter, however, some individuals with developmental stuttering might exhibit interiorized stuttering. This type of stuttering is the result of a skilled avoidance response of an experienced PWS. These individuals substitute words or descriptions in place of the target word which they wished to avoid for fear of stuttering. Gradually, experiences of success in hiding their stutter make them more adept at using these alternatives. This success and the apparent fluency, unfortunately, comes at the cost of anxiety and negative emotions they experience each time they need to hide their stuttering. We have had individuals confess to the clinician that they are almost exhausted at the end of a speaking experience, particularly when they need to substitute every other word. Some individuals that appear to have recovered spontaneously might, in fact, be cases of interiorized stuttering. Interiorized stutterers must be trained and counselled by the therapist to overcome their tendency of constantly hiding their stutter before it becomes a strong and unhealthy habit.

Another type of fluency disorder we had listed at the beginning of this chapter was acquired stuttering. The study of this condition is at its infancy, and we have limited studies reported on this topic. The two main types of acquired stuttering are neurogenic stuttering and psychogenic stuttering. As mentioned earlier, neurogenic stuttering will be discussed in Chapter 8. The present discussion will, therefore, be restricted to psychogenic stuttering.

Psychogenic stuttering

Psychogenic stuttering occurs when a psycho-emotional trauma leads to sudden abnormal disfluency. It must be noted that unlike neurogenic stuttering, the onset of stuttering is not associated with any organic etiology or neuropathology (Baumgartner, 1999). The foregoing statement makes it clear that psychological distressing event or a series of such events or emotional trauma can be the cause of the disorder. Commonly reported events are stresses related to a relationship, death of a family member or close friend, or any other sudden and tragic incident in the individual's personal life or family. As mentioned earlier, psychogenic stuttering is characterized by a sudden onset. Also, unlike developmental stuttering, psychogenic stuttering has a high likelihood of an adult onset (Yairi & Seery, 2023). The often-seen speech behaviours are sound and syllable repetitions, prolongations, hesitations, blocking, tense pauses, word repetitions, phrase repetitions and interjections (Duffy, 1995). The speech behaviours show less variability and predictability than developmental stuttering; they are neither affected by any of the fluency-inducing conditions, nor is any adaptation effect seen (Mahr & Leith, 1992). Another characteristic feature of psychogenic stuttering, in contrast to developmental stuttering, is that the person exhibits stuttering even though an utterance might be over-learned (such as a nursery rhyme). Similarly, disfluency is also observed for social responses such as "hi" or "good morning", which are usually automatic. In some individuals, however, speech fluency might vary according to task, environment, or time of day (Baumgartner, 1999). Persons with psychogenic stuttering do not seem to be emotionally affected or anxious. This is termed "la belle indifference" (Roth et al., 1989). Another characteristic feature is the presence of stuttering even when the person is asked to mime the intended utterance (Deal, 1982, as cited in Manning & DiLollo, 2018).

Assessment by a psychologist and/or a psychiatrist is a prerequisite for the diagnosis of psychogenic stuttering. Speech therapy for psychogenic stuttering involves the same strategies used for the treatment of adults with developmental stuttering. The response to treatment varies from individual to individual. It is important for the speech therapist to work in collaboration with a psychologist to try to resolve the psychological issues underpinning the stutter. The symptoms of psychogenic stuttering are likely to resolve as soon as the stress event resolves. A complete resolution of symptoms in a short period of time is common in persons with psychogenic stuttering. Some individuals might, however, need a longer duration of treatment. Spontaneous recovery can occur in psychogenic stuttering as a result of the process of grieving or through counselling, though in some cases, it does not recover irrespective of exposure to therapy (Ward, 2018).

In summary, stuttering is a multifactorial and complex speech disorder that consists of but is not limited to speech disfluencies. Knowing about its nature and development can aid a beginning clinician in performing a complete evaluation of all its facets and therefore, carry out efficient management of individuals who stutter.

Summary points to remember

- Fluency disorders may be of essentially three types – developmental stuttering, acquired stuttering and cluttering.
- Developmental stuttering consists of speech disfluencies in the form of repetitions, prolongations and hard blocks. These might be accompanied by secondary behaviours and negative attitudes towards communication.
- The progression of developmental stuttering is gradual, unlike acquired forms of stuttering which have a sudden onset.
- In some children, normal non-fluencies might progress to developmental stuttering while in some, these are just a phase of normal development.
- Various theories of development of stuttering have been put forth. Prominent among these are theories by Bluemel, Bloodstein, Van Riper, and Peters and Guitar.
- It is important to know about the different facts related to stuttering so as to understand the disorder in its entirety.

Study questions

1. Write an essay on variability and predictability of stuttering.
2. "Stuttering can be inherited". Do you agree with this statement? Support your answer by giving reasons.
3. What are the different aspects of stuttering in terms of the symptoms observed in individuals with stuttering?
4. What are the conditions that temporarily reduce stuttering?
5. Elaborate on the processes underlying each of the five stages of Peter's and Guitar's theory of stuttering development.

Notes

1 A sub group of stuttering known as interiorized stuttering also needs to be kept in mind by every clinician.
2 Readers unfamiliar with fluency disorders must note that the terms "stuttering" and "stammering" can be used interchangeably.
3 We prefer using the term "atypical" to refer to differences.
4 The terminology historically was "stutterer". However, in the present day, "person who stutters" is the preferred terminology to underline that stuttering is a behaviour displayed by the person, not something that colours their identity.
5 Family aggregation studies analyze the detailed distribution patterns of stuttering in the familial trees accounting for gender, family size, and degree of relatedness (e.g. first degree = siblings; second degree= cousins) (Yairi & Seery, 2014).

4 Theoretical perspectives in stuttering

Divya Seth and Santosh Maruthy

Introduction

The Oxford dictionary (n.d.) defines a *theory* as "a supposition or a system of ideas intended to explain something, especially one based on general principles independent of the thing to be explained". A theory cannot be mistaken to be permanent in nature and should be considered as a supposition that is enhanced and fine-tuned evolving into refined versions, particularly in the fields of behavioural and social sciences. The field of stuttering is no exception to this and has experienced significant paradigm shifts over time regarding the causal factors of stuttering.

Charles Van Riper (1971), in his classic work described stuttering as a "puzzle, the pieces of which lie scattered on the tables of speech pathology, psychiatry, neurophysiology, genetics, and many other disciplines . . . we suspect that some of the essential pieces are not merely misplaced but still missing" (p. 2). Through five decades of research and a plethora of empirical investigations exploring different dimensions of stuttering, one question that continues to persist, and is often asked by persons who stutter (PWS) or parents of children who stutter (CWS), is *What causes stuttering?* As Manning (2009) rightly pointed out, even the most experienced clinicians are at a loss for words when addressing this question. This is essentially owing to the wide range of explanations or reasoning available for the onset and development of stuttering. Over time several theories and models have evolved to explain the nature of stuttering. Understanding these theoretical aspects of stuttering is crucial, particularly for prospective clinicians and researchers. This would foster efficient decision-making regarding the assessment and management of stuttering in children and adults. The current chapter is an attempt to shed light on the historical perspectives or the early theories and provide a broader understanding of recent theories and models of stuttering.

Learning and psychological theories

Speech is a learned behaviour that is often influenced by environmental factors and thought processes of an individual who stutters. Stemming from learning and psychology principles, the following theories made a mark in the history of stuttering research.

DOI: 10.4324/9781003367673-4

Diagnosogenic theory

Proposed by Johnson (1942), the *diagnosogenic theory* is considered as one of the early popular theories of stuttering. Johnson asserted that stuttering and typical disfluency lie on a continuum; and that typical disfluencies are shaped into stuttering-like disfluencies (SLDs) when reinforced with negative reactions and labelled as stuttering by parents or significant others. His proposition led to several studies in the next two decades investigating differences between parents of children who do and do not stutter (Darley, 1955; Johnson et al., 1959; Moncur, 1952). However, in the later years, the theory witnessed a fall with emerging evidence regarding improved fluency skills when children were made aware of their stutter (Martin et al., 1972).

Classical and operant conditioning

The late 1950s and early 1960s witnessed a growing interest in the use of classical and operant conditioning principles to explain the cause of stuttering. Classical conditioning was implied within this context as emotional arousal while speaking that led to stuttering; however, the exact relation between negative emotions and speaking remained unclear. Operant conditioning gained more popularity when explaining stuttering moments. According to the principles of operant conditioning, reactions to fluency breaks of young children reinforce the occurrence of these breaks, often with a consequent increase in frequency and severity of disfluencies. The anticipation and associated struggle with stuttering leads to escape and avoidance behaviours; and it is believed that these behaviours are reinforced further by their consequence, that is, relief from the stutter and associated anxiety. Operant conditioning could successfully explain the development of stuttering through escape and avoidance behaviour. However, it failed to explain the onset of stuttering. Nonetheless, principles of operant conditioning continue to be the foundation for shaping evidence-based stuttering intervention programmes such as response cost and the Lidcombe programme (See Chapter 6 on the management of stuttering in children).

Personal construct theory

This theory emerged from the field of psychology based on Kelly's theory of personal construct (Kelly, 1955). Kelly proposed that people form notions or opinions about their environment and events. Based on their experiences, they note recurring patterns and similarities/differences between events and/or environments and form themes or constructs. They then use these themes to predict outcomes in the future when encountering similar situations. Within this context, Fransella (1972) suggested that individuals exhibit stuttering because they perceive it to be the most common or meaningful form of their speech. Further, they may also experience fear, anxiety, and guilt (Manning, 2009). Thus, the personal construct theory has been useful in explaining the anticipation of stuttering and the negative emotions associated with it. The theory also led to the development of *Personal Construct Therapy* – a cognitive restructuring approach for stuttering intervention. Through this therapy approach, clinicians help PWS change/discard their views or constructs associated with stuttering and form new constructs in the role of a fluent speaker.[1] Personal construct therapy has been reported to be effective for both children (Hayhow, 2018) and adults (Dalton, 2018).

Anticipatory struggle hypothesis

One of the most widely accepted explanations for stuttering was proposed by Bloodstein (1987) who surmised that children consider speaking to be a difficult task, and this anticipated difficulty leads to fluency breakdown. Although there existed some earlier evidence (Boome & Richardson, 1931; Freund, 1966; Gifford, 1940) that suggested stuttering to be caused by the anticipation of stuttering itself, the hypothesis gained popularity with the work of Bloodstein (1958). He suggested that the initial view of *speaking being difficult* develops as a result of communication failure that leads to tension and fragmentation in speech units. He also suggested that communication failure in the initial developmental years, owing to factors such as articulation difficulty, language delay, or even normal non-fluencies may cause frustration in a child. It was proposed that repeated communication failure in addition to negative listener reactions may induce anxiety, which in turn disturbs the speech motor activity. Other extrinsic factors such as high parental demands or intrinsic factors such as a perfectionistic personality were also said to influence the level of associated frustration and anxiety (Bloodstein & Bernstein Ratner, 2008).

Prior to Bloodstein's (1987) work, the concept of anticipatory struggle existed in alternate forms. Johnson (1942, as cited in Bloodstein, 2021) regarded stuttering as *anticipatory avoidance* and called it an "anticipatory, apprehensive, hypertonic avoidance reaction" (p. 150). In simple words, he suggested that stuttering is what an individual does when they anticipate it, dread it, and become anxious with an intention to avoid it. In an alternative explanation, Sheehan (1953, 1958) introduced stuttering as an *approach-avoidance conflict*, which is binary conflict between the need to speak and the urge to remain quiet. Though not directly stated as an anticipatory struggle, the *Preparatory set* of Van Riper (1937), famous as a therapeutic tool for stuttering, might have originated from Bloodstein's anticipatory struggle hypothesis.

Breakdown hypothesis

The physical breakdown in the speech execution has been elaborated in various forms earlier (Adams, 1974; Eisenson, 1958, 1975; Perkins et al., 1976; Travis, 1931; Van Riper, 1971; West, 1958). However, Bloodstein and Bernstein Ratner (2008) suggested that incoordination at the surface level, that is between the subsystems of speech, is a mere description of the behaviour (stuttering). The breakdown hypothesis includes an additional component in the form of specific environmental factors which act as precipitating agents and exert pressure on the subsystems of speech leading to a breakdown. These environmental factors, according to proponents of the hypothesis, include emotional and psychosocial stress as well as cognitive-linguistic demands. Owing to its deep-rooted belief in emotional and psychosocial involvement, this hypothesis has been influential in cognitive behaviour therapy-based treatments for stuttering. From the perspective of therapy, clinicians teach strategies and assist PWS in coping with external stress factors.

Repressed need hypothesis

The repressed need hypothesis originated with the psychoanalytic viewpoint of a few treating physicians. The psychoanalytic view proposed underlying psychopathology or neurosis and stuttering as the overt symptom of the same. While some suggested the source of this neurotic conflict to be psychosexual (Glauber, 1982), a few others attributed it to inadequate interpersonal relationships (Barbara, 1965; Wyatt, 1969). Other psychosocial issues where stuttering might be the overt symptom include gaining attention and sympathy, escaping from failure, and coping with other problems in life (Bloodstein et al., 2021). This hypothesis paved the way for research investigating personality and temperament differences between those who do and do not stutter. While several studies report between-group differences (Anderson et al., 2003; Choi et al., 2013; Eggers et al., 2013; Eggers et al., 2022; Iverach, Jones, et al., 2009; Iverach et al., 2010; Rocha et al., 2019; Rodgers & Jackson, 2021; Tichenor & Yaruss, 2020; Wakaba, 1997), a few others provide evidence that refutes the hypothesis and suggests that PWS do not vary in their personality and temperament traits than individuals who do not stutter (Alm, 2014; Eggers et al., 2010; Embrechts et al., 2000; Reilly et al., 2009; Reilly et al., 2013; van der Merwe et al., 2011; Williams, 2006). Further, it was also found that psychoanalysis or any other form of psychotherapy has not been significantly effective in treating stuttering (Andrews et al., 1983).

Organic theories

Organic theories represent a group of theories that consider stuttering to be a biological or physiological disorder. Based on these theories, the cause of stuttering could range from neurological (structure and/or function) to hormonal and biochemical differences, as well as differences in processing auditory, linguistic, and motoric information. What follows is a description of theories, models, and evidence, providing an account of the physiological underpinnings of stuttering.

Cerebral dominance theory

Another theory that made its mark in the history of stuttering research was the *cerebral dominance theory* proposed by Orton (1927) and Travis (1931). Proponents of the theory asserted that for smooth execution of speech, the nerve impulses sent to the left and right sides of different articulators need to be synchronized. They suggested that this synchronization was led by the dominant hemisphere (left hemisphere in most individuals), and the non-dominant hemisphere followed its lead. Based on this premise, the theory posited that the nervous system of PWS fails to mature completely, thereby leading to failure in achieving left hemisphere dominance for speech functions. Lack of dominance probably leads to a conflict between the two hemispheres, disrupting the synchronization process and culminating in a fluency breakdown. Several potential reasons for this maturational failure were suggested which included genetic influence, disease, injury or trauma, and emotional factors.

To verify the theory, a series of experiments were conducted which started with studies determining handedness in those who stutter versus those who do not stutter. Several of the initial investigations were in the favour of the theory (Fagan, 1931; Jasper, 1932; Orton & Travis, 1929; Travis, 1928; Travis & Herren, 1929; Van Riper, 1935). Thus, according to the "handedness theory" ambidextrous or left-handed individuals who were forced to shift handedness to the right were predisposed to and had a greater likelihood of developing stuttering. However, studies in the later years showed conflicting findings (Andrews & Harris, 1964; Johnson et al., 1959; Pierce & Lipcon, 1959; Records et al., 1977; Striefler & Gumpertz, 1955). By the late 1970s, handedness studies were replaced by newer experiments in which more precise procedures were conducted to determine cerebral laterality. One such famous experiment was the *Wada test* which involved the injection of sodium amytol in the left and right carotid arteries inducing a temporary loss of speech. The experiment revealed that PWS exhibited loss of speech when injected on either side indicating a lack of cerebral dominance for speech (Wada & Rasmussen, 1960).

Another paradigm that gained much popularity in assessing cerebral dominance was the *dichotic listening task*. A dichotic listening task involves the simultaneous presentation of different stimuli to the two ears and the participant is asked to repeat the stimuli presented to either one or both ears. According to literature, those with fluent speech exhibit a right-ear advantage on the dichotic listening task (Broadbent & Gregory, 1964; Kimura, 1961), indicating left hemisphere dominance for speech and language functions. Orton and Travis speculated that this situation would lead to a conflict between the hemispheres and consequently, a breakdown in the control of speech movements. Hence, based on the cerebral dominance theory, many researchers presumed that those who stutter might exhibit no ear advantage or may show a left-ear advantage. Successive studies showed a left-ear advantage in PWS in contrast to the right-ear advantage observed in the control group (Brady & Berson, 1975; Curry & Gregory, 1969; Foundas et al., 2004; Moore, 1984; Quinn, 1972; Sommers et al., 1975). However, these findings were noted only for verbal tasks and not in the context of non-verbal tasks. They suggested that these differences in the auditory system and cortical lateralization are in some way related to the disruption of critical feedback processes that permit the uninterrupted forward flow of speech. In contrast, several other studies reported no difference in performance on dichotic listening tasks between those who do and do not stutter (Dorman & Porter, 1975; Meyers et al., 1989; Newton et al., 1986; Pinsky & McAdam, 1980; Strub et al., 1987; Sussman & MacNeilage, 1975). Some studies suggested the presence of brainstem-related CAPD in PWS rather than hemispheric lateralization deficits (Dietrich, 1997; Hall & Jerger, 1978; Toscher & Rupp, 1978). The discrepancy in these findings was later explained by Moore (1984) as the result of the difference in stimuli used across studies.

In addition to these studies with adult subjects, several dichotic listening studies have compared stuttering and non-stuttering children. Studies with CWS are essential in order to develop a better understanding of the role that any factors of interest might play in the etiology of stuttering. A few of the early studies that conducted dichotic listening tasks using digits and monosyllables in children with and without stuttering indicated no significant group differences. In fact, either a right-ear advantage was detected in both groups (Slorach & Noehr, 1973) or no ear advantage was found in either of the two groups (Gruber & Powell, 1974; Liebetrau & Daly, 1981). In contrast, Sommers et al. (1975) and Cimorell-Strong et al. (1983) found between-group differences where a greater percentage of children with no stuttering showed a right-ear advantage in comparison to CWS. Further, a few researchers suggested that similar to adults, there exists a sub-group of CWS who exhibit a left-ear advantage or no ear advantage on dichotic listening tasks (Blood & Blood, 1984; Blood, 1985).

Although the cerebral dominance theory witnessed a decline in its popularity, subtle hemispheric differences continued to emerge with the development of newer and advanced measures such as imaging studies and advanced auditory processing investigations as discussed below.

Evidence from neuroimaging studies

The role of various cortical and subcortical structures for language formulation and speech production is well established in literature. Within this context, it is reasonable to assume that those with speech production deficits such as stuttering might exhibit structural and functional differences in these areas. Advancements in technology and research methods have been useful in determining the neuroanatomical and neurophysiological underpinnings of stuttering. The commonly used structural measures include computed tomography (CT), magnetic resonance imaging (MRI), and diffusion tensor imaging (DTI). Functional procedures consist of functional magnetic resonance imaging (fMRI), regional cerebral blood flow (rCBF), positron emission tomography (PET), and single-photon emission computerized tomography (SPECT). The main purpose of the neuroanatomical and neurophysiological investigations in PWS has been to determine the structural differences and variations in brain activity, particularly for speech perception and production when compared to their fluent peers. Extensive research has been carried out through the past three to four decades. A few of these investigations are summarized in Tables 4.1 and 4.2 below.

Overall, it has been observed that PWS exhibit structural differences when compared to typically fluent individuals across a wide range of anatomical sites. There have been consistent reports indicating increased activation of right hemisphere regions and hypoactivity in the left hemisphere of those with stuttering. Further, atypical neural activity in those who stutter has been primarily mapped on to regions of speech motor planning and execution along with areas responsible for maintaining feedback (De Nil, 2004; De Nil et al., 2007). A few differences have also been reported between children who persist and recover from stuttering (Chang et al., 2008; Koenraads et al., 2020). Chang et al. (2008) observed relatively greater grey matter volume in bilateral superior temporal gyri of children in the persistent group than children who recovered. Similarly, Koenraads et al. (2020) noted reduced

Table 4.1 Summary of neuroanatomical findings in those who stutter

Structure/regions & deficits identified	Population	Imaging technique	Source
Larger left and right planum temporale areas Reduced planar asymmetry	AWS	MRI	Foundas et al. (2001)
Reduced white matter in left hemisphere	AWS	DTI	Sommer et al. (2002)
Increased white matter volume in planum temporale, anterior and inferior frontal gyrus, precentral gyrus of right hemisphere and reduced cerebral asymmetry	AWS	MRI	Jancke et al. (2004)
Activation of right frontal operculum	AWS	fMRI	Preibisch et al. (2003)
Bilateral overactivity in anterior insula, cerebellum and midbrain Bilateral underactivity in rolandic operculum, sensorimotor cortex, ventral premotor area Underactivity in left Herschl's gyrus	Adolescents and AWS	MRI and fMRI	Watkins et al. (2008)
Reduced grey matter volume in left frontal inferior gyrus and bilateral temporal lobes Reduced white matter volume in left rolandic operculum, motor regions for face and larynx	CWS	MRI and DTI	Chang et al. (2008)
Lack of cortical asymmetry or Increased cortical volume in left frontal and right temporoparietal regions	AWS	MRI	Foundas et al. (2003)
Reduced white matter volume in ventral perisylvian region and corpus callosum	AWS	DTI	Cykowski et al. (2010)
Reduced white matter volume in ventral premotor cortex, cerebral peduncles, bilateral arcuate fasciculus, posterior corpus callosum, left corticospinal and cortibulbar tracts	Teenagers who stutter and AWS	DTI	Connally et al. (2014)
Reduced white matter volume in left inferior frontal gyrus, premotor cortex, motor cortex, middle/superior temporal gyrus, inferior parietal regions Reduced white matter volume in corpus callosum, cingulum, and cerebellum	CWS	DTI	Chang et al. (2015)
Right frontal aslant tract (cortico-striatal network)	CWS	DTI	Misaghi et al. (2018)
Larger right nucleus accumbens	AWS	MRI	Neef et al. (2018)

(*Continued*)

Table 4.1 (Continued)

Structure/regions & deficits identified	Population	Imaging technique	Source
Reduced grey matter volume in left superior and frontal regions	CWS	Structural MRI and DTI	Koenraads et al. (2020)
Reduced white matter volume in right inferior cerebellar peduncle	CWS	Diffusion MRI	Johnson et al. (2022)

(*Note:* CWS – *children who stutter*; AWS – *adults who stutter*)

Table 4.2 Summary of neurophysiological findings in those who stutter

Structure/regions & deficits identified	Task	Population	Imaging technique	Source
Reduced blood flow to frontal lobe and left temporal lobe	–	AWS	SPECT eliciting rCBF data	Pool et al. (1991)
Reduced blood flow to left and middle temporal region, right cerebellum Increased blood flow to substantia nigra and limbic system	Laryngeal reaction time task	AWS	SPECT eliciting rCBF data	Watson et al. (1992)
Increased blood flow to supplementary motor area (left > right) and superior lateral premotor cortex (right > left)	Resting, solo reading, choral reading	AWS	PET eliciting rCBF data	Ingham et al. (1994)
Decreased cerebral activation in left Broca's and Wernicke's areas along with several other regions	Solo and choral reading	AWS	PET scans	Wu et al. (1995)
Increased activation of cortical and cerebellar motor regions, lack of cerebral motor dominance, reduced transmission between left frontal and temporal cortices	Solo reading, choral reading, eyes-closed rest	AWS	PET scans	Fox et al. (1996)
Bilateral activation of speech and language areas (posterior superior temporal gyrus, inferior frontal gyrus, superior, mid-lateral precentral gyrus, association cortex)	Word description task for lexical access and lexical generation	AWS	fMRI	Blomgren et al. (2003)

(*Continued*)

Table 4.2 (Continued)

Structure/regions & deficits identified	Task	Population	Imaging technique	Source
Increased activation in left auditory and somatosensory cortices, left insula, dorsal precentral gyrus, midline SMA and anterior cingulate regions	Paced speech and singing	AWS	PET scan	Stager et al. (2003)
Increased activation of bilateral basal ganglia and posterior insula in resting state Reduced activation of left globus pallidus and bilateral posterior insula during speech	Oral reading and monologue	AWS	PET scan	Ingham et al. (2012)
Reduced white matter volume in left arcuate fasciculus and left middle cerebellar peduncle Higher diffusivity in bilateral frontal aslant tract	Sensorimotor synchroniza-tion task	AWS	Diffusion MRI	Jossinger et al. (2022)

(*Note:* CWS – *children who stutter;* AWS – *adults who stutter*)

left superior frontal grey matter volume in pre-adolescents who persisted to stutter than the recovered and control groups. In contrast to the above evidence, there were a few studies that found no significant structural or functional differences between individuals with and without stuttering (Cykowski et al., 2010; Gough et al., 2018; Ingham et al., 1996; Pinsky & McAdam, 1980). Nevertheless, most researchers agree that there are some underlying brain structure and function differences. Support may also be drawn from investigations that reported change in neural structure and/or function as a function of treatment, particularly under the influence of fluency-inducing conditions. Studies reported shift to typical left hemisphere laterality in PWS under fluency-inducing conditions, such as biofeedback (McFarland & Moore, 1982), choral reading (Ingham et al., 1994; Stager et al., 2003), on medication (Wood et al., 1980), and post fluency-shaping treatment (Kroll et al., 1997; Neumann et al., 2005).

Evidence from auditory processing studies

Although the overt symptoms of stuttering manifest themselves as breakdowns in speech fluency, one long-standing hypothesis suggests that those symptoms may result from underlying deficits in auditory processing that would disrupt speech production by affecting self-monitoring of the acoustic feedback signal (Cherry et al., 1955; Cherry & Sayers, 1956). Over the years, this suggestion appears to have found at least partial support in observations of (a) a reportedly lower prevalence of stuttering in the hearing-impaired population (Harms & Malone, 1939; Montgomery & Fitch, 1988), and (b) improvements in speech fluency when stuttering individuals speak while hearing delayed auditory feedback (DAF), frequency-altered auditory feedback (FAF), masking noise, or the simultaneous presentation of a second speaker's voice (unison or choral speech) (Ingham & Packman, 1979; Kiefte & Armson, 2008; Macleod et al., 1955; Martin & Haroldson, 1979; Martin et al., 1985; Max et al., 1997; Soderberg, 1969; Stuart et al., 2008; Stuart et al., 1996). Published studies in this area have used a wide variety of experimental approaches, and the results are often not easily integrated. These studies can be grouped into two categories representing distinct experimental approaches: Behavioural studies and auditory-evoked and event potential studies.

BEHAVIOURAL STUDIES

Early attempts to uncover abnormalities in the peripheral or central auditory system of PWS relied mainly on behavioural data. In general, various categories of behavioural tests can be distinguished based on the specific auditory processes being assessed, the types of auditory stimuli presented to the subjects, the nature of the test procedures, and the neural level at which the central auditory pathway is being evaluated. Categories of behavioural tests that have been used with PWS include dichotic listening tasks, monaural low redundancy speech tasks, binaural interaction tasks, temporal processing tasks, and other auditory tasks, such as sound localization, auditory tracking, and loudness matching. As discussed above dichotic listening tasks are observed to report mixed findings for both children and adults. The findings for other behavioural studies are summarized in Table 4.3 below. Overall, behavioural studies of auditory processing have not consistently found differences between those who do and do not stutter.

AUDITORY-EVOKED AND EVENT-RELATED POTENTIALS

Auditory-evoked potentials are used as objective measures to evaluate the brain's response to auditory stimuli at different levels along the auditory pathway. Using stimulus-locked epochs of electroencephalographic (EEG) recordings, both brainstem and cortical potentials have been recorded from stuttering and non-stuttering individuals as they listen to auditory stimuli. The findings of a few auditory-evoked and event-related potential studies are summarized in Table 4.4 below. Overall, a general agreement is noted among researchers for the delayed auditory brainstem responses in PWS. However, a delay in middle and late latency responses is seen inconsistently, and it remains unclear whether there exists any difference in signal transmission (and thus presumably information processing) at later stages of the central auditory pathways in PWS.

Genetic influence on stuttering

It has long been observed that stuttering frequently runs in families. Evidence from twin studies (Andrews et al., 1991; Bloodstein, 1961; Howie, 1981), adoption studies

Table 4.3 Summary of auditory behavioural task findings in those who stutter

Author (Year)	Task	Findings
Blood (1996) Hall and Jerger (1978)	Staggered Spondaic Word (SSW) test	Greater proportion of AWNS demonstrated a right-ear advantage than did AWS
Blood and Blood (1984)		Overall, no difference between CWS and CWNS; however, individual data indicated poorer performance in CWS than CWNS
Anderson et al. (1988)		CWS obtained relatively lower scores than CWNS in the left-competing condition
Hall and Jerger (1978) Toscher and Rupp (1978) Molt and Guilford (1979)	Synthetic Sentence Identification Contralateral Competing Message test (SSI-CCM)	Both PWS and PWNS obtained 100% scores with no group difference or indication of any deficits in central auditory processing
Kramer et al. (1987)	Synthetic Sentence Identification	No group difference between AWS and AWNS
Hall and Jerger (1978) Toscher and Rupp (1978) Molt and Guilford (1979)	Ipsilateral Competing Message test (SSI-ICM)	PWS obtained poorer scores than PWNS for both right and left ears
Gregory (1964)	Discrimination of monaurally- and binaurally-presented distorted speech	Decreased performance for AWS than AWNS
Bonin et al. (1985) Anderson et al. (1988)	Binaural fusion task	No difference in scores between PWS and PWNS (both for children & adults)
Kramer et al. (1987)	Masking level difference (MLD)	Lower MLDs for AWS than AWNS
Rousey et al. (1959)	Sound localization task	Poorer performance in CWS than CWNS
Meyers et al. (1989)	Auditory temporal ordering task	No significant difference in scores between AWS and AWNS
Barasch et al. (2000)	Duration pattern sequence task	
Blood (1996)	Pitch pattern sequencing test	
Howell and Williams (2004)	Temporal masking tasks	No significant difference in scores between PWS and PWNS (children and adolescents)
Howell, Rosen, et al. (2000) Howell et al. (2006)	Backward masking task	Lower scores for backward masking in CWS than CWNS

(Note: CWS – *children who stutter;* CWNS – *children who do not stutter;* AWS – *adults who stutter;* AWNS – adults who do not stutter)

Table 4.4 Summary of auditory-evoked and event-related potential findings in those who stutter

Author (Year)	Task	Findings
Blood and Blood (1984) Khedr et al. (2000) Stager (1990)	Auditory brainstem responses (ABR)	Prolonged latency and reduced amplitude in PWS than PWNS (children & adults)
Decker et al. (1982) Newman et al. (1985)		No significant difference in latency and amplitude between AWS and AWNS
Dietrich et al. (1995)	Auditory middle latency response (AMLR)	No significant difference for the P_a latency, although a shorter P_b latency was seen in AWS than AWNS
Finitzo et al. (1991)	Auditory late latency response (ALLR)	Reduced N1 and P2 amplitude in AWS than AWNS
Khedr et al. (2000) Hampton and 　Weber-Fox (2008)		No significant difference in latency and amplitude between AWS and AWNS
Morgan et al. (1997)	P300	Greater P300 amplitude in the left hemisphere for AWS unlike greater amplitude in right hemisphere for AWNS
Ferrand et al. (1991) 　Hampton and 　Weber-Fox (2008) Khedr et al. (2000)	P300	No significant difference in latency and amplitude between AWS and AWNS

(Note: PWS – person who stutter; PWNS – person who do not stutter; AWS – adults who stutter; AWNS – adults who do not stutter)

(Bloodstein, 1961), and aggregation and segregation studies (Viswanath et al., 2004) is consistent with a genetic etiology, although not all cases of stuttering are familial, and when they are, environmental factors play a role as well. A total of nine twin studies have been conducted with sample sizes varying from less than 100 subjects to greater than 2000 participants (Andrews et al., 1991; Dworzynski et al., 2007; Felsenfeld et al., 2000; Godai et al., 1976; Howie, 1981; Ooki, 2005; Rautakoski et al., 2012; Van Beijsterveldt et al., 2010). Evidence from twin studies suggests that monozygotic (MZ) twins have higher a concordance[2] than dizygotic (DZ) twins, highlighting there are strong role of genetic components in the development of the disorder. MZ twins share 100 % DNA, whereas DZ twins share 50% DNA. Further, results from these studies also estimate high heritability (0.80). When compared to twin studies, adoption studies are fewer in number (Bloodstein, 1961; Felsenfeld & Plomin, 1997) and suffer from methodological limitations in terms of limited sample size. Results from adoption studies suggest that stuttering does not develop through imitation of parents' speech. A few studies have also investigated the mode of inheritance in the family. It is known that over two-thirds of children who develop stuttering report a positive family history. Aggregation and segregation are done to investigate whether a positive family history increases the risk of developing stuttering and to trace the mode of inheritance in the family. One of the largest aggregation studies was conducted by Andrews et al. (1983). They included 725 probands and reported that females are less affected by the disorder if one of the family member stutterers. However, they have higher chances of having a child who stutters. Recently, Darmody et al. (2022) recruited 739 participants and their results suggested that males and females have higher chances of having a father who stutters than having a mother who stutters. They also reported that there was greater impact of stuttering for females than males with a family history of stuttering. However, there is no consensus with regard to mode of inheritance. Studies have failed to suggest whether stuttering has a dominant, recessive or sex-linked inheritance (Riaz et al., 2005; Viswanath et al., 2004; Wittke-Thompson et al., 2007). Under the common disease/common variant (CD/CV) model, the same genetic variants, each with a minor effect but acting together in an additive or multiplicative way, are assumed to underlie all cases of inherited stuttering. Under an alternate model, common disease/rare variant (CD/RV), stuttering is assumed to be heterogeneous, and in different families, different rare variants with major effects cause stuttering. It has been debated whether stuttering follows Mendelian inheritance patterns (i.e., is caused by a single gene) (Viswanath et al., 2004), or whether it is a complex trait (i.e., it is caused at the confluence of various genes). Furthermore, various modes of inheritance in stuttering have been proposed, including a sex-modified model (Kidd et al., 1978; MacFarlane et al., 1991). It has also been suggested that persistent and non-persistent forms of stuttering might be distinctly different disorder subtypes from the point of view of genetic contribution (Viswanath et al., 2004).

Recent molecular studies of stuttering (Table 4.5), building on each other's findings, have suggested candidate regions of moderate evidence of linkage when samples of unrelated families were studied, candidate regions with statistically significant evidence of linkage when a sample of unrelated families had high levels of consanguinity, and the identification of a causal gene when the candidate region was sequenced in single extended kindred (Kang et al., 2010). The results suggest genes on chromosomes 3, 12, 16 (Raza et al., 2010; Riaz et al., 2005) and on chromosomes 2, 3, 14, and 15 (Raza et al., 2013) cause stuttering. In 68 families (n=226) from the US and UK, a genome-wide linkage analysis (GWLA) using a 396-marker microsatellite panel suggested a region of interest on chromosome (chr) 18 (Shugart et al., 2004). This study focused largely on the affected members of the families and assumed a dominant mode of inheritance. Based on the hypothesis that stuttering is a complex trait influenced by several genes, a subsequent study (Riaz et al., 2005) focused on 44 Pakistani families with high inbreeding coefficients, where one may reasonably assume that only one or very few genes are causative for the phenotype shared in each of these families. Linkage analyses based on microsatellites with 366 markers resulted in four regions of interest on chrs 1, 5, 7, and 12, with the largest and statistically significant linkage signal at chr 12. Strong contributions to the linkage signals came from three extended kindreds within the sample. Suggestive evidence for the locus on chr 12 was also found in a study of 100 Caucasian families from the US, Sweden, and Israel (n=585). Linkage analysis was based on single nucleotide polymorphism (SNP) chip with 9,144 markers (Suresh et al., 2006). The

Table 4.5 List of studies that attempted to identify genes in stuttering

S. No	Chromosome Region	Gene Identification Method	Gene Identified	Author (Year)
01	1q	GWLA	N/A	Riaz et al. (2005)
02	2q	GWLA	N/A	Suresh et al. (2006)
03	3q	GWLA	N/A	Wittke-Thompson et al. (2007)
04	5q	GWLA	N/A	Riaz et al. (2005)
05	7q	GWLA	N/A	Riaz et al. (2005)
06	9p	GWLA	N/A	Suresh et al. (2006)
07	12q23	GWLA Targeted candidate gene sequencing	GNPTAB	Kang et al. (2010); Riaz et al. (2005)
08	13q	GWLA	N/A	Wittke-Thompson et al. (2007)
09	15P	GWLA	N/A	Suresh et al. (2006)
10	15q	GWLA	N/A	Wittke-Thompson et al. (2007)
11	16p13	Targeted candidate gene sequencing	GNPTG	Kang et al. (2010)
12	16p13	Targeted candidate gene sequencing	NAGPA	Kang et al. (2010)
13	18p	GWLA	N/A	Shugart et al. (2004)
14	21p	GWLA	N/A	Suresh et al. (2006)

authors argued that SNP panels have greater statistical power to detect linkage, compared to microsatellites, depending on selected densities. Phenotypes were classified into a broad (ever stuttered) and a narrow (persistent stuttering) definition. Results were suggestive of linkage to a locus on chr 9 for the broad definition of stuttering, a locus on chr 15 for the narrow definition of stuttering, a locus on chr 7 for male-only cases, a locus on chr 21 for female-only cases, and an increased signal on chr 12 conditional on the signal from chr 7.

A linkage analysis with a 5 centimorgan (cM) microsatellite panel was performed on an extended 232 persons family of Hutterite origin that included 48 biologically related individuals affected with stuttering (Wittke-Thompson et al., 2007). Microsatellite genotypes with an average density of 5 cM were obtained. Four types of analyses, nonparametric genome-wide linkage analysis, transmission disequilibrium testing (TDT), family-based association testing (FBAT), and a meta-analysis of two Caucasian genome screens (105 families plus the Hutterites) did not yield any statistically significant results, although some of the signals with nominal significance overlapped with linkage signals for previously reported speech and language disorders. The chr 12 locus was examined by sequencing a 300 kb region centred on the PAH (phenylalanine hydroxilase) gene (Kang et al., 2010) in one of the Pakistani families investigated in the Riaz et al. (2005) study reporting that a marker near this gene was linked to stuttering. Sequencing this region led to the discovery of a mutation in a gene in this region, GNPTAB. The same mutation was also found in 5 of

123 unrelated other Pakistani individuals who stutter and one of 270 Asian Indian individuals who stutter in the UK and US. Two other genes, GNPTG, and NAGPA, which are functionally related to GNPTAB, were identified as causative in four and six cases, respectively, in North America. Sequencing of these genes in controls showed that they explain stuttering in rare families with geographic ancestry in the Asian subcontinent but not in North American or British controls. In another study based on a functional hypothesis related to hyperactive dopamine metabolism in PWS, SNPs in the DRD2 gene were shown to be associated with stuttering in 112 Han Chinese individuals who stutter (Lan et al., 2009). Together, these studies show that the traditional view of stuttering as a common clinical entity with many common genetic variants of minor effects (CD/CV model) may be an accurate assumption for only some cases. Single extensive families contributed substantially to the linkage signal on chr 12, and a rare causative gene was identified when one of these families was studied. Given that worldwide, persistent stuttering affects 1% of the population and that the GNPTAB variant was observed in 6 of 123 unrelated kindreds of East Asian geographic ancestry and not at all in other ancestries, this variant occurs at a rate of approximately .0004 in East Asians only. This is consistent with a common disease/rare variant (CD/RV) model positing rare variants in individual families that, in aggregate, explain many cases of stuttering. The rare but highly penetrant disruptions in the FOXP2 gene causing severe difficulties with speech, receptive and expressive language, reading, writing, cognition, and oral praxis (Fisher et al., 1998; MacDermot et al., 2005; Vargha-Khadem et al., 1995; Watkins et al., 2002) are an example of such a rare variant. The CD/RV hypothesis for stuttering is in line with a general paradigm shift in thinking about genetic variation in complex diseases (McClellan & King, 2010), and in synergy with new approaches in gene discovery, most recently exome sequencing. This new wave of research endeavours follows in the wake of massive efforts to discover common genes, each with moderate to small effects, using genome-wide association studies (GWAS) in samples of thousands of unrelated cases and controls, an approach designed for gene discovery following the CD/CV model.

In addition to this problem of heterogeneity, a number of aspects complicate identification of genes associated with stuttering: Stuttering appears to have variable penetrance, which can confound the genotype/phenotype characterization. Stuttering is also variable in its expression, spanning a spectrum from mild to severe and forms that resolve (i.e., spontaneous recovery) as well as those that persist, and with different expression patterns in males and females. To advance our knowledge of genotype/phenotype relationships in PWS, future approaches and methodologies must be optimized to overcome these difficulties.

Speech motor control theories

The proposition that stuttering is a motor speech disorder is not recent. It has, in fact, surfaced as a component of several theories, old and new, explaining the causal factors of stuttering. These theories majorly focus on atypical neural processing, particularly in the context of motor control for speech movements. The emerging neuroimaging findings over the past few decades (as described under organic theories) have contributed significantly to validating the claims of speech motor control theories. We will now proceed to explain a few of the significant theories or models in this domain.

Zimmermann's model

Zimmermann (1980) was one of the earliest to propose speech motor control deficits in stuttering. He suggested that spatiotemporal processing of speech movements is highly variable in those who stutter and susceptible to instability in the motor system. Thus, when a movement variability surpasses the *critical threshold*, corrective feedback is sent to the motor control centres to initiate reprogramming, which in turn makes the motor system unstable and leads to a fluency breakdown. Zimmermann proposed that those who stutter either have an inherently unstable speech motor control system or exhibit low tolerance to speech movement variability. His findings were based on the cinefluorographic observations of reduced articulatory velocity and displacement measures in PWS. He argued that these reduced movement parameters ensured that the neural centres for speech motor control are stable and movement variability does not cross the critical threshold triggering fluency breakdown. His model could also provide a physiological explanation for stuttering under the influence of psychological factors such as anxiety and fear. He reasoned that intense emotions such as anxiety, fear, and at times even excitement could lead to increased activation of brainstem pathways crossing the critical threshold, thereby causing stuttering.

Cyberkinetic or servosystem model

Primarily based on Fairbank's model of speech production (Fairbanks, 1954), more popularly known as the "speech as servosystem mechanism", cyberkinetic theories imply feedback deficits in those who stutter. The servosystem model of the speech mechanism suggests that a part of the speech output is fed back to the system to be compared with the intended output. In case the feedback received does not match the intended output, it indicates an error in the production, and reprogramming is initiated. Based on this premise it was suggested that in those who stutter, disrupted feedback interrupts the smooth flow of speech. Major support for this model was derived from delayed auditory feedback (DAF) studies that found improved fluency in PWS under the influence of DAF (Bohr, 1963; Daliri & Max, 2018; Fiorin et al., 2021; Kalinowski et al., 1993; Lotzmann, 1961; Soderberg, 1969; Stuart & Kalinowski, 2004; Stuart et al., 1997; Van Borsel, Reunes, et al., 2003).

Interhemispheric interference model

Considered by some as an extension of the Orton-Travis theory, the interhemispheric interference model is a two-factor model proposed by Webster (1987). The two factors suggested by the model are an underlying inefficient supplementary motor area (SMA) and an over-reactive hemispheric activation. The model also proposes that both factors are independent, necessary, and sufficient to cause stuttering. In other words, stuttering may not occur in the absence of any one of the two factors. Unlike cerebral dominance theory, the model suggests left dominance even in PWS; however, it proposes that the SMA of those who stutter is susceptible to other ongoing neural activity, particularly to the over-activation of the right hemisphere often associated with negative emotions. Thus, its negative emotions such as fear or anxiety may lead to over-activation of the right hemisphere which in turn interferes with the activity of left SMA leading to stuttering. The stuttering moment may further reinforce the negative emotions, and thus this cycle of right hemisphere over-activation and left SMA disturbance may continue.

As discussed by Packman and Attanasio (2017), a variety of tasks have been used to verify this model such as index and sequential finger tapping, bimanual tasks, and key pressing; however, none of the investigations involved any speech-based task. Despite this, the model holds some logic and offers a reasonable explanation for stuttering. Support may also be drawn from some recent neuroimaging studies that report white matter differences between those with and without stuttering (Chang et al., 2015). The model attempts to explain natural recovery and attributes it to the maturation of the speech motor control system including SMA. Further, the variability in stuttering was reasoned to be dependent on the degree of interhemispheric interference (Webster, 1993). However, the model does not provide any explanation for different types of disfluencies associated with stuttering. Clinically, the model has been supportive in understanding outcomes of fluency-shaping procedures. For example, the commonly used *prolongation technique* in stuttering management focuses on simplifying the act of speech production facilitating SMA to function within its stability zone, hence managing the first factor proposed by the model. The second factor finds applications in a number of treatment programmes that utilize counselling and other structured methods to manage fear, anxiety, and other negative emotions, thereby restricting the over-activation of the right hemisphere.

The variability model

The variability model or the V-model came into existence during attempts to explain the favourable outcomes of prolonged speech and rhythmic speech techniques. Packman and colleagues framed the V-model and proposed that stuttering is a result of a breakdown of an unstable speech motor control system under the influence of increased syllabic stress variability (Packman et al., 2000; Packman et al., 1996). In simple words, those who stutter have an inefficient and susceptible speech motor control system that easily gets perturbed when placed with greater demands of motoric variability in terms of increased syllabic stress. The syllabic stress variability is suggested to be a trigger and not the cause of stuttering. The model explains the onset and development of stuttering by highlighting the overlap of stuttering onset (2 to 5 years of age) and the period of language development when a child starts communicating using longer utterances that demands using syllabic stress. According to the V-model, the initial symptom of syllable repetition noted in developmental stuttering represents the attempts of a child to restore the unstable speech motor system; and the struggle to avoid stuttering manifests as fixed postures and physical concomitants. Based on empirical investigations, Packman and colleagues suggested that therapy approaches such as prolonged speech and rhythmic speech reduce the syllabic stress variability demands, thereby facilitating fluent speech (Packman et al., 1997).

The model also explains that natural recovery from stuttering could be due to maturation of the speech motor control system; however, proponents of the model accept the possibility of other influencing factors. Further, the model proposes that cognitive and emotional factors influence the threshold at which the unstable speech motor system is thrown off balance, hence explaining the variability in the frequency and severity of stuttering across situations. Though logical, the model did not further the research in this domain. However, it did contribute to the development of another multifactorial model – the Packman and Attanasio 3-factor model (P&A model) discussed in later sections of the chapter.

DIVA/GODIVA model

Two recent additions to causal models of stuttering are the DIVA and GODIVA models. These are neuro-computational models, not specific to stuttering but rather explaining speech acquisition and speech production in neurotypical individuals. The DIVA or *Direction into Velocities of Articulators* model was proposed first. It was later revised and renamed as *Gradient Order Direction into Velocities of Articulators* (GODIVA). Both versions focus on the role of sensory information in speech motor control in the form of *feedforward* and *feedback* mechanisms. A detailed explanation of these models is beyond the scope of this chapter and it is suggested that readers refer to the original source for the same (Bohland et al., 2010; Guenther et al., 2006). However, as a prerequisite to understanding the role of DIVA/GODIVA in stuttering, the major components of the two models are described hereunder.

The DIVA model (Figure 4.1) accounts for neural processes underlying a single speech motor programme. According to the model, speech is initiated by the activation of a speech sound map (SSM) (neuroanatomically located in the inferior and posterior regions of Broca's area). The activation of the SSM leads to the relay of motor commands to the motor cortex via two systems – *feedforward* and *feedback control systems*. The feedforward commands further follow two routes, first, directly to the motor cortex, and second, via cerebellar and subcortical circuits. The model emphasizes that during the initial stages of speech development, a child is largely dependent on the feedback control system (auditory and somatosensory feedback). However, over time the feedforward commands are fine-tuned and are sufficient to produce speech. With a completely developed and accurate feedforward control system, the role of the feedback control system is restricted to error monitoring and adjustments of articulatory velocities and position maps (Tourville & Guenther, 2011).

The revised version of the model, namely, the GODIVA model, was proposed to account for higher-level processes involved in the temporal sequencing of speech sounds (Bohland et al., 2010) necessary for fluent speech. The GODIVA model

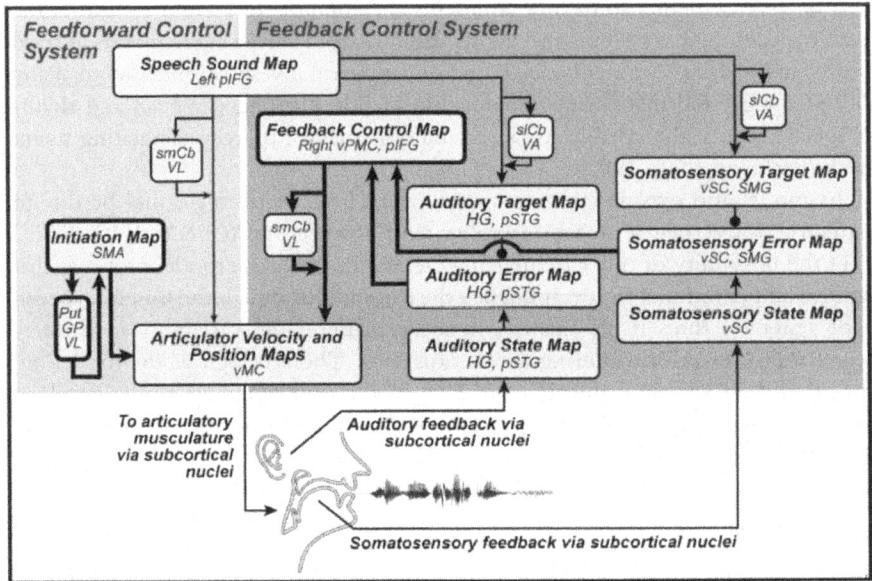

Figure 4.1 The DIVA model

Note. The DIVA model of speech acquisition and production. Recently added modules and connections are highlighted using black outlines. Model components associated with hypothesized neuroanatomical substrates. Abbreviations: GP = globus pallidus; HG = Heschl's gyrus; pIFg = posterior inferior frontal gyrus; pSTg = posterior superior temporal gyrus; Put = putamen; slCB = superior lateral cerebellum; smCB = superior medial cerebellum; SMA = supplementary motor area; SMG = supramarginal gyrus; VA = ventral anterior nucleus of the cerebellum; VL = ventral lateral nucleus of the thalamus; vMC = ventral motor cortex; vPMC = ventral premotor cortex; vSC = ventral somatosensory cortex.

Source: "The DIVA model: A neural theory of speech acquisition and production," by J. A. Tourville and F. H. Guenther, 2011, *Language and cognitive processes, 26*(7), p. 23 (https://doi:10.1080/01690960903498424). Copyright 2011 by the Taylor & Francis.

suggests two important loops, *the planning loop* and *the motor loop*. While the motor loop is shared with the DIVA model (including cortical and subcortical regions generating coordinated articulatory movements), the planning loop acts as a storage buffer and is responsible for the temporal sequencing of upcoming speech sounds. The planning loop includes regions of the left posterior inferior frontal sulcus, pre-supplementary motor area, basal ganglia (caudate nucleus and globus pallidus), and ventral anterior thalamic nucleus.

Within the context of stuttering, Civier et al. (2013) proposed two hypotheses based on the GODIVA model. The first hypothesis suggests that stuttering is caused by elevated dopamine levels in PWS. The second hypothesis proposed impaired white matter connectivity in the brain underlying the speech motor control deficits in stuttering. They found support for both these hypotheses from their simulations and suggested that stuttering is exhibited as a combined result of elevated dopamine levels and impaired white matter connectivity. The model explained loci of stuttering (predominantly initial position) and moments of stuttering. Blocks and prolongations reflected the execution of the initial syllable and a delay in commands for subsequent syllables. The initial sound or syllable repetition was reasoned to be a result of impaired execution of feedforward commands due to underlying deficits in white matter connectivity. Further, the variable nature of stuttering and the influence of environmental factors were also linked to increased dopamine levels. Civier et al. (2013), however, suggested that their model and simulations warranted more research in furthering our understanding of causal factors for stuttering.

Psycholinguistic theories

While the proposed organic origin of stuttering gained popularity across decades with strong literature support as discussed above, researchers from another school of thought highlighted disrupted psycholinguistic processes underlying stuttering. Psycholinguistic theories suggest deficits in the encoding of phonological, lexical, syntactic, or suprasegmental information. Studies in this domain indicate deficits in lexical retrieval, lexical decision-making, and phonological processing, particularly phonological encoding, in children and adults who stutter (Newman & Bernstein Ratner, 2007; Pellowski & Conture, 2005; Zhao & Lian, 2021). Further, language-related factors have also been said to determine the loci of stuttering. Based on the constellation of research done across languages, stuttering frequency is said to be higher in the initial position, on content words, for longer words, and for linguistically complex utterances (Aryal & Maruthy, 2022; Brown, 1945; Dayalu et al., 2002; Howell & Au-Yeung, 2007; Maruthy et al., 2015; Masumi et al., 2015; Seth & Maruthy, 2019).

Fault-line hypothesis

Proposed by Wingate (1988), the *fault-line hypothesis* suggests a disrupted synchronization in arranging linguistic elements in a word. The hypothesis suggests the existence of a fault-line, usually at the juncture of phonological and prosodic encoding. Wingate described stuttering as a "prosodic disorder" or a "phonetic transition defect" (Yairi & Seery, 2023), where the underlying difficulty is to string the linguistic elements together or transition from one element to the other rather than the production of these elements. Wingate also suggested that most of the moments of stuttering occur at stressed syllables that require pitch and loudness adjustments at the laryngeal level. Based on these observations, he proposed that PWS have deficits at the central processing levels that control and coordinate the production of stress. This theory did receive some criticism as it failed to explain the course of developmental stuttering. Further, stuttering does not always occur on stressed syllables; however, the hypothesis failed to explain the stuttering that might occur on unstressed syllables (Yairi & Seery, 2023). Nevertheless, the hypothesis has been of some clinical utility and supports the "speak slowly" strategy for PWS. It is believed that speaking at a slower rate allows more time for the synchronization of linguistic elements and hence reduces the likelihood of a fluency breakdown. Another technique that draws support from this hypothesis is "gentle voice onset" that might ease the process of phonetic transition.

Covert repair hypothesis

Postma and Kolk (1993) and subsequently Kolk and Postma (1997) based their hypothesis on the Levelt's model of speech production (Levelt, 1989). They proposed that stuttering occurs due to underlying phonologic encoding deficits. It was suggested that there exists an internal monitor in the speech production system that keeps track of any errors in phonological encoding. On encountering an error, the system stops the overt speech and initiates a covert repair. This interruption, re-initiation, and covert repair of the phonetic plan leads to a breakdown in fluency. Kolk and Postma (1997) proposed that the covert repair mechanism is not unique to PWS and takes place in typically fluent individuals as well. However, what differentiates the two groups are their phonological skills in terms of the frequency of errors (higher in the stuttering group) and the time taken to revise the plan. Hence, the current hypothesis is in line with the continuity hypothesis that suggests typical disfluencies and SLDs to be on the same continuum.

The hypothesis utilized the "interrupt rule" and "restart hypothesis" from Levelt's model. The interrupt rule suggests that speakers interrupt their speech as soon as they encounter an error and hence SLDs are within-word disfluencies. An immediate interruption of the phonetic plan is followed by attempts to revise and re-execute the phonetic plan (i.e., restart hypothesis). Kolk and Postma (1997) used the restart hypothesis to describe the type of disfluencies. They suggested that *early-occurring errors*, or in other words, phonologic errors that occur before the initiation of the word or the initial syllable, lead to silent or tense pauses and blocks. Similarly, errors occurring beyond the initial syllable are referred to as *intermediately occurring errors*. These might lead to sound repetitions or sound prolongations (*p-p-p-p or p . . .* for the word pen). Lastly, *late-occurring errors* are those that occur in the syllable coda or the later part of a word and these may be exhibited as part-word repetitions (*pe-pe-pe-pen*). The covert repair hypothesis gave way to substantial research, testing the proposed hypothesis in both children and adults. The hypothesis draws support from a range of studies alongside evidence not in its support. Table 4.6 summarizes the findings of evidence supporting and contradicting the *covert repair hypothesis*.

As observed in Table 4.6, the covert repair hypothesis is noted to have both supporting and refuting evidence. Kolk and Postma (1997) admit that the hypothesis does not provide an explanation for the onset and course of stuttering or for natural recovery. Despite these limitations, the hypothesis has been of clinical utility, particularly in the context of stuttering treatment in addition to explaining the repetitive movements and fixed postures observed as key features of the condition. The hypothesis supports treatment techniques that promote rate reduction with the rationale that reducing the rate of speech provides increased time for phonological encoding, thereby reducing fluency breaks. It also offers an explanation for the adaptation effect and fluency-inducing conditions such as choral reading and shadowing (Packman & Attanasio, 2017). It was suggested that the adaptation effect (reduction in stuttering on reading or repeating over and over again) is a result of increased activation of correct phoneme selection. Similarly, choral reading and shadowing are related to the concept of priming, wherein the activation level of the

Table 4.6 Summary of findings from studies evaluating the covert repair hypothesis

Evidence supporting the Covert Repair hypothesis

Author (Year)	Findings
Louko et al. (1990)	CWS exhibited relatively greater number and variety of phonological processes than fluent peers
Byrd, McGill, et al. (2015) Pelczarski and Yaruss (2014) Sasisekaran and Byrd (2013)	Poor performance for phoneme blending and phoneme elision tasks in CWS than CWNS
Anderson et al. (2019) Gerwin et al. (2022) McGill et al. (2016) Sakhai et al. (2021) Sugathan and Maruthy (2020)	Poor phonological memory and poor verbal short-term memory in CWS than CWNS
Sasisekaran et al. (2013) Sasisekaran and Weisberg (2014) Sugathan and Maruthy (2020)	Poor performance on phoneme monitoring, non-word repetition, and non-word identification tasks
Yang et al. (2018)	Atypical neural processing (greater activation in the right inferior frontal gyrus extending up to the middle frontal gyrus) while performing a syllable repetition task in AWS
Pelczarski et al. (2018)	Significantly higher number of fixations and longer dwell times on eye-tracking measures in AWS during a non-word reading task

Evidence contradicting the Covert Repair hypothesis

Author (Year)	Findings
Yaruss and Conture (1996)	No difference in the self-repair behaviour between CWS with disordered phonology and CWNS
Yaruss (1997b)	No correlation between articulation rate and stuttering severity in CWS
Brocklehurst and Corley (2011)	No correlation between number of errors and stuttering severity in AWS while saying tongue twisters
Vincent et al. (2012)	No significant difference in the speed of phonological encoding between AWS and AWNS
Bakhtiar et al. (2007) Sasisekaran and Weathers (2019)	No significant difference in performance on a non-word repetition task between CWS and CWNS

(*Note: CWS – children who stutter; CWNS – children who do not stutter; AWS – adults who stutter; AWNS – adults who do not stutter*)

target utterance is increased by external supplementation in the form of auditory (choral reading and shadowing) and visual (choral reading) aids. These explanations stand strong with literature supporting efficacy of the above-mentioned fluency-inducing conditions (Bowers et al., 2012; Dechamma & Maruthy, 2018; Healey & Howe, 1987; Park & Logan, 2015; Ritto et al., 2016).

Execution and planning (EXPLAN) model

After the covert repair hypothesis, another psycholinguistic model that has its origins in Levelt's model of speech production is the recent EXPLAN model. Proposed by Howell and colleagues (Howell, 2004; Howell & Au-Yeung, 2002), the model suggests stuttering to be a result of deficits in either planning (-PLAN) or execution (EX-) of speech or in the synchrony of the two processes. Similar to the covert repair hypothesis, EXPLAN supports Bloodstein's continuity hypothesis and agrees that typical disfluencies in childhood later develop into stuttering. According to the model, if the linguistic plan for the target utterance is delayed and arrives late for execution, it leads to a fluency breakdown. Specifically, the model centres around the production of content words. According to the EXPLAN model, content words are difficult to plan, owing to their underlying phonetic and semantic complexity as well as word length in comparison to function words. Hence, stuttering tends to occur more on content than function words (Au-Yeung et al., 1998). The model suggested two forms of disfluencies, *stalling* and *non-stalling*. The stalling is observed during the early phases wherein children stall the production of the content word for which the plan is delayed, and in the process, they repeat the preceding function word (whole-word repetitions) or pause. Over time, stalling reduces, and they attempt to produce the target word even though the complete plan for the same may not be available. In this scenario, non-stalling disfluencies are seen which include initial syllable repetition, prolongation, or within-word pause. Thus, the model successfully explains why stuttering does not occur on every word or utterance (it occurs only when the linguistic plan is delayed and does not arrive on time for motor execution). In addition, SLDs can also be explained clearly based on this model.

The model has been empirically tested and has shown mixed findings. As discussed above, there is abundant literature suggesting increased stuttering on function words in children (Dworzynski et al., 2003; Howell, Au-Yeung, et al., 2000; Natke et al., 2004; Richels et al., 2010; Rommel, 2001) and on content words in adults who stutter (Au-Yeung et al., 1998; Brown, 1945; Dayalu et al., 2002; Jayaram, 1981; Maruthy et al., 2015). Further, the transition from function to content words is said to occur around school age and complete by 10–12 years (Howell et al., 1999). In contrast, a few studies reported higher stuttering frequency on content words or no difference between content and function words for children who stutter in languages such as Japanese or Kannada (Seth & Maruthy, 2019; Smith & Howell, 2013). These discrepancies were majorly attributed to the differences in the linguistic structure across languages. The model also draws support from studies indicating phonetic, lexical, and syntactic encoding deficits in children who stutter (Anderson & Conture, 2000; Anderson & Conture, 2004; Anderson et al., 2006). Further, SPECT rCBF data from another experiment agreed with the model indicating significant differences in rCBF in adults who stutter with poor linguistic skills when compared to matched fluent adults (Watson et al., 1992). The findings of the study showed atypical neural processing in the middle temporal and inferior frontal regions. In addition, Weber-Fox and colleagues in a series of event-related potential experiments have successfully established significant differences in lexical and syntactic processing between children with and without stuttering (Cuadrado & Weber-Fox, 2003; Usler & Weber-Fox, 2015; Weber-Fox, 2001; Weber-Fox et al., 2004).

The EXPLAN model, however, fails to explain the phenomenon of natural or spontaneous recovery. It does not provide satisfactory answers to why stuttering shows a sudden onset in some individuals and a gradual onset in others. It does not shed light on individual and situational variability observed in stuttering. Another limitation of the model is its inability to justify why stuttering occurs on non-words where lexical processing is not involved. Nonetheless, similar to the covert repair hypothesis, the EXPLAN model does stand in support of rate reduction strategies for the management of stuttering. It suggests that reducing the rate of speech provides greater time for linguistic planning to occur and helps avoid a delay in motor execution.

Multifactorial models

It is evident from previous sections of this chapter that there exist several perspectives regarding causal attributions of stuttering. However, it may be agreed upon that a majority of the above-mentioned theories or models are one dimensional and fail to explain the multidimensional nature of stuttering. Within this context, Smith and Kelly (1997) suggested that "workers in the area of stuttering should adopt a multifactorial, nonlinear, and dynamic framework" (p. 205) for the disorder. Multifactorial models propose that stuttering is a result of a complex interaction between several internal (such as temperament, cognitive and linguistic capacity) and external/environmental factors (such as listener reactions). We discuss some of the common multifactorial models of stuttering below.

Demands and Capacities Model (DCM)

The concept of demands and capacities dates back to the 1970s (Sheehan, 1970, 1975); however, it was elaborated with considerable detail by Starkweather (1987) who proposed that stuttering occurs when there's an imbalance or mismatch between the capacities of a child and the demands placed. Capacities may be defined as the dynamic and evolving abilities or skills of the child. The DCM talks about four major types of capacities: *Motoric* (ability to perform smooth and coordinated articulatory movements with minimal effort), *linguistic* (ability to express using age-appropriate language), *socio-emotional* (ability to express emotions and speak fluently when under stress), and *cognitive* (ability to use metalinguistic skills). Demands are broadly classified as internal and external. Internal demands refer to demands placed by children on themselves, such as the need to use a specific vocabulary, the need to be able to form complex utterances, and feelings of anxiety and excitement. External demands imply demands placed on the child by the environment. These include, but are not restricted to, the parents' rate of speech, parents' expectation of specific linguistic complexity in the child's utterance, time pressure to respond, and competition with peers. According to Starkweather, when capacities of a child surpass demands, the resulting speech is fluent. In contrast, when demands surpass capacities, the outcome is a fluency breakdown or stuttering. This imbalance might be triggered at a point that varies across individuals and could be considered as a threshold. Thus, the DCM helps understand the variability observed between PWS. Also, the fluctuating nature of stuttering, particularly in children, could be explained based on the DCM. Guitar (2019) suggested that children have growth spurts, and that their capacities grow manifold during these spurts. Likewise, environmental demands also vary over time. The day-to-day variability in stuttering, then, reflects the interaction between the growing capacities and demands in a child.

The DCM gained substantial support from several researchers who reported fluency breakdowns in children undergoing therapy focused on improving expressive language and phonological skills (Hall, 1977; Meyers et al., 1990). Winslow and Guitar (1994) found that stuttering in a child reduced when turn-taking was made a rule at the dinner table in contrast to when no turn-taking was followed during the interaction. Yaruss et al. (1995) lent support to the model by demonstrating positive correlations between diadochokinetic rate (DDK) and articulation rate in children who do and do not stutter. The model did receive its share of criticism in the form of a few researchers questioning its testability (Ingham & Cordes, 1997; Siegel, 2000). They argued that there is no direct measure of *capacities* or the *threshold*. Siegel (2000) suggested that proponents of model could consider revising the concept of *capacities* into *performance* and the model be renamed the *Demands and Performance model*. Nonetheless, the DCM continues to be a robust theory. Recent evidence for its popularity comes in the form of the RESTART-DCM[3] intervention programme (de Sonneville-Koedoot et al., 2015). The programme is an indirect treatment approach that focuses on teaching parents strategies to facilitate an increase capacities and reduction in demands for children who stutter.

Neurophysiological model

The neurophysiological model is credited to De Nil and his colleagues who attempted to provide a comprehensive view of stuttering (De Nil, 1999). This model is similar to the DCM in terms of discussing the capacities or skills of an individual. It proposes that fluent speech is influenced at three levels and the dynamic interaction between the three. The first, the *processing level*, represents the neurophysiological processes at the central level; the second, the *output level*, is associated with motor, cognitive, language, social, and emotional factors; and the third is the *contextual level* that reflects the influence of environmental factors. In addition, the model also proposes a bidirectional feedback loop at each of the three levels that are said to affect the final output. Proponents of the model suggested that external or environmental factors influence the output as well as neurophysiological processes. Further, environmental information is filtered within an individual, and thus, central level neurophysiological processing varies across individuals. These central-level processes also change over time, based on environmental filtering and feedback with every experience of a stuttering moment. Thus, they concluded that stuttering is a result of interaction between the neuropsychological and neurophysiological processes that vary across individuals. This individual variability helped explain differences observed between PWS in response to stressful situations as well as intervention.

CALMS model

The CALMS model was developed by Healey et al. (2004) who stated that their model was inspired by the preceding multifactorial models. They included five major domains or factors in this model – *cognitive, affective, linguistic, motor, and social.* They reasoned that stuttering occurs as a result of a complex interaction between these factors as represented in Figure 4.2. The degree of influence of each of the five factors may vary across individuals and across time, and this determines the frequency, type, and duration of stuttering. According to the researchers, the model facilitates qualitative and quantitative assessment of each of the five domains based on the performance of the PWS.

According to the model, the relationship between thoughts, perceptions, feelings, and attitudes of an individual, and the processes of linguistic formulation and motor execution, is bidirectional. The model suggests individually assessing each of these domains when conducting an evaluation and determining performance level across these domains as outcome measures post intervention (Healey et al., 2004). Following the conceptual and organizational framework of the model, the CALMS assessment scale (Healey, 2007) was developed – which has specific items under each of the five domains. Each item is rated on a 5-point scale and the ratings assume different meanings depending on the domain being assessed. The ratings are averaged for each domain and represented graphically providing a CALMS profile for a child who stutters. Proponents of the model suggest that the CALMS profile could help frame treatment goals, select appropriate treatment approaches and measure therapy outcomes.

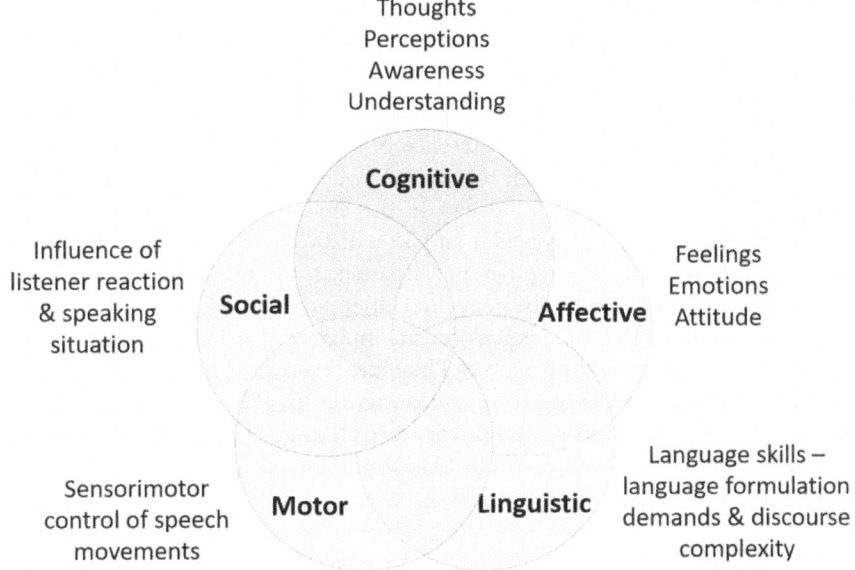

Figure 4.2 Schematic representation of the five factors of CALMS model and their complex interaction

Communication-Emotional (C-E) model

Proposed by Conture and colleagues (Conture et al., 2006; Richels & Conture, 2010), the *Communication-Emotional (C-E)* model of stuttering attempts to determine the likelihood of stuttering in an individual. In those with already established stuttering, the model attempts to identify which factors contribute to overt instances of stuttering-like disfluencies (SLDs). The model describes its two major components – the *distal and proximal contributors* of stuttering. Distal contributors are factors that help determine individuals who are likely to develop stuttering. The model proposes two distal contributing factors – the first is *genetics* and the second, the *environment* (communicative, emotional, and social environment). Proximal contributors represent factors that might have an immediate impact on stuttering. These include *speech motor control abilities of speakers* (planning and programming skills at a given point in time) *life experiences of speakers*, and *emotional functioning* (emotional reactivity and regulation). The model proposes that individuals who are genetically predisposed to stuttering have an inefficient speech production system and are more likely to exhibit stuttering. Early communicative experiences of a speaker have a significant influence on the likelihood of developing stuttering as well as its severity. Individuals who experience relatively more negative communicative experiences, particularly in the moments of stuttering, are likely to persist with stuttering and exhibit greater severity. Environmental factors that increase demands on the speaker, also referred to as fluency stressors, might exacerbate stuttering. High emotional reactivity and poor emotional regulation in PWS might further influence SLDs.

Dual-diathesis stressor model

Monroe and Simmons (1991) presented a diathesis-stress theory to explain the interaction between an individual's ability (or inability) to regulate emotions and external stressors. Walden et al. (2012) adapted this model to explain the manifestation of SLDs. According to the model, the presence of an emotional diathesis (high emotional reactivity and low emotional regulation) coupled with an emotional stressor such as a change, excitement or novelty in the environment precipitates stuttering. Similarly, the presence of a speech-language diathesis, which implies difficulties related to expressive and/or receptive speech-language coupled with a stressor such as a demand for a spontaneously generated utterance, would manifest stuttering (Walden et al., 2012). The model goes on to emphasize that for those who do not stutter, such diatheses would be absent. Therefore, even an increase in the number of external stressors would not precipitate stuttering. In PWS, on the other hand, even a small increase in stressors would worsen stuttering. The model found support in multiple studies (Ntourou et al., 2013; Zengin-Bolatkale et al., 2015) among children who stuttered.

Multifactorial dynamic model and multifactorial dynamic pathway theory

The multifactorial dynamic model emerged based on more than two decades of work by Smith and colleagues (Smith, 1999; Smith & Goffman, 2004; Smith &

Kelly, 1997; Smith & Weber, 2017; Zimmermann et al., 1981). The original version of the multifactorial dynamic model (Smith & Kelly, 1997) proposed that stuttering is a result of a nonlinear interaction between five internal factors (cognition, emotion, genetics, language, and speech motor) and one external (environment) factor. They also suggested that the extent of influence of each of the factors varies both between and within individuals over time and across situations. Based on it they could explain the individual and day-to-day variability in stuttering. Recently, the Smith and Kelly (1997) model was extended and revised as *multifactorial dynamic pathway theory* (Smith & Weber, 2017). In its revised form the model proposes stuttering as a motor speech disorder or a disorder of speech motor coordination at its core that is influenced by several other factors. The theory attempts to explain the onset and development of stuttering as well as the persistence and recovery in PWS. As described by Logan (2020), in its current form the theory has four major tenets as shown in Figure 4.3.

In simpler words, *multifactorial dynamic pathway theory* suggests that breakdowns in fluency occur during the developmental phase of a child when the speech motor control system is unstable. The occurrence of these disruptions or disfluencies leads to behavioural and physiological responses within the child as well as reactions from people in their environment. These may act as epigenetic influences on the expression of genes underlying the development of speech motor control. As noted in literature (Andrews & Harris, 1964; Sheehan & Martyn, 1966; Yairi & Ambrose, 1992; Yairi & Seery, 2014), 80% of children recover from these disruptions as their brain adapts to the disrupted neural activity; however, in 20% of children, the brain adaptations are inadequate and their speech motor control system remains unstable

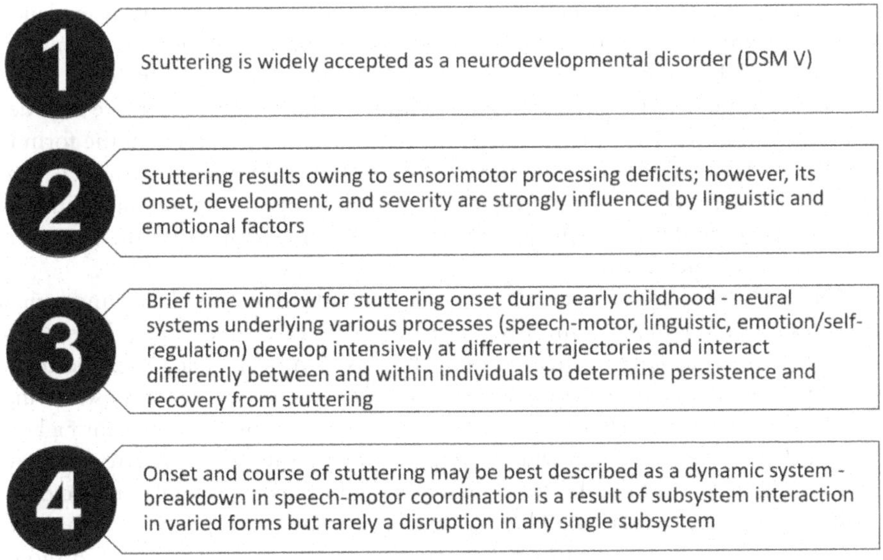

1 Stuttering is widely accepted as a neurodevelopmental disorder (DSM V)

2 Stuttering results owing to sensorimotor processing deficits; however, its onset, development, and severity are strongly influenced by linguistic and emotional factors

3 Brief time window for stuttering onset during early childhood - neural systems underlying various processes (speech-motor, linguistic, emotion/self-regulation) develop intensively at different trajectories and interact differently between and within individuals to determine persistence and recovery from stuttering

4 Onset and course of stuttering may be best described as a dynamic system - breakdown in speech-motor coordination is a result of subsystem interaction in varied forms but rarely a disruption in any single subsystem

Figure 4.3 Tenets of multifactorial dynamic pathway theory

and vulnerable to disruptions. An exposure to increased linguistic demands or psychosocial stressors acts as a trigger and disrupts the already unstable speech motor system, thereby leading to the persistence of stuttering in the latter group. Within this context, proponents of the theory suggest that assessment protocols for stuttering should be multidimensional and include assessment of speech motor skills, linguistic skills and temperament. Likewise, the implications in the context of management of stuttering focus on early intervention. As mentioned earlier, SLDs are a result of disrupted speech motor behaviour, and repeated occurrence of the same might strengthen the underlying neural patterns which are difficult to alter in late childhood and adolescence. Hence, the current theory is not in favour of the wait-and-see approach for children who stutter, particularly for those who are at a higher risk of persistence. Instead, it emphasizes on utilizing the critical period of development and neural plasticity to strengthen neural connections that facilitate fluent speech simultaneously reducing SLDs (Smith & Weber, 2017).

Packman and Attanasio 3-factor (P & A) model

An extension of the variability model, the Packman and Attanasio 3-factor model, or the *P & A model* (Packman & Attanasio, 2010) is a multifactorial model that proposes three factors under necessary and sufficient conditions to be underlying the moments of stuttering. The first factor listed under this model is *neural underpinnings* (i.e., impaired neural processing for spoken language). Based on the growing evidence on neuroanatomical differences between those with and without stuttering, the model specifically favoured the impaired myelogenesis hypothesis of Cykowski et al. (2010). The second factor proposed by the model is *triggers* that are characteristics of the spoken language, placing higher demands on the speech motor system and renders it to be perturbed easily. Based on the available empirical evidence, the model proposes two triggers – variable syllabic stress and linguistic complexity. The model also suggests that other triggers identified could be included in the model upon empirical verification. Neural underpinnings and triggers are regarded as necessary but not sufficient to cause stuttering. The third factor is in the form of *modulators*. According to the proponents of the model, the critical threshold is variable and influenced by environmental factors, referred to as the modulators in the model. These modulators influence the critical threshold to perturb the inefficient speech motor control system.

The explanation for the onset of stuttering under the P & A model is same as their previous variability model. Similarly, natural recovery is reasoned to be the result of delayed maturation of the neural system. The P & A model went a step ahead and suggested that children in whom neural maturation occurs recover from stuttering, while those in whom such maturation does not occur continue to stutter throughout life. Further, the model also provided an explanation for the variable nature of stuttering. Within-individual variability was said to be influenced by modulators (factor 3), while between–individual variability was suggested to be a function of the severity of underlying neural impairment (factor 1). Similar to earlier models, the P & A model justifies the efficacy of various stuttering treatment approaches. Fluency-shaping methods (prolongation, syllable-timed speech) and reducing the linguistic complexity of utterances is known to reduce stuttering (i.e., reduce the frequency of triggers). Likewise, therapy approaches such as cognitive behaviour therapy or indirect approaches for CWS help manage the environmental factors or modulators. It may be noted that any of the behavioural treatment approaches target either the second and third factors of the model or both; however, whether the first factor, neural impairment, can be addressed by any of the treatment approaches remains unclear.

Although the numerous theories and models of stuttering might baffle a student of fluency disorders at the outset, getting gradually acquainted with them facilitates progression to higher levels of understanding and gives the student a view of stuttering from a vantage point. Multifactorial models have further extended our understanding of the disorder as they emphasize the interaction of several factors that constitute the mosaic of stuttering. Knowledge of theoretical perspectives of stuttering makes one appreciate the heterogenous nature of the disorder and explains the variability observed for an individual who stutters across time and situations. It enables prediction of persistence or recovery to a fair degree of accuracy; and it justifies the efficacy and outcomes of various treatment approaches used with children and adults who stutter. On the whole, it enriches our understanding of the disorder and guides assessment and management of stuttering.

Summary points to remember

- The early learning and psychological theories of stuttering imply that stuttering is a learned behaviour. They proposed that breakdowns in fluency during the developmental period may take the shape of stuttering based on the listener's reactions and environmental factors.
- Organic theories suggested that a lack of hemispheric dominance or the influence of genetic factors could play a role in the manifestation of stuttering.
- Empirical investigations reveal neuroanatomical and neurophysiological differences between those with and without stuttering, predominant differences in the size of the planum temporale, reduced white matter volume, reduced blood flow, and reduced activation of regions for speech and language in the left hemisphere.
- Genetic influence in stuttering has been studied for decades. Recent empirical investigations have also helped identify a few genes that are strongly implicated in stuttering.
- Speech motor control theories emphasized that an impaired or inefficient speech motor control system is easily perturbed under the influence of external factors, resulting in the emergence or exacerbation of stuttering.
- Another school of thought included proponents of psycholinguistic theories who postulated deficits in linguistic processing to be the underlying cause for stuttering.
- The most recent approach has been of a multidimensional perspective giving rise to the multifactorial models. These models attempt to bridge the gap between neural underpinnings, psychological traits and temperament, environmental factors, and genetic influences in stuttering.

Study questions

1. Compare and contrast organic and psychological theories of stuttering.
2. Discuss speech motor control theories and models highlighting the empirical evidence.
3. Highlight the neuroanatomical and neurophysiological differences between individuals with and without stuttering.
4. Elaborate on the CALMS model.
5. Describe the role of linguistic factors in stuttering drawing support from psycholinguistic theories.

Notes

1 For a detailed explanation refer to Ward (2018).
2 The concept of concordance and discordance has been introduced in Chapter 3 under Twin studies.
3 For more details on RESTART-DCM refer to Chapter 6 on management of stuttering in children.

5 Assessment of stuttering

Amudhu Sankar, Anjana B. Ram,
Pallavi Kelkar and Santosh Maruthy

Introduction

Children show a wide degree of variation in the way they learn to speak and the rate at which their speech development occurs. Just as a child stumbles while learning to walk, repeating a sound or syllable or restarting a sentence because they are unsure of how to put their thoughts across are common occurrences during the mastering of speech and language skills. Of the children that display disfluency, some experience typical disfluency as a developmental phase, while others experience the beginnings of stuttering. In a young child, making a decision about whether they belong to the former category or the latter is possible only after detailed assessment. Assessment also gives crucial information about the degree of stuttering (if the child exhibits stuttering) and the extent to which stuttering affects the child or adult with disfluency.

The World Health Organization's International Classification of Functioning, Disability and Health (ICF) (WHO, 2001), provides an ideal framework for assessment of the experience of stuttering in its entirety. It is a clinical tool that speech-language pathologists (SLPs) and other health care practitioners can use to create detailed descriptions of people's health. Yaruss and Quesal (2004, 2006) suggested an ICF-based approach for stuttering assessment and intervention. Fitting the phenomenon of stuttering into the ICF framework, core behaviours and physical concomitants of stuttering represent the "impairment in function"; the individual's affective, cognitive and behavioural reactions to stuttering represent personal contextual factors; and the attitudes and support (or lack of it) from others around them constitute environmental factors. The speech behaviours, personal and environmental factors influence each other bidirectionally and as a result, affect the degree to which the individual participates in various activities, and consequently their quality of life. Some authors (Logan, 2005; Yaruss & Quesal, 2004) have highlighted how ICF-based tools can be used to holistically assess fluency disorders. Assessment of cluttering is discussed in detail in Chapter 9 of this book. The present chapter focuses on the assessment of stuttering.

The assessment process

Stuttering can be described in terms of three components – *core speech behaviours, secondary behaviours* and *feelings and attitudes* (Guitar, 2019). Chapter 3 elaborates on

DOI: 10.4324/9781003367673-5

each of these with examples. The relative proportion of these components might differ across individuals who stutter. Further, even for the same absolute values (in a manner of speaking) of each of these components, there might be individual differences in experiences, cognitive evaluations, and consequently *impact* on the person's life (Yaruss & Quesal, 2006). In addition, persons in the immediate environment of an individual who stutters, further affect and are affected by the above-mentioned components of stuttering. The assessment process, therefore, necessitates careful planning, observation, and analysis. It begins with the clients receiving assistance and ends with a rehabilitation plan. Assessment is a personal encounter that entails getting to know the client as well as their significant others by tuning your antennae as a clinician to pick up on subtle signals they might send out about their needs and how you might be able to help them.

Very broadly speaking, the assessment process is divided into three major stages – data collection, analysis, and interpretation. All of these are directed towards some common objectives the stuttering assessment must aim to achieve, which are as follows:

1. Rapport building to facilitate a smooth interaction during subsequent sessions
2. Obtaining a detailed case history
3. Observing speech production in multiple contexts
4. Describing the client's overall speech characteristics
5. Analyzing the nature and frequency of disfluencies
6. Noting the presence of concomitant speech, language, motor or general health problems, if any
7. Understanding the client's present environment
8. Identifying different factors that might affect stuttering in that individual
9. Getting an idea of the degree of impact stuttering has on the individual's life

Collating all this information, finally, would aid the clinician in arriving at an accurate diagnosis and planning intervention in an efficient manner. We will now go over each of the steps in the stuttering assessment process in detail.

Case history

The first step in any assessment protocol is a detailed case history. During the case history taking process, a skilled clinician is able to get preliminary data pertaining to all the nine objectives listed above. A well-taken case history gives the clinician valuable diagnostic information. For example, the sudden onset of stuttering could give the clinician clues to the presence of acquired forms of stuttering.

The preschool child

For a preschool child with stuttering, case history gives information about how parents currently perceive the child's problem, the onset and course of the problem, and the child's medical, family and academic history. This is obtained through parent interview and observation of parent–child interaction. This gives an opportunity to assess the child in a natural situation. Enquiring whether the preschool teacher has noticed the problem and knowing the nature of the interactions that happen in pre-school is also valuable information for attaining objectives 7, 8 and 9 of assessment. Some important questions that may be asked while assessing environmental pressures and demands on a child have been delineated by Guitar (2006).

a) Rate of speech of persons who are usually around the child
b) Parents tending to use complex sentence constructions and a linguistic repertoire beyond the child's current level of comprehension and processing (e.g. Kloth et al., 1999)
c) Is the child being given ample opportunity to speak?
d) Reactions of parents or others towards the child's disfluency
e) The child being interrupted frequently (maybe by a sibling or cousin) during conversations
f) The environment around the child (anxious versus calm)
g) Is there competition for speaking? (If the child does not speak up fast, they lose their chance to speak.)
h) Is a lot of value placed on achievements and fluency?

The clinician must remember that such a young child may or may not be aware of their disfluencies. It is, therefore, crucial that conversations describing the child's speech do not take place in the child's presence. It helps to have both parents, or a parent and a caregiver accompany the child, so that while the clinician elicits information about disfluencies, the other parent or caregiver engages the child in another activity out of earshot of the conversation. The detailed format for eliciting information can be referred to in the Appendix A.

The school-age child

For a school-age child, in addition to information about the child and the parent-child or family-child dyad, it is important to enquire into communicative situations that the child might engage in outside the home environment (e.g. daycare, hobby class, neighbours and other people in the neighbourhood). In cases of developmental stuttering (Chapter 3), the stuttering could have emerged some years back. Asking how the problem has changed since it was first noticed, reactions of significant others towards the child's problem and how the problem has been dealt with so far, therefore, becomes crucial. The child's academic history would now include information about his academic performance, attention and behaviour in the classroom.

A school-going child with normal cognitive development is usually well aware of the presence of disfluencies and might even say the phrase "I stutter" or "I stammer" in response to the question, "Do you know why your mommy/daddy brought you here today?". This is often due to having overheard parents or caregivers use the label while speaking to someone else. Nonetheless, it is important to ask this question for several reasons. First, because it gives us a lot of insight into how much, if at all, the child is aware. Awareness may range from just knowing that there is something different about their speech to knowing exactly when and how they stutter. Second, it gives us an insight into whether the child has begun to feel self-conscious about their speech, a very important variable while planning intervention. If the child seems well aware, questions regarding the variability in stuttering with people, content and situations can be asked simultaneously to the parent as well as the child. Knowing both perspectives can add valuable information for planning intervention as well. Specific questions for case history taking are given in Appendix A.

The adolescent or adult who stutters

In case of an adolescent or an adult who stutters, the clinician must remember that the environment around the individual has now expanded manifold, compared to childhood. In addition to the developmental, medical, family and academic history, the initial interview must now also include information about social participation and relationships, intimate relationships, as well as employment and professional relationships (if applicable). It is usually established by adolescence whether the individual exhibits stuttering or typical disfluency. Typical disfluency seen during the developmental period would, by now, either have abated or developed into stuttering. Questions to this age group would therefore pertain largely to the following:

1. The nature and severity of stuttering
2. The reactions of the adolescent to their stuttering
3. Presence and nature of avoidance behaviours and emotional reactions
4. The degree to which stuttering tends to affect their life

The detailed case history format can be found in Appendix A along with the assessment protocol for stuttering.

It helps if the clinician speaks to the adolescent and their parent or caregiver separately. This enables the adolescent as well as their caregivers to voice their concerns in an uninhibited manner. An additional benefit of this practice is that it gives the adolescent a sense of agency and a feeling of being involved in the intervention process and being treated as an equal. In case of adults, too, a choice may be given to the individual and their partner, spouse or accompanying person to have separate conversations with the clinician. Even though they choose not to do so, the questions in the case history must be asked to both the person who stutters and their caregiver in order to know both perspectives. This also gives the clinician some information about the relationship that the adolescent/adult and their caregiver share. If the caregiver is a strong support system for the client, this can be a valuable resource in the intervention process. If the caregiver seems to be creating barriers to progress, this aspect would need to be addressed through counselling in future.

The case history session can end by informing the client and caregiver about what is to follow in the assessment process, that is, recording of speech samples and administration of standardized tests and checklists to quantify stuttering and its impact.

Speech sample recording

The speech sample gives the some understanding of client's overt behaviour of stuttering. It is advisable to collect an in-clinic sample as well as a sample from an actual speaking situation. It is preferable to do both, an audio as well as video recording. Video recording of speech samples is preferred as the client's core as well as accessory behaviours can be seen. Missing accessory or secondary behaviours might lead to an underestimation of the severity of stuttering (Rousseau et al., 2008). A video recording is also useful at the beginning of the intervention process to help the client understand the nature of their stuttering in its entirety.

Picture description, narrating an event or familiar story can help obtain speech samples for analyses. In school-going children, adolescents and adults, a reading task is recommended as well. However, the material used for eliciting the reading sample must not be at the child's present level of reading proficiency. Recall that disfluency can also be linguistic in nature, that is, when language processing takes longer. Thus, if a child finds a reading passage difficult, a greater number of disfluencies might result, and we would end up overestimating the severity of stuttering. We recommend using a reading passage which is a level or two below the present academic grade, or a reading passage that the child has read before. Similarly, asking the child to recite a poem or sing a rhyme might not elicit the usual amount of stuttering, and might lead to underestimation of severity. Recording speech when the child is delivering emotionally laden content, on the other hand, might lead to overestimation of stuttering severity.

Riley (2009) recommends eliciting a 300-syllable sample in order to represent the range of stuttering behaviours as well as physical concomitants. However, stuttering in children might vary to a greater extent than adults, even through a single task. Speech samples elicited from children must therefore, be longer (Sawyer & Yairi, 2006). Also, it is recommended that speech samples from children be elicited in multiple settings, contexts and with different communication partners, to get a true idea of their degree and types of disfluency. Such assessment also aids in assessing the environmental influences on the child's fluency levels.

Speech sample transcription

The recorded speech must be transcribed orthographically for further disfluency analysis. Trained clinicians transcribe speech in an online mode while the client speaks. However, this type of transcription could lead to difficulties such as keeping pace with the client's speech, missing out on subtle disfluent episodes and missing out on observing secondary behaviours while the clinician focuses on the core behaviours. Hence, offline transcription of the recorded speech sample is preferable. The advancement of video analysis software allows clinicians to play the video back to identify disfluencies and conduct an offline analysis (Table 5.1) with a higher degree of accuracy.

Table 5.1 Offline analysis of disfluencies

Transcribed sentences	Number of syllables	Stuttering-like disfluencies	Other disfluencies
I go to my office by nine thirty in the morning	14 syllables	0	0
I like /ba/ /ba/ blue colour	5 five syllables	1 (PWR)	0
I feel ashamed of mmmmmyself when I /ca/ /ca/ can't even say /ma/ /ma/ /mmmmmm/ my name correctly	18 syllables	3 (2 prolongations, 2 PWR)	0
/ssss/ /ssss/ Suzanne said /you know/ she /ummm/ may /c/- ome home this weekend	10 syllables	2 (1 PWR, 1 broken word)	2 (1 parenthetical remarks, 1 filled pause)
/Saturday/ /Saturday/ Saturday is a working day for us	10 syllables	0	1 (multisyllabic word repetition)
Total number of syllables	55 syllables	6	2

Note: *PWR – Part-word repetition*

Assessing concomitant problems

Apart from collecting and transcribing the speech sample for fluency assessment, there are other parameters that must be assessed by a speech-language pathologist.

1) Oro-motor skills: Measures of articulation and diadochokinetic rate may help to differentiate between stuttering and developmental apraxia of speech.
2) Language ability: Recalling again, the concept of linguistic disfluency mentioned in Chapter 1, if a child has a delay or deficit in language, it might increase the number of disfluencies due to problems in retrieving words and constructing sentences (Anderson & Conture, 2000; Boscolo et al., 2002). Along similar lines, detecting a language delay and working on it would make stuttering intervention easier.
3) Articulation and overall speech intelligibility: This especially aids in differential diagnosis of stuttering and cluttering. The reader is referred to Chapter 9 for a detailed account of speech intelligibility problems in cluttering.
4) Voice: Assessment of pitch, intensity and quality of voice should routinely be conducted as a part of speech assessment.
5) Hearing: The fact that the reported complaint is disfluent speech does not conclusively rule out the presence of a hearing loss. Especially in a child, a subtle hearing deficit or auditory processing deficit might be missed, and might consequently make the prognosis poorer.
6) Intellectual ability: Intelligence shows a positive association with the possibility of spontaneous recovery from stuttering (Yairi, Ambrose, Paden, et al., 1996). A lower than normal intelligence quotient would also influence a clinician's choices of intervention approaches and the simplicity of counselling.

Once the presence of concomitant deficits is accurately documented or conclusively ruled out, the clinician can proceed to assessing fluency in terms of its various concomitants.

Assessment of core behaviours

Accurate assessment of core behaviours, or the actual stoppages or blocks experienced while speaking, is essential to differentially diagnose typical disfluency from a fluency disorder and to further differentially diagnose between the different fluency disorders. Three aspects of core behaviours hold crucial information for diagnostic process, the frequency, type and duration of disfluencies.

Frequency of disfluencies

The frequency of stuttering not only aids diagnostic decisions (Andrews & Ingham, 1972), but also acts as a snapshot indicator of progress throughout treatment (Guitar, 2019). Frequency of stuttering can be calculated per 100 words or per 100 syllables. Syllable-based measurements are considered more accurate as they help in identifying multiple disfluencies within multisyllabic words.

What disfluencies to count

Part-word repetitions, syllable repetitions, monosyllabic whole-word repetitions, prolongations, hard blocks at the beginnings of words, or broken words (hard blocks in the middle of a word), are counted as indicative of stuttering (Johnson et al., 1959; Conture, 1990a) as these are most likely to be judged by listeners as stuttering (Boehmler, 1958; Williams & Kent, 1958).

How to count disfluencies

Table 5.1 gives multiple examples of disfluencies and how they must be counted across syllables for the benefit of beginning clinicians.

The first example in Table 5.1 has no disfluent episodes to give the readers a baseline as an example for counting syllables in an utterance. It must be noted that only intended syllables are counted and not ones that are repeated during production. For example, in the second example there are only five syllables, and the two part-word repetition units are not included while counting the syllables. In the third example, for the word "my", the speaker has produced a part-word repetition as well as a prolongation of the syllable "my". Note that this is counted as one disfluent episode because irrespective of the types of disfluencies, the person has experienced struggle for production of that one syllable. It is clear from the fourth and fifth examples that while counting the percentage of syllables stuttered, non-stuttering-like disfluencies or other disfluencies (ODs) are excluded.

In the clinic, clinicians may also be able to perform real-time analysis of stuttering instances. A table can be made to count the disfluencies in a hundred-syllable sample (as shown below). Place a dot (.) for each fluent utterance in each box and (/) slash mark for a disfluent utterance. Disfluencies can additionally be marked as repetitions, prolongations, broken words, etc., using codes such as R = repetitions (Syl R, WR, PR, Sen R), P = prolongations, B = blocks, AP = audible pause, IP = inaudible pause, Rev = revision, F= filler, etc. Multiple iterations of the same disfluency should not be represented on separate boxes but on the same box. Several

Table 5.2 Real-time analysis of disfluencies

.	/ (B)	/ (P)	.	
.	.	.		/ (B)
.	/ (AP)	/ (WR)	.	

measures can be computed from this documentation, such as percent syllables stuttered (%SS), percent type disfluency, and speech rate (which would also require the use of a stopwatch).

Percentage of disfluencies is calculated using the formula:

$$\frac{Total\ number\ of\ disfluencies \times 100}{Total\ number\ of\ syllables\ spoken}$$

While many researchers recommended using a criterion value of 10% disfluencies or more to diagnose stuttering (Bloodstein & Bernstein Ratner, 2008; Yairi, 1997; Yaruss, 1998), Yairi and Ambrose (2005) also suggested presence of >3% stuttering-like disfluencies (SLDs) to make a decision about the presence of stuttering. They also provided criteria for each type of disfluencies, namely, >1.5% part-word repetitions, >2.5% single-syllable word repetitions, >0.5% instances of disrthythmic phonation, a weighted SLD > 4, and >1% repetitions with two or more extra units. Overall, the general clinical impression across the globe seems to be that greater than 5% disfluencies must alert a clinician to the presence or emergence of stuttering (Hegde &Hartman, 1979a;1979b).

The process of counting syllables and disfluencies can also be accomplished using a variety of software such as TrueTalk (www.synelec.com.au/synergy/) or an online counter freely available at www.natkeverlag.

Types of disfluencies

Although children who stutter produce more disfluencies than their non-stuttering peers, sometimes it is difficult to differentiate stuttering from normal disfluencies based only on the frequency of stuttering. Identifying the types of disfluencies aids in determining the presence as well as severity of stuttering. The percentage of a particular type of disfluency among the total number of disfluencies is calculated using the following formula:

$$\left(\frac{Total\ number\ of\ a\ particular\ type\ of\ disfluencies}{Total\ number\ of\ disfluencies} \right) \times 100$$

As mentioned in Chapter 2 of this book, the proportion of SLDs to ODs will differ significantly between children who do and do not stutter. The different stuttering-like and non-stuttering-like disfluencies have been discussed with examples in Chapters 2 and 3. In the words of Meyers (1986), persons who stutter were quantitatively and qualitatively different in their stuttering compared to their non-stuttering peers. According to the findings of Yairi (1997), 3 to 4 SLDs were seen in preschoolers who stutter, while the number of SLDs in children who did not stutter was less than 3, for every 100 syllables spoken.

Ambrose and Yairi (1999) also proposed the use of a weighted SLD score. The formula for weighted SLD given in Chapter 2 is reproduced here for the readers' convenience:

$$\frac{\left(Repetitive\ disfluencies \times Mean\ number\ of\ repetition\ units\right) + \left(Disrhythmic\ phonations \times 2\right)}{100}$$

The duration of sound/syllable part-word and whole-word repetitions is expressed in terms of number of repeated units (RU) (e.g. p-p-p-pencil has three RUs). Ambrose and Yairi (1999) asserted that a weighted SLD threshold of 4 could correctly classify children as those who stuttered (score of 4 or more) and those who did not; Anjana and Savithri (2013) found this threshold to be at a weighted SLD score of 3.

Clustering of disfluencies

When two or more disfluencies occur on the same word, they are called cluster disfluencies. Literature reveals a higher likelihood cluster disfluencies in children who stutter compared to typically speaking children (Hubbard & Yairi, 1988; LaSalle & Conture, 1995; Logan & LaSalle, 1999). In fact, Zebrowski and Kelly (2002) asserted that if a child exhibited at least three instances of cluster disfluencies per 100 syllables, the child could be at risk for developing stuttering.

Duration of disfluencies

Zebrowski (1994) suggested using both stuttering duration and frequency when rating the severity of stuttering. The duration of a moment of stuttering has been seen to vary between 1 to 5 seconds (Bloodstein, 1987). In instances of sound, syllable and word repetitions, the number of RUs has been identified as a distinguishing characteristic of early stuttering. Ambrose and Yairi (1995) studied the absolute number of repetition units as well as the ratio of single-unit to multiple-unit repetitions in children who stutter in comparison with controls. The control group showed a significantly lower number of RUs and a higher ratio of single- to multiple-unit repetitions (6.58) compared to the ratio seen in children who stutter (2.06). The duration of the blocks can give us important information about how it may interfere with communication. The duration is measured by taking the average of three longest stuttering instances in a speech sample (Preus, 1996; Van Riper, 1982; Riley, 2009).

Assessment of rate of speech

The relationship between speech rate and stuttering was further described by Onslow (1996). He suggested that speech rate and stuttering can have a direct or inverse relation. First, stuttering may reduce with a decrease in speech rate (direct). It is observed in a few treatment strategies like prolonged speech therapy that the rate of speech is slowed down. In such instances, speech rate would prove to be an effective measure to comment on the efficacy of the treatment. The second relation is an inverse relation, wherein the speech rate increases as stuttering reduces or vice versa. This can be explained in terms of the proportion of fluent and disfluent utterances. When stuttering reduces, the percentage of disfluent utterances will reduce, and fluent utterances will increase, thereby increasing the speech rate. Speech rate is estimated as either syllables per minute (SPM) or words per minute (WPM). A fast and/or irregular speech rate can also alert the clinician to the possible presence of cluttering (see Chapter 9). Speech rate should, therefore, be a part of the fluency assessment protocol.

The formula for speech rate is reproduced below:

$$\text{Speech Rate} = \frac{\textit{Total number of words or syllables read}\left(\textit{excluding disfluent utterances}\right)}{\textit{Total time taken to read the passage}}$$

Although most of the studies investigating speech rate have included SPM as a measure (Druce et al., 1997; Koushik et al., 2009; Kully & Boberg, 1991; Lincoln et al., 1996; Onslow et al., 1994; Vong et al., 2016; Wilson et al., 2004), few others have used WPM (Smits-Bandstra & Yovetich, 2003; Wagaman et al., 1993). It must be noted in the above formula that the total speaking time, inclusive of disfluencies is considered while calculating speech rate. However, only intended syllables are counted, and not those syllables, while additional repeated units are excluded. One limitation of this measure is that it is highly variable depending on language, dialect and age, especially in young children.

Some studies also emphasize computation of articulation rate calculated as syllables spoken per second (Lattermann et al., 2008; Onslow et al., 2009). Note that in contrast to rate of speech computation, the formula for articulation rate excludes unfilled pauses from the total time taken. The formula for calculation of articulation rate is as follows:

$$\text{Articulation rate} = \frac{\textit{Total number of syllables}\left(\textit{without pauses and disfluent utterances}\right)\textit{read}}{\textit{Total time taken to read the passage}\left(\textit{without unfilled pauses}\right)}$$

Similar to overall speech rate, articulation rate may vary with age due to differences in the rate of articulation of speech sounds in children and adults. However, language specific prosody affects articulation rate to a lesser extent as compared to speech rate, as we exclude both, disfluent episodes as well as unfilled pauses during analysis.

Assessment of speech naturalness

As defined in Chapter 1, naturalness refers to how acceptable the speech sounds to listeners and is affected largely by fluency and prosody. The various tools that may be used to measure speech naturalness are mentioned in Chapter 1. Of these, the most commonly used tool uses the 9-point speech naturalness rating scale by Martin et al. (1984). A rating of 1 on this scale indicates highly natural speech. The rating would progressively increase towards 9 if the person exhibits disfluencies or is fluent but the speech lacks prosody. Literature reveals that mean naturalness ratings can vary between 2.12 to 2.39 for adolescents and adults, while for children it is slightly higher (3.0). (Martin et al., 1984; Ingham et al., 1985).

A tool of Indian origin for assessing speech naturalness is the multi-dimensional speech naturalness scale for stutterers (Kanchan, 1997), which assesses seven parameters – rate, continuity, effort, stress, intonation and rhythm, articulation, and breathing pattern at a natural and unnatural level. It is a binary choice scale consisting of a 2-point scale as "1" or "0" for natural or unnatural, respectively.

Thus, if an individual's disfluencies reduce after using a particular intervention approach but the speech still sounds unnatural, it would indicate that therapy goals must now target prosodic aspects of speech. Another variable that affects speech naturalness is the struggle that accompanies disfluencies in the form of audible secondary behaviours.

Assessment of secondary behaviours

A secondary behaviour, also called an accessory or associated behaviour, often begins as an involuntary movement that coincides with a release from a moment of stuttering. This might covertly convince the individual that its occurrence led to the release from stuttering, thus increasing their frequency through a self-reinforcing cycle. It is natural, then, that these behaviours may not begin at the onset of stuttering, but emerge as stuttering progresses (Eichorn & Fabus, 2018). However, there is a large degree of individual variation in the time taken for these behaviours to appear, with some children exhibiting them one month post stuttering onset (Zebrowski & Kelly, 2002). Secondary behaviours also have diagnostic value, as they are not a characteristic feature of typical disfluency (Chapter 2). During assessment, the clinician must carefully observe the client's secondary behaviours while taking case history or during the recording process. In the case of children, information can be obtained from the caregivers as well for secondary behaviours that may be missed during the limited duration of an assessment session. Accessory behaviours observed during assessment can be checked off on the checklist given in Table 5.3.

A pertinent point that beginning clinicians must note is that the above behaviours must be present only at or just before the moment of stuttering. If they are habitually present at all times, they would not be counted as secondary behaviours. For example, a habitual leg shaker would keep shaking his leg at all times, whether or not he stutters. A person with an eyebrow tic would keep involuntarily raising his eyebrows at regular intervals. This is not a marker of struggle occurring during a moment of stuttering.

A look at the variety and subtlety of the behaviours listed in Table 5.3 is another reason why video recordings of speech samples are a must. These enable the clinician to carefully observe and note secondary behaviours, ensuring that their presence is not overestimated or underestimated during assessment. An accurate count

Table 5.3 A checklist of secondary behaviours

Occurrence on the part of the body	Secondary behaviours
Head and torso	Rapid and tense eye blinks
	Shutting of eyelids
	Looking around, not making eye contact
	Knitting of the eyebrows
	Flaring of nostrils or wrinkling the nose
	Lip movements such as puckering, pursing, tremors, etc.
	Tongue extension or protrusion
	Gritting teeth
	Increased amount of tension in the muscles of the face
	Raising eyebrows to wrinkle the forehead
	Jaw jerks
	Tensing jaw muscles
	Head movements (turns, shakes, lateral, upward and downward movements)
	Tension in the chest, shoulder and neck muscles
Hands	Hand or finger tapping
	Wringing hands
	Clenching one or both fists
	Covering face/mouth with hand(s)
	Using the palm to tap on the thigh
	Pressing the palm against the stomach
Legs	Foot tapping
	Tense and jerky leg movements
	Rubbing or pressing the feet together
	Making circular movement with toes
Audible secondary behaviours	Increase in pitch
	Increase in loudness
	Tongue clicking
	Whistling
	Sniffing
	Blowing

of secondary behaviours as well as core behaviours also enables the clinician to administer formal assessment tools to quantify the severity of stuttering.

Tools for quantification of core behaviours and secondary behaviours

Various standardized tools have been published to measure different aspects of stuttering in children and adults. Some of the commonly used tools are discussed below.

The Stuttering Severity Instrument - 4 (SSI-4; Riley, 2009)

This is, by far, the most widely used standardized instrument to quantify the severity of core behaviours and secondary behaviours seen in stuttering. It is composed of three subsections, namely, frequency, duration and physical concomitants (secondary behaviours).

To assess *frequency*, the clinician calculates the %SS. This value is then matched against a set of task scores which are given on the record form, to find the task score that corresponds to that frequency of stuttering. There are two task scores for clients who can read: A task score for %SS during reading and one for %SS during narration. For those who are unable to read, a non-readers table with a single set of task scores can be referred to. Thus, a score can be obtained for the frequency subscale which may be the addition of the reading and narration task scores or simply the non-readers task score.

To assess *duration*, the clinician needs to measure the length of the three blocks perceived as longest in the recorded sample with a stop watch. An average of the three durations is calculated and the corresponding task score is noted for this subscale.

The last subscale*, physical concomitants,* classifies secondary behaviours into four types, distracting sounds, facial grimaces, head movements and movements of extremities, each category being rated on a scale of 0 to 5. A score of 5 indicates that the secondary behaviours in that category are very severe. The total score for this subscale is computed after adding the ratings for the four categories of secondary behaviours.

The three subscale values are then added, yielding a total score. The SSI-4 gives three tables with percentile ratings for total score ranges, for preschoolers, school-going children and adults. The appropriate percentile range is found from the total score, and the corresponding degree of stuttering is noted. This can range from very mild to very severe.

The SSI-4 manual also has valuable material for eliciting speech samples, such as reading material according to grade levels for children and at a greater level of difficulty for adults. The SSI-4 also contains a software called the Computerized Scoring of Stuttering Severity (CSSS 2.0; Bakker & Riley, 2009) which can be used to compute stuttering frequency and duration.

However, there is a high possibility of human error while using the CSSS 2.0, as it involves rapidly clicking a key or a mouse for counting syllables, while simultaneously clicking another key/right clicking the mouse for noting disfluencies. The SSI-4 has other limitations as well. For instance, it cannot be used to diagnose typical disfluency. Also, types of disfluencies are not documented in the SSI-4.

Iowa scale of severity of stuttering (Sherman, 1952, as cited in Silverman, 1992)

This is an 8-point rating scale to perceptually evaluate stuttering severity. Although more subjective than the SSI-4, it ensures the inclusion of stuttering frequency, duration and the amount of secondary behaviours while deciding on a severity rating. Values on the scale range from 0 to 7, 0 being indicative of no stuttering and 7 indicative of very severe stuttering. The scale can be used for frequent and periodic assessments by the clinician or by the individual who stutters, due to its ease of administration. However, it shows greater variability among clinicians rating the same sample, compared to the SSI-4. It may, therefore, be used as an adjunct to another standardized assessment instrument.

The Test of Childhood Stuttering (TOCS; Gillam et al., 2009)

The TOCS, though not as widely used as the SSI-4, is becoming increasingly popular among clinicians for assessing the severity of stuttering in children. It can be used with children in the age range of 4 to 12 years.

The first component of the TOCS assesses speech fluency through tasks such as picture naming, sentence construction in response to pictures, narration and conversation. The second part of the tool consists of two rating scales, namely, the *speech fluency* rating scale and the *disfluency-related consequences* rating scale. These scales require the clinician to gather information from individuals in the child's immediate environment at home and school. The third part of the tool consists of detailed assessments of different aspects of speech such as rate, naturalness, frequency and type of disfluencies, number of repetition units, secondary behaviours, etc.

The TOCS has many advantages over the SSI-4, especially for assessment of children. Firstly, it can be used to differentially diagnose typical disfluency from stuttering. Secondly, it takes into account the types of disfluencies, thus giving the clinician an idea of how stuttering might change or evolve over time in a child. Lastly, it appears to have greater face validity because of inclusion of tasks such as conversation and the addition of information about the child's environment.

The Stuttering Prediction Instrument (SPI; Riley, 1981)

This assessment instrument is useful for evaluation of children aged 3 to 8 years. Assessment using the SPI would involve eliciting a detailed history, observing for different types of disfluencies, and the frequency of disfluencies. In addition, the SPI also documents information about the child's reactions to their stuttering. The SPI thus enables a clinician to measure stuttering severity as well as predict the tendency of stuttering to be chronic or persistent. It also helps determine if a child is a candidate for stuttering intervention. The SSI-4 can also be used in conjunction with the SPI while assessing children who stutter.

The Pindzola Protocol (Pindzola & White, 1986)

Like the TOCS, the Pindzola Protocol can also be used for the differential diagnosis of typical disfluencies from stuttering. For this purpose, the protocol includes measurement of frequency and type of disfluencies, duration of disfluencies, secondary behaviours as well as avoidance behaviours that the client might engage in.

Careful assessment and quantification of core behaviours and secondary behaviours thus helps the clinician differentially diagnose stuttering from other fluency disorders, and document a baseline from which intervention for speech-related concomitants of stuttering can begin. Recall from the beginning of this chapter, however, that the assessment of stuttering cannot be complete without the quantification of all the components of the ICF (WHO, 2001), including personal contextual factors or the person's own reactions to their stuttering. Assessment of this variable is discussed below.

Assessment of feelings and attitudes accompanying stuttering

The presence of negative emotional and cognitive reactions to communication can worsen the impact of stuttering on an individual and adversely affect prognosis. An assessment protocol without the quantification of this concomitant of stuttering is, therefore, incomplete. The development of assessment tools to measure attitudes was initiated during the 1960s. The past six decades have seen a rapid increase in the number of scales and checklists to measure attitudes and feelings (Andrews & Cutler, 1974; Craig et al., 1984; Ornstein & Manning, 1985; Woolf, 1967; Wright & Ayre, 2000). Each of these instruments has unique strengths and specific areas of focus. Some of them measure attitudes directly, while some indirectly indicate a change in cognitive and affective aspects of stuttering.

Direct measures of attitudes and feelings

A beginning clinician can identify these instruments from their names (which refer to attitudes, perceptions, etc.) or the items they contain, which describe how an individual feels or thinks about their speech or about their stuttering.

THE PERCEPTIONS OF STUTTERING INVENTORY (PSI; WOOLF, 1967)

This tool examines the struggle, avoidance, and expectancy of stuttering as experienced by the PWS. It consists of 60 first person statements which the PWS must check off as applicable. Twenty of these are representative of struggle, represented by an S in brackets next to the statements; 20 represent avoidance (A) and 20 represent expectancy (E) or how much a person anticipates stuttering. The resultant score profile can be used to help clients view their problem more objectively, to develop treatment goals, and assess progress in therapy. A limitation of the PSI is the absence of norms, or cut-off values to decide whether a certain score is representative of attitudes that need intervention. The PSI, however, is very easy to administer and is freely available online. Its simple wording renders it useful for assessing attitudes of adolescents as well.

THE MODIFIED SCALE OF COMMUNICATION ATTITUDES; S-24, ANDREWS & CUTLER, 1974)

The original version of this tool was the S-scale (Erickson, 1969), a 39-item scale for measuring attitudes related to speaking. The S-scale was revised to give the 24-item S-24. This scale consists of statements that reflect negative attitudes to communication. The respondent either agrees or disagrees with each statement. Each agree response gets scored as one. A score closer to 24 is thus indicative of a higher degree of negative attitudes towards communication. An improvement in S-24 scores has been associated with positive treatment outcomes (Andrews & Craig, 1988; Guitar & Bass, 1978).

COMMUNICATION ATTITUDE TEST FOR ADULTS; BIGCAT, VANRYCKEGHEM & BRUTTEN, 2011)

This 35-item test reflects the self-perception of a PWS as a communicator and their attitude toward communication in general. The responses are in the form of "True" or "False". Its advantage over the S-24 scale is that a "True" response does not necessarily indicate a negative attitude towards stuttering. It thus encourages a respondent to read each item before deciding a response. A key given with the tool indicates whether a particular response indicates a negative attitude and is to be scored as 1. The test manual gives mean and SD values of scores indicative of negative attitudes to communication.

Its variant for school-age children and early adolescents is the CAT (Brutten & Dunham, 1989). The CAT has 35 items with a same True/False response format and can effectively differentiate children who stutter from those who do not, based on mean scores. It is recommended for use with children in the age range of 6 to 15 years.

Similarly, the Kiddy CAT assesses communication attitudes of preschool children who stutter (Vanryckeghem et al., 2005). It comprises of 12 yes/no questions that the clinician asks after a few practice items. Children are engaged in play activities such as putting a marble in a carton after each response. Scores of 5 or more indicate attitudes similar to children who stutter.

The CAT, BigCAT and KiddyCAT have also been translated and validated to other languages. For example, Kannada versions, the CAT-K (Veerabhadrappa, Vanryckeghem, et al., 2021a) and BigCAT (Veerabhadrappa, Krishnakumar, et al., 2021) have recently been validated for use with Kannada-speaking school-going children and adults, respectively.

STUTTERERS' SELF-RATINGS OF REACTIONS TO SPEECH SITUATIONS (SSRSS; SHUMAK, 1955)

A unique and useful attitude assessment instrument, the SSRSS requires a respondent to rate each of 40 speaking situations along four aspects: Avoidance of the situation, reaction to the situation, stuttering within the situation and frequency of encountering the situation. Each rating scale is a Likert type scale from 1 to 5. A separate key for each of the four aspects is given along with the tool. A set of 40 Likert ratings is obtained for each of the four aspects tested. These 40 ratings are added and divided by 40 to get an average score. Thus, four average scores are obtained, one each for avoidance, reaction, stuttering and frequency. The score profile helps the client get a better insight into their speech–related attitudes and helps the clinician plan goals for therapy. The tool is freely available online. However, its major drawback in the present day is that its items are dated. An adapted Indian version of the SSRSS, called the SSRSS(I), was therefore created by Kelkar (2017). This version was applicable to the current cohort of adolescents and adults in India, making it culturally appropriate for use in the country.

THE SPEECH SITUATION CHECKLIST (SSC; BRUTTEN & VANRYCKEGHEM, 2003, 2007)

Similar to the SSRSS but without the "Frequency" profile, the SSC requires the client to rate their emotional reactions to a set of speech situations, followed by rating the degree of speech disruption they face, for the same set of situations. This is done using two sections of the SSC, namely the Speech Situation Checklist-Emotional

Reaction (SSC-ER) and Speech Situation Checklist-Speech Disruption (SSC-SD), respectively. Its revised version, the SSC-R (Vanryckeghem et al., 2017) consisted of 38 items and yielded significantly different scores for PWS and typical speakers.

There is also a version of the SSC for children. This is included in the Behaviour Assessment Battery (BAB; Brutten & Vanryckeghem, 2003, 2007; Vanryckeghem & Brutten, 2018; Vanryckeghem & Brutten, 2020). Studies related to the BAB indicate a clear difference in scores obtained by children who stutter (CWS) and children who do not stutter (CWNS), those obtained by CWS being consistently higher, indicating a greater degree of speech-related anxiety in CWS. Similar results were also obtained in India for a Kannada version of the SSC (SSC-ER) (Veerabhadrappa, Vanryckeghem, et al., 2021b). The authors concluded that the SSC was a value addition to the assessment protocol for stuttering among Kannada-speaking children in India.

THE A-19 SCALE (GUITAR & GRIMS, 1977)

Useful for assessing school-age children who stutter, this 19-item scale requires the child to respond to each statement with a yes or a no. An answer that matches the key (indicative of negative attitudes) given with the tool, gets a score of 1. The higher the score, the more negative the attitude to communication (Guitar, 2013).

Indirect measures of therapy outcome

Apart from the above tools that directly measure attitudes to communication, there are scales that measure related constructs such as self-efficacy, locus of control or communicative competence. An improvement in their scores thus indicates positive therapy outcomes. Some of these tools are discussed below.

THE LOCUS OF CONTROL OF BEHAVIOUR SCALE (LOC-B; CRAIG ET AL., 1984)

A locus of control is defined as either internal or external, depending on the extent to which a person is self-directed or seeks external gratification. A more internal locus of control would, therefore, indicate self-reliance and a better ability to cope despite external adversity, as would be required for those who stutter to maintain long-term positive outcomes of therapy. A high score on the scale indicates a more external locus of control. Thus, effective therapy must lead to a reduction in scores on the LOC-B scale. A lack of shift in locus of control post-treatment, or a reduction of less than 5%, has been demonstrated as indicative of a relapse (Craig & Andrews, 1985; Craig et al., 1984). Along similar lines, McDonough and Quesal (1988) also gave the Speech Locus of Control Scale (Sp-LOC).

UNHELPFUL THOUGHTS AND BELIEFS ABOUT STUTTERING (UTBAS) SCALES
(ST CLAIRE ET AL., 2009)

This comprehensive checklist of 66 items helps the clinician assess the negative thoughts experienced by adults who stutter. Therapy directed to modifying cognitive and affective aspects of stuttering would lead to a reduction in UTBAS scores and indicate an increased ability to cope with negative or challenging communicative experiences.

THE SELF-EFFICACY SCALE FOR ADULT STUTTERERS (SESAS; ORNSTEIN & MANNING, 1985)

The SESAS is very similar to the SSC, in that the PWS rates 50 speaking situations along two aspects, approach attitude and fluency performance, on a 10-point scale. Furthermore, for approach attitude, the PWS gives two ratings, one representing whether they would enter the situation and the second representing the degree of confidence they have in their response. Similarly, fluency performance gets two ratings, one representing whether they will be fluent in the situation and the second indicating their degree of confidence in their response.

SELF-EFFICACY SCALE FOR ADOLESCENTS WHO STUTTER (SEA; MANNING, 2001)

The SEA consists of 100 speaking situations that are rated by an adolescent who stutters on a 10-point scale. The ratings reveal the adolescent's self-perception of their ability to enter the speaking situation and their ability to speak in that situation.

TEACHERS' ASSESSMENT OF STUDENTS' COMMUNICATIVE COMPETENCE (TASCC; SMITH ET AL., 2000)

As the name suggests, the TASCC is a teacher-administered tool which helps assess a student's overall communicative abilities in a classroom situation. Naturally then, benefit from stuttering therapy would translate to better communicative abilities and consequently better scores on the TASCC. For detailed information on the TASCC, the reader can refer to Guitar (2013).

Assessing impact of stuttering

The assessment protocol described so far helps the clinician document the various concomitants of stuttering. However, holistic assessment must also include the client's perception of how much their stuttering impacts their life. This impact, then, would be a culmination of all the three concomitants and their interaction with the environment. As mentioned in the beginning of this chapter, the ICF helps collate and quantify each individual's own experience of their stuttering and its impact on their life. Tools to measure impact are, therefore, largely based on the biopsychosocial model of the ICF. These are discussed below.

THE WRIGHT AND AYRE STUTTERING SELF-RATING PROFILE (WASSP; WRIGHT ET AL., 1998)

One of the earliest tools to measure impact of stuttering, the WASSP has items distributed among five subscales: Behaviours, thoughts, feelings, avoidance and disadvantage. The behaviours subscale essentially measures core behaviours, secondary behaviours and speech rate. The thoughts and feelings subscales address cognitive and affective aspects of stuttering, respectively. The avoidance subscale pertains to the activities and participation that an individual indulges in (or avoids indulging in), and disadvantage subscale delves into social, educational and other barriers faced by the adult who stutters. Recently, a Turkish version of the WASSP (WASSP-TR) was developed by Uysal and Kose (2021) and found to be a reliable and valid tool.

OVERALL ASSESSMENT OF THE SPEAKER'S EXPERIENCE OF STUTTERING (OASES; YARUSS & QUESAL, 2006)

One of the first impact assessment instruments to closely mirror the structure of the ICF, the OASES, consists of 100 statements. These are drawn from codes in the ICF pertaining to stuttering and communication. The scale is divided into four sections. The first section, general information, elicits detailed information about the client's speech as perceived by the client. The second section elicits the client's responses for their reactions to stuttering. The third section titled communication in daily situations, contains an exhaustive list of different scenarios that the client might face in his day-to-day interactions and requires the client to quantify the degree of difficulty faced in these scenarios. Finally, the quality of life section elicits information about the extent to which the client's academic, vocational, social and family life is affected by his or her stuttering. With 20 items in section I, 30 in section II, and 25 each in sections III and IV, the OASES consists of a total of 100 items.

Each item is rated by the client on a five-point Likert type scale. The scores on all the Likert scales are then totalled to give a total score. A higher score indicates a higher impact. Total scores can also be calculated separately for each of the four sections. The total score then needs to be converted to an impact score. After calculating the total score, the clinician must count the total number of items the respondent completed and multiply this number by 5 to obtain the total possible score. The impact score then is the total score divided by the total possible score. The value thus obtained is multiplied by 100. Impact scores can also be computed separately for each section in a similar manner. The impact score can then be used to interpret the degree of impact ranging from mild to severe.

There are, at present, three versions of this tool, meant for children (OASES-S; Yaruss, Coleman, et al., 2010), adolescents (OASES-T; Yaruss, Quesal, et al., 2010) and adults (OASES-A; Yaruss & Quesal, 2006). The latest addition is the OASES for caregivers (OASES-C) meant to be filled by parents of preschoolers (Guttormsen et al., 2020).

Although the OASES seems to be a comprehensive impact assessment instrument, it does have its limitations. Firstly, it does not account for the presence of concomitant cluttering, which might be the case for some persons who stutter. Secondly, although it claims to mirror the ICF, it does not emphasize enough on the contribution of the environment in the form of the caregiver's perspective of impact. The self-report versions of the OASES for school children, teenagers and adults report impact only as perceived by the PWS. It is, however, common knowledge that the way others perceive a PWS might, in turn, influence the thoughts and feelings of the PWS towards their own stuttering (Boyle, 2018). This is not accounted for by the OASES.

The ISACS was constructed in order to account for the entire experience of stuttering, including the client's immediate environment and also to account for the concomitant presence of cluttering. As it originates from the ICF just like the OASES does, the structure of the two instruments is similar, and so is the scoring process. The ISACS has four subscales: Body functions (12 items), personal contextual factors (28 items), activities and environmental factors (42 items) and participation/ quality of life (18 items). The ISACS has two parallel versions, (A) which measures the self-reported impact of stuttering from the perspective of the PWS and (B), to which the significant other responds, by estimating the impact of stuttering on the PWS. Overall, higher scores on the ISACS indicate higher perceived impact. Discrepancies in the two versions indicate a need for appropriate counselling. For example, if a 16-year-old who stutters does not seem to experience a lot of impact as seen on ISACS(A) scores, but their parent perceives the impact to be very high as seen on ISACS(B), the therapist needs to speak to the parent about the fact that the adolescent needs to be given agency to decide whether he would like to take therapy for his stuttering. The adolescent, on the other hand, can be informed about the pros and cons of starting or deferring therapy. Apart from this, the ISACS also has the added advantage of an indigenous normative and is an appropriate impact assessment tool for the Indian population (Kelkar et al., 2020). It has also been translated to Marathi, one of the local Indian languages, so as to reach out the rural areas in the Maharashtra state of India, and the English and Marathi versions have been found to be equivalent (Kelkar et al., 2018). The ISACS is reproduced in Appendix B.

For those who might find it difficult to choose the appropriate tools for assessing attitudes and impact, Table 5.4 summarizes these by classifying them according to age and utility.

The closing interview

At the end of an assessment session, the clinician must define the roles of the client and caregiver(s) in the intervention process. This should not be a directive interaction, but more of a mutual discussion in order to reach a point of agreement. This gives the client a sense of confidence in their ability to be an agent of change. It also draws subtle boundaries for caregivers, especially of adolescents, to be a support system for the adolescent without being excessively directive or instructional in their approach.

Assessment along the ICF framework

In order to ensure that the assessment process has covered all the information necessary for diagnosis, severity estimation and intervention planning, the beginning

Table 5.4 List of attitude and impact assessment instruments for those who stutter

	Direct assessment of communicative attitudes	Indirect assessment of communicative attitudes	Assessment of impact
Children	Communication Attitude Test for Preschoolers (KiddyCAT) Communication Attitude Test (CAT) SSC (for children) A-19 scale	Teachers' Assessment of Students' Communicative Competence (TASCC)	Overall Assessment of the Speaker's Experience of Stuttering for Students (OASES-S) Overall Assessment of the Speaker's Experience of Stuttering for Caregivers (OASES-C)
Adolescents	Perceptions of Stuttering Inventory (PSI) Stutterers' Self-Ratings of Reactions to Speech Situations (SSRSS) S-24	Self-Efficacy scale for Adolescents who stutter (SEA)	Overall Assessment of the Speaker's Experience of Stuttering for Teenagers (OASES-T)
Adults	Speech Situations Checklist (SSC) Communication Attitude Test for adults (BigCAT)	Self – Efficacy Scale for Adult Stutterers (SESAS) Locus of Control Behaviour Scale (LOC-B) Unhelpful Thoughts and Beliefs about Stuttering (UTBAS)	The Wright and Ayre Stuttering Self-Rating Profile (Wright et al., 1998) Overall Assessment of the Speaker's Experience of Stuttering for Adults (OASES-A) Impact Scale for Assessment of Cluttering and Stuttering (ISACS)

clinician can use Figure 5.1 below. This figure represents the assessment protocol discussed in this chapter in the light of the ICF model.

Note that names of some of the assessment tools are repeated under different components of the ICF. This is because one tool might serve multiple purposes. This also makes us realize that different parts of the assessment protocol overlap to some extent, and this redundancy in assessment procedures is important. Such a test battery approach increases the validity of our assessment and resultant diagnosis.

Diagnosis

A diagnosis should give an accurate idea of the presence/absence of the fluency disorder, the type of fluency disorder and the severity of the disorder, so as to give a direction to therapy. Firstly, the diagnostic label should convey the presence and type of fluency disorder. Based on the differential diagnostic criteria given in Chapter 2, the clinician would first determine if the client exhibits typical disfluency or stuttering. If the presence of typical disfluency is ruled out, the clinician would then

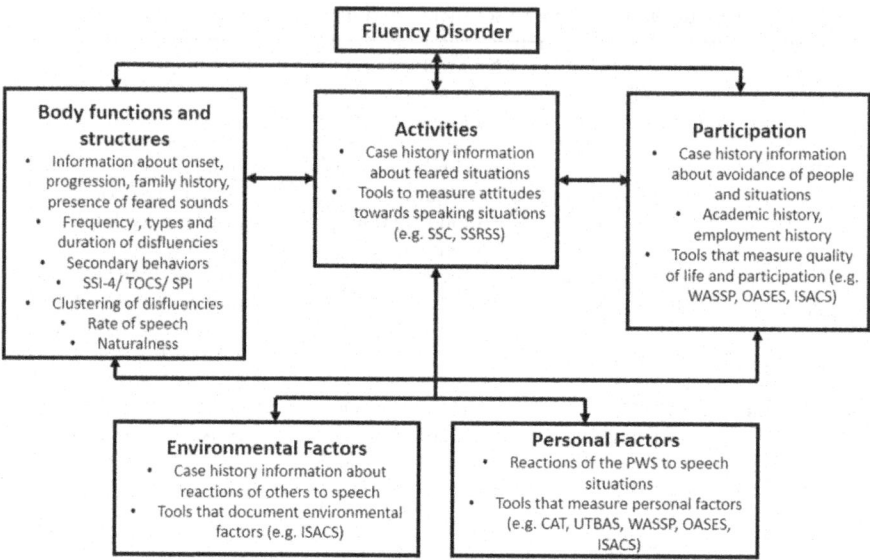

Figure 5.1 Stuttering assessment in the light of the biopsychosocial model

proceed to decide whether the client exhibits developmental or acquired stuttering (see Chapter 8 for differential diagnostic criteria). Also, the concomitant presence or absence of cluttering needs to be ascertained by the clinician (see Chapter 9). Each step in the assessment protocol should be taken into account before arriving at a diagnosis. For instance, the clinician can get clues to the presence of neurogenic stuttering from the case history (sudden onset, neurotrauma), the assessment of loci of stuttering (not necessarily at word initial position), and the absence of secondary behaviours as observed on the video recording. Based on these diagnostic decisions, the clinician would decide if the client exhibits developmental stuttering, neurogenic stuttering, psychogenic stuttering, or a combination of stuttering and cluttering.

Secondly, the diagnostic label must include the severity of stuttering. Several different nomenclature systems may be used for this purpose. Riley (2009) advocates the use of the terms mild, moderate, severe, etc., to diagnose the degree of stuttering, if stuttering is present. This, however, seems to be a unidimensional diagnostic label. For instance, when would we term stuttering as severe? Would speech and secondary behaviours alone determine the severity of stuttering? A slightly better diagnostic system is the one used by Guitar (2013) that uses the terms normal non-fluency and borderline, beginning, intermediate or advanced stuttering, to give a broader description not only of the core behaviours and physical concomitants but also the feelings and attitudes accompanying stuttering. However, there are two problems with this labelling system. It is often difficult to find a PWS who perfectly fits one of the five profiles of core behaviours, secondary behaviours and attitudes towards stuttering. There might be a PWS who exhibits beginning stuttering but has attitudes mirroring those of an intermediate stutterer. What, then, would be the diagnostic label? Also, core behaviours and secondary behaviours are assessed by the clinician. How severe does the client perceive their own stuttering to be? What is the impact of stuttering as perceived by the PWS? Would the severity be determined by the clinician's ratings or the client's? These are questions that still need answers. Until then, we recommend that the clinician include only the type of fluency disorder in the diagnostic label, and accompany it with a diagnostic summary or diagnostic formulation (Appendix A) of four to five lines to give a broad idea of the severity of core behaviours and secondary behaviours as quantified by the clinician, as well as the client's self-reports of attitudes and impact. This would ensure that a teacher or caregiver who reads the report does not overestimate or underestimate the severity by relying on a single label. It would give a true idea of severity of stuttering and also help chalk out an appropriate intervention plan.

Summary points to remember

- Holistic assessment of stuttering is aided by the ICF model (WHO, 2001).
- The case history and initial interview needs to be modified based on the age of the person who stutters.
- Assessment of core behaviours must include the frequency, type and duration of disfluencies, the rate of speech and speech naturalness.
- Tools to measure client-reported attitudes and feelings are an essential part of assessment.
- Assessing impact of stuttering increases face validity of our assessment and serves as a valid and holistic outcome measure of the effectiveness of intervention.
- The diagnostic label must give the reader of the report a true and complete picture of the nature and severity of stuttering.

Study questions

1. Write a short note on assessment of secondary behaviours.
2. Describe any two tools to assess the severity of stuttering.
3. Elaborate on the various scales that measure negative attitudes of children with stuttering.
4. List the tools that can indirectly measure stuttering therapy outcomes.
5. Why is impact assessment important? Describe one impact assessment tool for adults who stutter.

6 Management of stuttering in children

Gagan Bajaj and Divya Seth

Introduction

Treating stuttering among children warrants several additional skillsets for clinicians when compared to adults with stuttering (Blomgren, 2013). This is specifically due to the rapid psychosocial and developmental changes during childhood, an increased influence of the environment around the child, the dynamic nature of stuttering itself, and concerns about the potential long-standing impact of the disorder on children who stutter (CWS) (Rousseau et al., 2007). A clinician, therefore, has several important questions to consider when dealing with childhood stuttering. Some of these critical questions include the following: "How severe is this child's stuttering?"; "Does he/she need treatment?"; "When would it be ideal to initiate treatment?"; "How intense should the treatment be?"; "What treatment options are available for different scenarios?" etc. This chapter on the treatment of stuttering in children is an attempt to get closer to answering some of these questions. It highlights critical issues such as decision-making in treatment planning, choice of treatment options, and protocol of suitable treatment approaches.

Decision-making in the treatment of childhood stuttering: walking a tightrope

Clinicians face fewer dilemmas about the initiation and nature of treatment when dealing with school-aged children, who usually have established or advanced stuttering, unlike preschoolers (Nippold, 2018). Treatment-related decisions for preschoolers are difficult because fluency often appears to be on the borderline between normal developmental trends and stuttering-like disfluency (SLD). The decision on the initiation and nature of treatment for borderline/emerging stuttering has been an issue of debate for decades (Bernstein Ratner, 2018). Although there are schools of thought that believe initiating treatment in such a scenario might prove to be counterproductive for the child, there is also emerging evidence suggesting positive benefits from early treatment. However, several factors that influence the nature of stuttering and its likely course in early childhood (Rousseau et al., 2007) must be considered by clinicians while deciding on appropriate treatment options.

DOI: 10.4324/9781003367673-6

Factors that might influence management decisions

As seen in Chapter 5, the assessment protocol includes a detailed case history, followed by keen observation and formal assessment tools being administered to get the complete picture of the stuttering mosaic. Once this is done, the clinician is equipped with knowledge about certain crucial variables that might help make decisions regarding management (Table 6.1).

Potential scenarios and suitable goals

Based on the findings obtained from the formal and informal assessments and parental interviews, the clinicians should be able to devise a risk profile of the child. Following are the five potential clinical scenarios into which a child may be placed, and accordingly, appropriate goals decided (Table 6.2).

Table 6.1 Factors that might influence management decisions

Factors	Influence on management decisions
1. Genetic predisposition	A positive family history of stuttering poses a higher risk of developing SLDs. It is essential to closely assess the fluency profile of such children and follow them up before clinical decisions.
2. Environmental Factors	Factors such as emotional irregularities in family dynamics, a moment of sudden psychotrauma, loss of a family member, the arrival of a sibling, bullying at playschool or in the neighbourhood, the nature of speech-language models in a child's environment, and psychosocial and emotional expectations from the child are important to note. Noting if manipulation of any of these environmental constraints brings a desirable change in a child's fluency is also essential.
3. General Development of the Child	Children with motor, speech and language delays, and advanced speech and language abilities may be at a higher risk of developing SLDs. It is important to consider the developmental status of the children while making decisions about their speech fluency.
4. Development of Fluency Breakdowns	Reduction in fluency breakdowns over time could be indicative of a better prognosis; whereas breakdowns that do not decrease in frequency post one year of the onset could be worrying.
5. Secondary Behaviours	Physical concomitants such as excessive eye blinking, facial grimacing, jerks in extremities, etc., are usually alarming. Consistent or increasing secondary behaviours might warrant urgent attention and a more direct stance towards the child's fluency.
6. Awareness and Attitude	A child who is aware of disfluencies and is beginning to exhibit social withdrawal with reduced conversational participation is likely to develop consistent SLDs.

Note: SLDs – Stuttering-like disfluencies

Table 6.2 Potential clinical scenarios and management options

Profile	Risk factor analysis	Management options
1. Observe profile	Infrequent disfluencies such as word revisions, interjections, and word repetitions with single iterations are present. The risk profile suggests a positive environment with the presence of no other significant risk factor. The child seems to be unconcerned about his speech.	Reassurance and resolution of the queries of a worried parent. Appropriate follow-up based on the child's chronological age to monitor speech and risk profile.
2. Conservative profile	The fluency profile is indicative of no SLDs. Analysis of the risk profile reveals the presence of one or more risk factors, such as a positive family history of stuttering, speech and language delay, negative modelling, and reactions in the immediate environment of the child.	Rather than direct intervention, appropriate measures are taken to transform the child's environment to become more facilitative and less demanding. Frequent follow-ups would be warranted here to closely monitor the environmental variables and track any changes in the child's fluency.
3. Indirect profile	The fluency profile is indicative of some early signs of SLDs with or without secondary behaviours. The risk profile of the child may or may not show the presence of any significant risk factor.	Initiate treatment that would help alleviate the early signs of stuttering and promote speech fluency. The treatment could include less intensive and indirect strategies along with some environmental manipulations. Ensure that early signs do not bring an undesirable change in a child's attitude towards speech and their social participation.
4. Early Direct profile	The fluency profile is indicative of established stuttering with one or more secondary behaviours that may or may not be accompanied by other high-risk factors. Here a child might be aware of his disfluencies with emerging behavioural and social implications.	This profile requires a relatively stronger action plan. One may choose to explore potential benefits of indirect therapy approaches, while at the same time being open to making a shift to more direct measures, if necessary.
5. Direct profile	The fluency profile shows an advanced stage of stuttering in which a child might exhibit severe disfluencies along with secondary behaviours and significant escape and avoidance behaviours.	The goal is to reduce the frequency and severity of stuttering and address avoidance behaviours of the child. For this, direct therapy with the child on a one-on-one basis at regular intervals is recommended.

Note: SLDs – Stuttering-like disfluencies

Treatment options: indirect vs. direct

Treatment approaches for children with stuttering are broadly classified into indirect and direct approaches (Nippold, 2018) (Figure 6.1). An indirect approach implies treatment measures in which there is no direct contact between the child and the clinician. The clinician indirectly works on improving a child's fluency by manipulating the immediate environment which could potentially be responsible for deviations in the child's speech. These measures include counselling parents to speak at a slower rate with simple linguistic content; advising parents to reinforce the child's fluent utterances and inhibit any negative reactions to child's disfluencies; facilitating teachers, friends, and relatives to be patient with child's speech, etc. An indirect approach operates on the assumption that reducing demands in the child's environment might bring about a balance between demands and capacities, as Starkweather suggested in his model (Starkweather & Gottwald, 2000). This kind of approach is more suited for the first, second, and third clinical scenarios described in the previous section.

A direct approach refers to the treatment measures in which a clinician directly deals with the child who has stuttering, over fixed schedules, in a therapeutic setting. There are multiple direct approaches, and each of them follows a different philosophy and rationale for treatment. The rationale is grounded in the theoretical understanding of stuttering based on either psychological, linguistic, or motor speech perspectives. Intervention strategies are implemented directly by the therapist with the child having stuttering. A direct approach is usually applied by clinicians when stuttering in children is established or advanced (Early Direct or Direct profiles in Table 6.2 above). A clinician might choose to teach a child strategies to modify moments of stuttering or strategies to speak fluently using methods such as a gradual increase in length and complexity of utterances (GILCU), stretched speech, soft

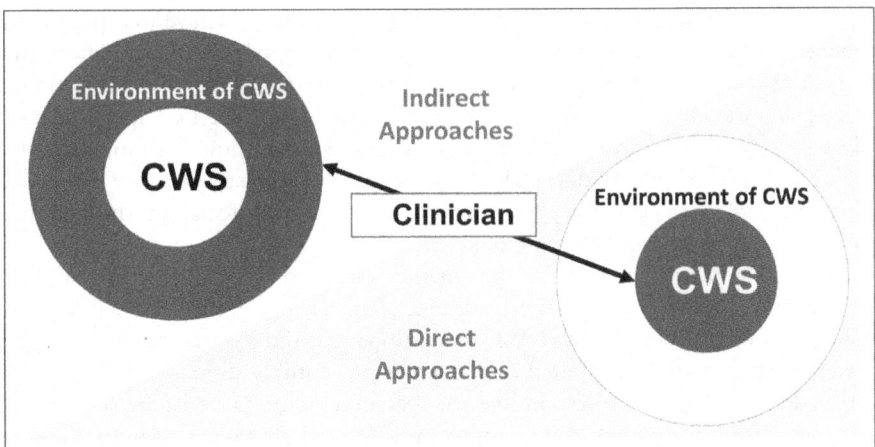

Figure 6.1 Schematic representation of the *Direct* and *Indirect* classification of treatment approaches for stuttering management in children

articulatory contacts, and airflow modifications. Some treatment strategies are classified as hybrid approaches. These have both indirect and direct components which may be initiated depending on the nature and extent of the child's disfluency. In the following section, some of the well-established and widely used indirect, hybrid, and direct treatment approaches for children with early stuttering have been described.

Indirect approaches

Indirect approaches, as discussed above, focus on modifying the child's environment. Until the 1930s, stuttering intervention for young children (2 to 6 years) predominantly involved indirect methods such as parent counselling (Bloodstein et al., 2021). Parent counselling majorly involved guidelines on modifying the parents' interaction style with the use of slow rate of speech, age-appropriate linguistic structure, facilitating pause time and turn-taking, reduced interruption or completing child's sentences, reduced demands and time pressure on the child to speak fluently, and acknowledging the difficulty with speech. Although parent counselling has been a common clinical practice in the management of stuttering for young children, it lacks documented literature on its efficacy. Only one structured programme following an indirect approach – the *Palin Parent-Child Interaction therapy* – provides well-documented evidence on its efficacy (Millard et al., 2008; Millard et al., 2009; Millard et al., 2018).

Parent-Child Interaction therapy

Parent-child interaction (PCI) based therapeutic approaches have been formulated and advocated by a group of researchers from the Michael Palin Centre for children with stuttering (Kelman & Nicholas, 2020). The PCI therapy approach operates on the rationale that stuttering in children is a heterogeneous condition. Multiple factors such as personality traits, speech/language skills, motor control, family dynamics and child-rearing practices play a crucial role in determining the speech fluency of the children. The proponents of the PCI approach strongly believe that the speech fluency of children with stuttering can be achieved optimally by modifying the immediate environment of the child and refining the style of parental interaction.

To plan individualized goals for the child with stuttering, the PCI approach considers assessment to be an integral component of the programme. It emphasizes that assessment must be done with the child and the parents alone followed by assessment of parent-child interaction. Key assessment components for the parent-child interaction have been shown in the Table 6.3.

A clinician then compiles the information obtained from various segments of the evaluation and formulates the treatment plan. Various contributing factors for child disfluencies are analyzed and shared with parents during a counselling session. Special care is taken that parental concerns are not entirely dismissed, and they are not made to feel guilty or responsible for the child's status. Parents are shown specific segments of the parent-child interaction video to help them understand certain modifications in interaction style that could facilitate desirable fluency in the child's

Table 6.3 Key aspects of the assessment process for a clinician who plans to use the PCI approach.

Assessment	Procedure	Key aspects assessed
Child	• Observation • Interview	• Speech fluency • Receptive-Expressive language status • General behaviours • Social skills • Pre-literacy/literacy abilities • Cognitive skills • General attitudes • Awareness of fluency deviations • Attitude to speech in different situations • Perception of the parental concerns and reactions
Parent	• Interview with each parent alone	• Concerns regarding the child's disfluencies • Perceived impact of the fluency breakdown on the family • Reaction to the child's speech
Parent-Child interaction	• 15-minute video of parental involvement with the child during a play activity	**Parental attributes** • Verbal and nonverbal communication style • Turn-taking • Rate of speech • Linguistic complexity • Listening skills • Tone of speech • Proximity with child • Reaction to disfluent moment **Child attributes** • Communicative autonomy • Turn-taking • Linguistic complexity • Speech fluency • Secondary behaviours • Avoidance behaviours • Coping strategies • Reaction to parental concerns

speech. Some of the interaction targets include following the child's lead, being more attentive and patient listeners, taking mindful turns during the conversation, implementing appropriate wait time to facilitate the child's response, using age-appropriate linguistic content and being a desirable speech model with an optimum rate of speech.

Treatment using the PCI approach is carried out in four phases:

1. Establishing Talk Time: Parents are instructed to set aside a brief talk time or special time of five minutes that occurs no more than three to six times a week. During this special time, parents are instructed to carry out a quality interaction while indulging in a play activity. Parents must be careful listeners during this special time and focus on the child's linguistic content rather than deviations in

speech. They must acknowledge the difficulty of the child's speech and avoid any form of negative reaction.

2. Weekly clinical sessions: In this phase, parents attend six weekly sessions with the clinician at the clinic. In each of these sessions, they discuss their experience during the special times of the previous week and receive appropriate feedback from the clinician. Then, a short parent-child interaction is video recorded, and parents are specifically instructed to keep the interactions during these recordings as similar as possible to the special times. The video recorded session is then played back to the parent, and the clinician instructs them to identify one segment of the video where they feel their interaction style was at its best and one area that could be improved further. The clinician then helps the parent to work on weak interaction domains and practice them in the clinical setting. The clinician also provides appropriate interaction targets to the parents for the special times of the upcoming week.

3. Consolidation period: Once the six weekly sessions with the clinician are completed, parents are instructed to continue the special time periods at home, update the clinician on weekly basis through structured progress reports, and contact the clinician if any regression in the child's fluency is observed during the consolidation period.

4. Follow-up: In the last phase of the PCI approach, parents are instructed to perform three-month follow-ups over a period of at least one year. If the child continues to be disfluent, additional interaction strategies and environmental modifications may be suggested by the clinician. Unsatisfactory progress in a child's fluency may even warrant the implementation of direct treatment approaches with the child.

Direct approaches

The past few decades have witnessed a paradigm shift from indirect to direct approaches for the management of stuttering for children. As described earlier, direct approaches focus on establishing fluent speech through direct interaction with a CWS. They comprise of treatments based on response-contingent stimulation and fluency shaping methods. Hereunder, we discuss a few popular traditional approaches, followed by more recent evidence-based treatment techniques.

Traditional approaches

Conventional stuttering treatment approaches have implications in the intervention of adults as well as children. A popular traditional approach is Van Riper's stuttering modification approach which focuses on modifying moments of stuttering by targeting muscle tension as well as associated fear and anxiety, thereby decreasing the severity of stuttering.

VAN RIPER'S APPROACH – MIDVAS

Van Riper (1971) suggested that individuals who stutter experience fear, avoidance and are in a constant struggle to escape from stuttering. Based on this premise, he proposed a stuttering modification approach/strategy or the non-avoidance approach, which focuses on reducing stuttering related fear and anxiety. In this approach, individuals who stutter are trained to overcome their fear and avoidance behaviour through graded steps, thereby transitioning from an *effortful stutter* to an *easy stutter*. The approach comprises of a set of strategies, commonly referred to as the *MIDVAS approach* (motivation, identification, desensitization, variation, approximation, and stabilization). It may be noted that this approach demands adult-like linguistic and cognitive skills, and is thus suitable for older children and adolescents. Table 6.4 below provides a summary of the six steps of the MIDVAS approach.

Table 6.4 Steps of Van Riper's MIDVAS approach

Step	*Description*	*Tasks/Activities*
Motivation	Gaining the confidence of the child and seeking compliance for treatment. In case of CWS, parents are active participants at this stage.	Use of success stories, video models or direct interaction with children who recovered from stuttering and their families helps motivate a CWS and gain confidence of parents/family towards the intervention programme
Identification	Self-awareness – identification of overt and covert features of stuttering	• Yes/No task (*"Do you think that was smooth or did you get stuck?"*) • Simultaneous use of a mirror to identify secondary behaviours • Analyzing audio-video recordings of speech samples for both overt and covert features
Desensitization	• Making a CWS understand that it is okay to stutter and that they can overcome it. • Important step for reduction of stuttering related anxiety and stress	• Stutter voluntarily (the clinician may mimic a stutter and ask the child to do it voluntarily) – fosters belief that they can gain control of their stutter • Other strategies – relaxation, adaptation, and anxiety reduction
Variation	Aims to facilitate control over stuttering rather than eliminating it	• Stutter slowly (slow the rate of repetitions) • Stutter less (reduce the number of iterations) • Starting a word with some audible airflow or voicing to release the block
Approximation	Aims at reduction in the struggle that accompanies a moment of stuttering Three strategies: a. Cancellation b. Pullout c. Preparatory set	Let the stuttering moment finish, then repeat that particular word slow and easy (cancellation) Alter the stuttering behaviour while it is occurring, for instance, adding a vowel segment, inserting a breath release, voicing, waiting till the articulatory posture relaxes rather than fighting a fixed posture, etc. (pullout)

(*Continued*)

Table 6.4 (Continued)

Step	Description	Tasks/Activities
		Modify the stuttering before it occurs (applicable only for those who anticipate stuttering). For example, voluntary release of air when starting the word or reducing the rate of speech in advance when stuttering is anticipated (preparatory set)
Stabilization	Aims at stabilizing use of the strategies learnt and maintain fluent behaviour across situations	• Continued and varied practice • Reduced frequency of monitored sessions and promoting self-monitoring

COMPREHENSIVE FLUENCY SHAPING PROCEDURES

Fluency shaping procedures are often a preferred choice of treatment for adults and can also be used for school-age children who stutter (Guitar, 2006; Shapiro, 1999). Fluency shaping procedure involves strategies such as airflow management and slow rate of speech achieved using syllable prolongation. Working on airflow has been found to be particularly useful in children with severe disfluencies and poor respiratory control for speech.

Airflow management   Two key components of airflow management are "inhalation" followed by "slight exhalation before the onset of phonation". The two may be taught as independent skills initially and later as steps on a continuum. When teaching inhalation, the child is taught abdominal breathing. It helps to ask the child to keep their hand on their stomach and inhale till there is a significant outward movement of the hand. Inhaling on count can also be tried, where the clinician counts to a specific number, say five, and the child is instructed to breathe in till the count is over. Inhaling through the mouth is preferable, as it mimics speech (inhaling orally followed by speaking on exhalation). When training on pre-phonatory exhalation, the clinician can model and ask the child to imitate. Here, the child is expected to exhale slightly and then initiate speech. The exhalation could be audible initially (said as syllable / ha/) and then transition to inaudible exhalation at later stages of therapy. This is followed by implementing the entire breath cycle in continuation, inhalation, slight exhalation and then initiating speech. Theoretically, it might sound simple and easy; however, when considered from a child's perspective, it requires monitored training and practice.

Slow rate of speech with syllable prolongation   The second fluency shaping strategy is to achieve a slow rate of speech by prolonging each syllable. This strategy is based on the premise that stuttering is a timing disorder. When speech is slowed and prolonged, the speech motor control system has sufficient time to plan and programme the speech signal, thereby reducing chances of disfluencies. Also, as mentioned ear-lier, fluency shaping strategies diminish the naturally occurring prosodic variations in speech. Hence, the risk of the speech motor control system getting disturbed is lower.

Conventionally, prolongation is done for each syllable. This can give speech a robotic and unnatural tone. As it is an unnatural way of speaking, it might take a while to establish a prolonged speech pattern. The clinician can start with reading tasks and progress gradually stepwise to spontaneous speech tasks. To begin with, the clinician prolongs every syllable by stretching the duration of the vowel component of the syllable. Once slow and fluent speech is achieved in this manner, prolongation on each syllable is gradually faded out so that the child prolongs only the first syllable of every word and finally the first syllable of a sentence. This progression will depend on the proficiency of the child in using the technique at the previous level and thus would vary across children.

Normalizing prosody while using fluency shaping A major limitation of the fluency shaping procedure is unnatural sounding speech post-treatment. Hence, Hegde (2007) suggests that once fluency is established using a fluency shaping procedure and the child can maintain it across settings, it is important to reinstate normal speech rate, intonation and loudness variation during therapy sessions. This would ensure that the child's speech is socially acceptable, thereby preventing psychosocial issues such as bullying and mockery.

Fluency rules programme

Fluency rules programme is a direct approach developed by Runyan and Runyan (1986) for young school-age children who stutter. At its conception, the programme had ten rules which have been revised since then (Runyan & Runyan, 1986, 1999), and in its current version (Runyan & Runyan, 2007), the programme comprises seven rules. These seven rules are further categorized as *universal rules (rules 1, 2, & 3)*, *primary rules (rules 4 & 5)*, and *secondary rules (rules 6 & 7)*. In the latest revision (Runyan & Runyan, 2007), the rules were re-ordered and a new component of accompanying gestures or nonverbal cues was included. Table 6.5 provides a brief overview of each of these rules along with the suggested accompanying nonverbal cues

When implementing the *fluency rules programme*, the recommended order as per the latest revision (Runyan & Runyan, 2007) suggests identifying the fluency rules that are broken and working on them. As a general guideline, the proponents of the fluency rules programme suggest implementing *universal rules 1 and 2*, first. Implementation of *universal rule 3 ("Say it short", formerly known as "Keep the Speech Helpers moving")* is advised in case of children who exhibit prolongations. The programme suggests using primary rules if stuttering persists even after the child has mastered the universal rules. The use of secondary rules is recommended only when child exhibits hard articulatory contacts and associated physical concomitants.

While implementing fluency rules, clinicians are advised to incorporate hand gestures or nonverbal cues as early as possible to avoid interrupting the child.

Table 6.5 Summary of fluency rules programme

Rules		Goal	Accompanying nonverbal cue
Rule 1 – Speak slowly/Turtle speech	Universal Rules	To teach the child to use an overall slow rate of speech	Moving hand up and down indicating to slow down
Rule 2 – Say a word only once		To explain to the child that repeating the word does not aid in being understood by others. Feedback is provided whenever the child encounters a part-word or syllable repetition.	Holding one finger up
Rule 3 – Say it short		To teach smooth transitions between sounds and words.	Keeping thumb and finger close as a reminder to keep utterances short and not prolong them
Rule 4 – Use speech breathing	Primary Rules	To teach the child coordinated and controlled inspiratory and expiratory cycles, particularly slow controlled exhalation while speaking.	Drawing breath curve with finger (indicating inspiration) followed by silent finger snap (indication to initiate speech)
Rule 5 – Start Mr. voice box running smoothly		To help the child differentiate between a hard and a gentle onset of phonation. Teach gentle onset with visual and tactile feedback.	Touching fingers of both hands together (representing vocal fold contact) and gently moving fingertips apart elevating one hand slightly (indicating gentle onset of phonation)
Rule 6 – Touch the "Speech Helpers" together lightly	Secondary Rules	To help the child differentiate between a hard and soft articulatory contact. Teach soft articulatory contacts with visual and tactile feedback.	Gently touching thumb to forefinger (indicating soft articulatory contact)
Rule 7 – Use only "Speech Helpers" to talk		To reduce secondary behaviours or physical concomitants. Visual feedback and negative practice can help.	No nonverbal cue/ gesture used

Also, the programme suggests targeting all disfluencies rather than focusing only on SLDs to expedite the therapy process. Further, the programme aims to facilitate self-monitoring as well as carryover and transfer of learnt fluency skills. During the generalization stage, discriminative stimuli (any symbol, sign, toy, or object) are placed in the home and classroom environment of the child as a reminder to use fluency rules.

Collaborative Oral Language Fluency (COLF) programme

Proposed by Cooper and Cooper (1991), the focus of the COLF programme is to establish fluent speech by teaching six specific speech techniques communicated to children as animated characters. These animated characters are referred to as *fluency initiating gestures or FIGS*. To make it interesting for children, the animated characters are introduced to the children as FIG man and his friends. Here the FIG man represents fluent speech, and his friends (the six techniques) are the helpers for achieving fluent speech. The six FIGS are as follows: *Slow FIG, Easy FIG, Deep FIG, Loud FIG, Beat FIG, and Smooth FIG.*

While *Slow FIG* tells the child to prolong each syllable and use a slow rate of speech, *Easy FIG* emphasizes pre-phonatory exhalation and the gentle onset of phonation. *Deep FIG* reminds the child to focus on inhalation before initiating speech. Further, *Loud FIG* insists on voluntary and sustained variations in the loudness levels while speaking. The fifth technique is explained by *Beat FIG* that suggests voluntary changes in the prosodic aspects (intonation, stress and rhythm) of speech. Lastly, *Smooth FIG* refers to smooth voicing and soft articulatory contacts to eliminate cessation of voicing and blocks.

Pause and talk

Pause and talk is one of the early conventional approaches used in stuttering intervention. It may be considered as a form of time-out. This technique is based on the principles of operant conditioning. The response of the clinician/listener is contingent on the speech of the child/speaker. *Pause and talk* is usually preferred for school-age or older children because conversational speech skills are essential for this technique. It is not recommended for young preschool children in whom eliciting continuous speech samples is often challenging.

The two major components of pause and talk, as suggested by Hegde (2007) are *reinforcement for fluency* and *reinforcement withdrawal for stuttering*. During the production of fluent utterances, the clinician reinforces fluency by maintaining eye contact, paying attention to the child's speech, presenting a pleasing facial expression, indulging in the conversation through questioning, prompting, and using other strategies to keep the conversation going. The clinician also ensures that the child is doing most of the talking, keeping their own utterances to a minimum. In contrast, when the child encounters a moment of stuttering, the clinician stops the child, terminates eye contact, and pauses the conversation for a count of five seconds. During the five-second pause, the clinician stays still, looks elsewhere and maintains a neutral expression. At the end of the five-second pause, the clinician re-establishes eye contact and provides gestural (e.g. a smile and a head nod) or verbal cues (e.g. please continue, go ahead, etc.) to resume the conversation. A five-minute time-out is considered to be optimum. Clinicians may vary this duration when necessary; however, it may be kept in mind that a prolonged time-out might have detrimental effects and should be avoided. Modelling correct speech, explicit instructions to imitate the clinician's production, introducing a slower rate of speech or modified airflow methods are usually avoided when strictly following the pause and talk method. The efficacy of pause and talk in school-age children who stutter has been evaluated by Rakesh (2021) as a part of his doctoral dissertation, the details of which are mentioned later in this chapter under the section on evidence in the Indian context.

Response cost

Another popular approach based on the principles of operant conditioning is the *response cost* technique. Unlike the above approaches, this treatment technique can be used for both preschool and school-age children who stutter. However, it is relatively popular for its efficacy in preschool children. This technique involves response-contingent reinforcement. Every fluent utterance is reinforced with a token and for every disfluent utterance the reinforcer/token is withdrawn. The tangible reinforcers (tokens) are accompanied by verbal contingencies and corrective feedback. For example, for a fluent production, the clinician may say, "That was a smooth production. Here's your token". Likewise, production of a disfluent utterance results in withdrawal of the token and corrective feedback such as "Oh, that was bumpy"! At the end of each session, a child gets to exchange the tokens collected for a reward of their choice. As the treatment progresses, the tangible reinforcers or tokens may be faded out, and only verbal contingencies can be used. In this technique, the clinician models fluent speech without any explicit instructions such as "speak slow" or "speak smoothly". CWS are encouraged to imitate the model and are reinforced for their fluent production. Hegde (2007) provides a structured step-by-step procedure for the administration of the response cost technique. The programme begins with *base-rating* or a baseline assessment during which speech samples are collected from different settings. The collected samples are analyzed for the frequency of stuttering (percentage of syllables stuttered; %SS) and the types of disfluencies. The treatment is then initiated at the sentence level and then progressing to continuous speech, narration and conversational speech levels. The criteria to move from one level to the next is the attainment of 98% fluency at the current level. For further reading on the details of the protocol, we recommend that readers refer to Hegde (2007).

Occasionally children might react negatively towards the withdrawal of tokens, particularly young children, more so during the initial sessions. One can try to overcome this issue by providing some tokens at the beginning of the session and avoiding total bankruptcy at any point. Clinicians can use a 2:1 ratio wherein two tokens are provided for every fluent utterance; however, a disfluent production costs the child withdrawal of one token only. Role reversals could also help, where the clinician or parent stutter intentionally and the child gets to withdraw their tokens. This would prepare the child for their turn and facilitate better compliance for therapy sessions. In order to ensure active participation of children and sustain their interest, Hegde (2007) also recommends using a variety of therapy stimuli, tasks and reinforcers (tokens).

Lidcombe Program

The *Lidcombe Program* was developed by Mark Onslow and his team at the Australian Stuttering Research Centre in the early 2000s. The development of the programme began much earlier; however, the structured protocol was proposed after the year

2000 and, since then, is one of the most popular intervention programmes for young children who stutter worldwide. It was initially proposed for preschool children who stutter up to the age of 6 years.

The Lidcombe Program is based on the principles of operant conditioning and is a parent-delivered intervention approach. It is different from other intervention programmes for children, as it does not require any change in speech production characteristics of children or any environmental modification. The programme is based on the use of verbal contingencies for fluent and disfluent utterances. It specifies five categories of verbal contingencies (Figure 6.2). The first three contingencies are given for stutter-free speech to promote fluent speech while the remaining two are in the form of corrective feedback for unambiguous stuttering moments (Onslow, 2021). The first verbal contingency is *praise*. Parents are trained to appreciate or praise their child's fluent utterances (e.g. "That was some smooth speech!"; "Oh! You did great there!"; "Good job!"). Parents are encouraged to keep it genuine and not exaggerate the praises making it unnatural. The second verbal contingency is *request self-evaluation* and is recommended for use only when the child has not stuttered for a specific period (ranging anywhere from one utterance to several hours). The parent can make requests such as "Were there any bumps there?"; expecting a "no" as a response or may ask "Did you say all that smoothly?" with a "yes" as the expected response. The third verbal contingency is *acknowledge* and unlike the earlier two verbal contingencies, this is usually given at the end of a practice session without interrupting the conversation. The parent can acknowledge the stutter-free productions by using statements such as "that was smooth", "no bumpy words". The next two verbal contingencies are used for the unambiguous moments of stuttering and are in the form of corrective feedback. These should be used less frequently and with caution as young children might start becoming apprehensive about them. The first verbal contingency for the unambiguous moments of stuttering is *acknowledge*, where the clinician points at the moment of stuttering by using phrases such as "that was bumpy" or "I heard some stuck word". The second verbal contingency for unambiguous stuttering is *requesting self-correction* using phrases such as "can you try that again"? or "see if you can say that without the bump".

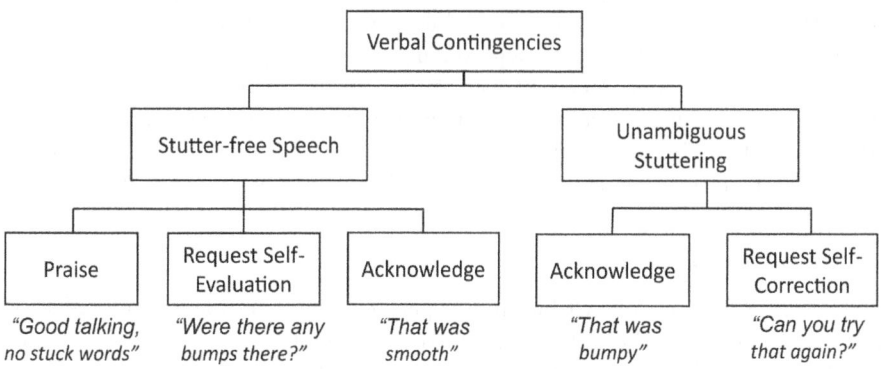

Figure 6.2 Classification of verbal contingencies in the Lidcombe Program

In addition to the above five contingencies, the Lidcombe Program recommends two optional contingencies: *Praise for spontaneous self-evaluation of speech* and *praise for spontaneous self-correction*. Occasionally the older children who stutter might self-evaluate their stutter and may comment, "I didn't say that right" or "Oh! That was bumpy". In such instances, the parents are encouraged to reinforce the self-evaluation with responses such as "*Good! You are listening for your smooth talking*". Parents should be clearly explained the difference between *praise* (for stutter-free speech) and *praise for self-evaluation* and should be trained to use them appropriately. The second optional contingency is *praise for spontaneous self-correction*, to be given when the child self-corrects or repeats the stuttered word fluently without any prompts by the parents, for example, "Good, you fixed that bumpy word all by yourself". A word of caution is to use optional verbal contingencies judiciously and not as frequently as verbal contingencies for *stutter-free speech* and *unambiguous moments of stuttering*. Parents are trained to identify moments of stuttering and correct delivery of appropriate verbal contingencies. They are informed that if they are at all unsure about a moment of stuttering, then they must refrain from delivering a contingency. A major consideration of the Lidcombe Program is to make the entire treatment process a positive experience for the child. Within this context, parents are trained to deliver contingencies for stutter-free speech first, followed by other types of verbal contingencies.

The Lidcombe Program is a structured programme and can be practised by certified professionals only. The treatment guide (Onslow et al., 2021) provides details on what is done in each clinic visit and how the treatment progresses. The programme is mainly divided into two stages, called the *establishment* and *maintenance* phases. The major components of the two phases are described in Table 6.6.

Proponents of the Lidcombe Program strongly believe in evidence-based practice. Currently, the Lidcombe Program has a relatively greater evidence base in comparison to any other treatment programmes designed for children who stutter. It is an effective treatment programme with long-term maintenance of fluency skills (Jones et al., 2008; Lincoln & Onslow, 1997; Rousseau et al., 2007). Keeping up with the pace of technological advancements, the researchers developed a teletherapy or web-based model of the programme that has proven to be equally effective (Bridgman et al., 2016; Lewis et al., 2008; O'Brian et al., 2014; Van Eerdenbrugh et al., 2016). The Lidcombe Program is also reported to be successful for school-age children who stutter (Bakhtiar & Packman, 2009; Koushik et al., 2009) when delivered as group therapy (Arnott et al., 2014). Although the programme originated in Australia, and a majority of the evidence comes from Australian data, it has been evaluated in other countries with sociocultural adaptations and has shown promising findings (Al-Khaledi et al., 2018; Bakhtiar & Packman, 2009; Hewat et al., 2018; Koushik et al., 2009; Lattermann et al., 2008; Murza & Nye, 2009; Vong et al., 2016).

The Westmead Program

The Westmead Program or syllable-timed speech is another popular intervention approach for children who stutter, particularly the school-age group. The technique dates back to the 1930s when it was referred to as syllable-timed speech or pacing and was initially used for adults who stutter. It involved speaking each syllable to a beat. In the 1980s, researchers attempted to use it with children who stutter and conducted experimental research; however, the findings remain unpublished. The technique requires a certain minimal level of cognitive and linguistic skills, and is therefore preferred for school-age children.

In the last two decades, researchers have attempted to generate evidence on its efficacy for children who stutter. Currently, this research is in its early developmental stages at the Australian Stuttering Research Centre. The Westmead Program involves training and encouraging parents to help their children use syllable-timed speech, also known as "robot talking". The goal of the programme is to establish fluent speech with a normal rate that sounds natural. Similar to the Lidcombe Program, the Westmead Program also has two stages: Stage 1 aims to establish *"no stuttering"* or *"nearly no stuttering";* stage 2 is the *"maintenance stage"* and aims to maintain fluent speech for a long time. Stage 1 is further divided into phase A and phase B. Phase A involves weekly clinical visits during which the clinician trains the parent to model syllable-timed speech and encourage the child to use the same. The clinician also guides parents on how to modify utterance length and complexity while interacting with the child. Every weekly visit is a 30–60 minutes session. Further, parents are encouraged to have five to six practice sessions (10–15 minutes/session) at home every day. Phase B of stage 1 consists of fortnightly clinic visits and regular practice sessions at home. The criteria for transition to stage 2 are the same as those in the Lidcombe Program (Table 6.6). During Stage 2, the frequency of practice sessions is reduced along with the frequency of clinic visits. The efficacy of the Westmead Program has been established through phase I and II randomized clinical trials (Andrews et al., 2016; Ilkhani et al., 2019; Trajkovski et al., 2006; Trajkovski et al., 2009; Trajkovski et al., 2011; Trajkovski et al., 2019).

Hybrid approaches

A hybrid approach, as the name suggests, combines principles of both direct and indirect treatments. Hybrid approaches are based on the premise that while direct approaches help establish fluent speech, reducing the environmental stressors as an indirect method might additionally facilitate fluency. Most of the practicing clinicians follow a hybrid approach, using parent counselling and environmental manipulation in addition to fluency shaping procedures. However, similar to indirect approaches, the evidence base for hybrid approaches is still in its infancy and only one structured programme – the RESTART treatment provides evidence in support of such an approach.

RESTART-DCM

RESTART-DCM is a highly structured approach based on the demands and capacities model (DCM). Treatment is oriented towards achieving and maintaining a balance between the communication demands of the child with early stuttering and their capacities across motoric, linguistic, socio-emotional, and cognitive domains (de Sonneville-Koedoot et al., 2015). Similar to the PCI approach discussed earlier, this approach begins with a detailed assessment of the child, the parents, and their interaction. Key assessment components for this approach have been shown in the Table 6.7.

Table 6.6 Summary of Phase I and II of the Lidcombe Program

Phase	Description
Phase I – Establishment	• Aim: To establish *"no stuttering"* or *"nearly no stuttering"* • Includes delivering verbal contingencies during practice sessions and natural conversations • Weekly clinic visit – clinician trains parent on delivering verbal contingencies; observes parent-child interaction and provides feedback • On average one to two beyond-clinic practice sessions, 10 to 15 minutes per session are recommended • The purpose of practice sessions is to train parents on delivering verbal contingencies and help the child get accustomed to treatment • Once parents' delivery of verbal contingencies is satisfactory, gradually interaction in natural settings takes over and practice sessions are faded out
Phase II – Maintenance	• Aim: Maintaining attained fluency skills for a long period • In order to progress from stage 1 to stage 2, children need to meet the following criteria for three consecutive weeks: *Parent severity ratings of "0" or "1" for at least four days in the week and a clinician severity rating of "0" or "1" during the clinic visit.* • Weekly clinic visits are reduced in steps with a gradually increasing gap between two consecutive visits. • At any given point in time, if the clinician feels that the child doesn't meet the criteria of *no* or *nearly no stuttering*, they are asked to step down to stage one and resume weekly clinic visits

Based on the results obtained during assessment, the first conference with parents is organized in which parents are briefed about the assessment findings. The clinician uses illustrations based on a demand and capacity weighing scale to explain the imbalance in environmental demands and the child's capacities to the parents. At this point, the clinician also introduces the concept of the special talk time to the parents. In RESTART-DCM, special talk time refers to a 15-minute block of time that occurs at least five times a week. During these 15 minutes, parents are instructed to provide complete undivided attention to the child and practice various strategies demonstrated by the clinician to reduce demands and increase the child's capacities across the target domains. Parents are also introduced to logbooks, where they can document their experiences during the special talk time along with progress, if any, in reducing demands and increasing the child's capacities during the special talk time.

The RESTART-DCM approach strongly recommends one-on-one demonstration sessions for parents at least once a week to ensure that desirable behaviour for demand reduction and capacity building has been learnt by the parent. Once this is learnt to the clinician's satisfaction, parents are permitted to implement this behaviour at home.

The first phase of its treatment segment deals with helping parents identify undesirable demands on the child and learn strategies to alleviate them. It is recommended that demand reduction be followed in the given order of motoric, linguistic,

Table 6.7 Key aspects of the assessment process in RESTART-DCM

Assessment	Procedure	Key aspects
Child	• Oral Motor Assessment Scale (OMAS; Riley & Riley, 1986) • KiddyCAT (Vanryckeghem & Brutten, 2007) • Stuttering Severity Instrument (SSI-4) (Riley, 2009)	• Language comprehension and expression • Oro-motor abilities for speech production • Speech sound production at phonologic and phonetic levels • Ability to control speech and language output across different pressure conditions • General attitude towards one's speech and listener reactions
Parent	• Parental interview	• Medical and other relevant developmental history • Progression of disfluencies • Environmental reactions • The child's understanding of their own speech
Parent-Child interaction	• Videotaping a 15-minute conversation between the child and the parent during a structured and an unstructured play situation	• Motoric, linguistic, socio-emotional and cognitive demands are identified, and their frequency of occurrence is noted.

socio-emotional, and cognitive demands respectively. Parents are asked to target the reduction of specifically those demands which are identified in the context of their child during assessment. An example of high motoric demand for a child may be family members talking at a fast rate of speech as compared to the child and frequent interruptions during conversations. In such a scenario, a parent is made aware that the goal would be to work on reducing the time pressure and rate of speech used by everyone in the family, to ensure that planning and execution of the child's verbal output (demand) does not overtake capacity. Parents are also taught strategies to lower their speech rate, increase latency time to avoid interruptions, and provide more time to the child to express themselves with optimum turn-taking to achieve the desired goal of reducing the motoric demands. Likewise, goals and strategies are prepared and implemented in the context of linguistic, socio-emotional, and cognitive demands. Sometimes, achieving mastery over one domain might show a transfer effect on other demands, and they might, therefore, not require active intervention. Such decisions are made during regular discussions with the clinician who monitors the skills of parents as well as improvement in the child's fluency.

It is possible that the child achieves good fluency levels after all target demands have been effectively reduced during phase 1. However, if not, then the clinician moves towards phase 2 of the programme in which efforts are made to improve the capacities of the child across motoric, linguistic, socio-emotional, and cognitive domains. Similar to the previous phase, the clinician models appropriate strategies for capacity enhancement to the parent and the child in the clinical setting once every week. Once parents seem to have mastered the strategies, they are asked to train the child using the same during special talk time at home. Unlike the previous phase, capacity building can be simultaneously worked on for any of the four domains. An example of building emotional capacity for children with a highly reactive temperament, anxiety, and fear about moments of stuttering would be to model desensitization. Clinicians and parents may also model voluntary stuttering in their speech followed by self-talk indicating it is okay to stutter. Likewise, strategies for capacity building are trained for other domains.

If the clinician and the parent feel that the fluency of the child's speech is yet to reach acceptable levels after the completion of phase 1 and phase 2, then a more direct approach towards the child's fluency is adopted in phase 3. Maintaining a positive attitude towards stuttering continues but parents may be trained in certain fluency shaping and stuttering modification methods which the child could incorporate during special talk time at home. The child is encouraged to use strategies such as smooth and easy speech, soft articulatory contacts, gentle speech onset, etc., during game-based activities with an assumption that the child would be able to naturally adopt these methods in their speech outside of the special talk time.

Whenever during the programme a child attains acceptable levels of fluency, the clinician tapers the therapeutic involvement and empowers parents to maintain the attained balance of demands and capacity with the child. Parents are also made aware of the possibility of a relapse and ways to reinstate the strategies if such a need arises. A need to revisit the clinician in case disfluency increases is also discussed. At present, two clinical trials have revealed that the RESTART-DCM programme is as effective as the Lidcombe Program in improving fluency in CWS (de Sonneville-Koedoot et al., 2015; Franken et al., 2005). For further reading related to this approach, we recommend that interested readers refer to the latest and revised version of the document by Franken and Laroes (2021).

Evidence in the Indian context

Despite abundant evidence regarding efficacy of programmes such as Lidcombe and RESTART, there are a few cultural and linguistic challenges one might face in their implementation. Direct implementation of these approaches might often be difficult in the Indian context owing to several reasons. First, in order to practice some of these standard programmes such as Lidcombe and Westmead, clinicians need to be certified. Getting certification might not be possible for all practicing clinicians owing to financial, geographical, and technical factors. To the best of our knowledge, currently there are no online certification programmes available and going overseas is not a feasible option for every clinician. Second, programmes such as Lidcombe and Westmead were designed for children who belong to cultural and linguistic backgrounds with extremely few, if any, similarities with the Indian linguistic and sociocultural scenario. Hence, generalizing efficacy data on these treatment programmes to the Indian scenario must be done with caution.

Although stuttering intervention for children has been practised clinically since decades in India, empirical investigations assessing efficacy of specific treatment approaches are still in their infancy. In a recent study, Seth (2020) investigated the efficacy of response cost in Kannada-speaking preschool children who stutter (3 to 6 years). Treatment was delivered to 27 CWS using Hegde's (2007) protocol. Speech samples were recorded in both within-clinic and beyond-clinic conditions and multiple outcome measures such as percentage of syllable stuttered (%SS), clinician and parent severity ratings, speech naturalness, speech rate, articulation rate, and parent perception of impact of stuttering. Their findings indicated significant improvement in all participants with near normal fluency (<2 %SS), reduced stuttering severity ratings and impact of stuttering as perceived by parents. Although speech naturalness ratings and the overall speech rate improved post-therapy, no difference was seen in the articulation rate. All changes observed were maintained up to six months post-discharge. In another investigation, Rakesh (2021) evaluated the efficacy of prolongation and pause and talk in 6- to 10-year-old school-going children who stutter. They compared spontaneous speech samples (within- and beyond-clinic) taken before and after therapy and conducted follow-up evaluations for up to three months. Similar to the previous study, they included multiple outcome measures, %SS, stuttering severity ratings, speech naturalness ratings, speech rate, physical concomitants, and attitude assessments such as the Communication Attitude Test in Kannada: CAT-K and the Speech Situation Checklist in Kannada: SSC-ER-K (Veerabhadrappa, Vanryckeghem, et al., 2021a, 2021b). Findings of their study revealed a significant reduction in %SS, severity ratings, physical concomitants, as well as associated negative attitudes and anxiety. In addition, there was an improvement in naturalness ratings, no significant difference in speech rate, and maintenance of fluency skills up to three months. The study concluded that both prolongation and pause and talk are equally effective in treating stuttering in school-age children. These investigations add substantially to evidence-based practice in the Indian context. All three techniques – response cost, prolongation, and pause and talk are time- and cost-effective and clinicians can be readily trained. These preliminary studies can be regarded as the beginning of many more efficacy studies and randomized controlled trials in future.

Analogies

A discussion on the management of stuttering in children would be incomplete without a mention of analogies. Analogies are not direct therapeutic strategies to shape fluency or modify stuttering. They are simplified examples or references to explain concepts related to speech in general or stuttering in particular. Analogies help to bring the child and the clinician on a common platform, where a child is taught in a simple manner about speech subsystems and ways to manipulate them in order to attain optimum fluency. Analogies may also be used to help parents understand the nature of stuttering. Conture (1990b) proposed several analogies, each with a purpose of attaining specific goals pertaining to management of stuttering in children. A summary of various analogies along with their applications is provided in Table 6.8 below.

Some analogies can be explained better using illustrations. Figures 6.3 and 6.4 illustrate two commonly used analogies.

Table 6.8 A summary of analogies proposed by Conture

Analogy	Description	Applications/Goals
Out of sight, out of mind	• Questions such as "How does your heart look like?"; "What is it doing right now?" are asked to the parent • Speech movements are equated to the cardiac function • It is reasoned that akin to heart movements embedded deep within the chest cavity, speech movements are embedded within the vocal tract • In case of stuttering, there is a difficulty in speech production, but most of the time it is treated like the heart – *out of sight, out of mind*	• Helping parents to understand the speech production mechanism • Helping parents and the child understand why a child is having difficulty in something that is taken for granted as easy or requiring minimal effort (i.e., speech)
Jumping into a swimming pool	Parents are asked to imagine jumping into a pool of ice-cold water while expecting warm or room-temperature water. The *unexpectedness* and *suddenness* one feels on encountering ice-cold water is reasoned to be similar to the feeling a child experiences when they encounter a moment of stuttering. Forced inspiration, a feeling of being stuck, and the struggle to get out of the cold water are explained to be similar to struggles of a child during a moment of stuttering (sudden inspiration, physical tension in vocal tract and/or body)	• Helping parents empathize and understand the experiences and challenges of a child when they stutter • Helping parents understand the *unexpectedness, suddenness, fear, and out of control* feelings during moments of stuttering
Touching a hot stove burner	Parents are asked to imagine accidently touching a hot stove burner. The *unexpectedness* and *suddenness* one feels on encountering a hot stove is reasoned to be similar to the feeling a child experiences when they encounter a moment of stuttering. The sudden recoil, forced inspiration, and tensing of the muscles are likened to struggles of a child with a moment of stuttering (sudden inspiration or gasping, physical tension in vocal tract and/or body)	• Helping parents empathize and understand the experiences and challenges of a child when they stutter • Helping parents understand the *unexpectedness, suddenness, fear, and struggle* during moments of stuttering
Garden hose (Figure 6.3)	The mechanism of speech production is equated to water flowing out of a garden hose. A smooth flow out of the hose signifies easy flowing speech. An obstruction at the nozzle of the hose implies an articulatory arrest at the level of the lips as seen during a labial block. An obstructed flow due to a constriction somewhere along the length of the hose implies an undesirable constriction in the vocal tract or oral cavity as experienced during a velar or alveolar block. A scenario in which the flow in the hose is seized at the level of the faucet signifies an undesirable glottal constriction as experienced in form of laryngeal tension.	• Helping the child understand the speech mechanism and how blocks in speech come about • Explaining concepts such as "*air stoppers, tightness due to air pressure versus muscle tension, feelings of tension versus feelings of fear*" (Conture, 2001; p. 195–198)

Blown-up balloon	The clinician blows up a balloon and makes the child feel the stretched sides of the balloon to explain the tension created by air pressure in the lungs and vocal tract. The child is then asked to figure out the most efficient way to ease the pressure out of the balloon. For example, a child may slowly release air out of the blown–up balloon by slightly separating the finger and the thumb at the opening of the balloon. This way he/she understands the gentle onset of voice with a gradual release of air pressure from the lungs.	• Helping the child understand how to regulate aerodynamics in the lungs and vocal tract for gentle speech onset
Lily pad/ Barrel bridge (Figure 6.4)	A lily pad or barrel bridge is drawn, and a frog/a boy is made to hop on the lily pads/barrel bridge one by one to cross over from one bank of the river to the other. Each hop on the lily pad/barrel accompanies every syllable uttered by the child. So, a prolongation in the child's speech is illustrated by staying too long on a lily pad/barrel, too hard a jump on the lily pad/barrel signifies a hard contact and up-down hopping movement on the same pad/barrel depicts a repetition. It can also be emphasized that the chances of the frog/boy falling into the water are lower if they jump slowly and carefully from one lily pad to the next. *Note: The Lily pad analogy is preferred for very young children (preschoolers); a barrel bridge can be used with older children.*	• Helping the child and/or parents understand the smooth continuous movement from one syllable to another for fluent speech • Teaching the importance of using and maintaining a slow rate of speech for better coordination and control and minimal disfluencies
Thumb and opposing finger	Each finger symbolizes a speech unit, and the opposing thumb represents the articulator used to produce that speech unit. A smooth sequential and easy movement of the thumb from one finger to another represents fluent speech. A moment of stuttering is represented by a long, strong, or repeated force between the opposing finger and the thumb as observed during a prolongation, block, or repetition, respectively. Also, slower movements from one finger to the next increases chances of the movements being smooth and sequential. *Note: This analogy is preferred for older children, teenagers or adults*	• Helping the child and/or parents understand the smooth continuous and coordinated movement from one syllable to another for fluent speech • Emphasizing the importance of a slow rate of speech to reduce the demands on the speech motor coordination system
Clenched-fist-to-relaxed-hand	A parallel is drawn between *fist* and *speech.* A moment of stuttering is equated to a tightly closed fist. The clinician gradually releases the fist, transitioning from a tightly clenched fist to an open palm. The child is made to understand that physical tension in speech can also be released over time. *Note: A word of caution is to discourage extensive use of this analogy, especially outside the clinic, as there is a risk of the child beginning to clench and unclench the fist as a secondary behaviour or coping mechanism in an attempt to release the physical tension in articulators*	To teach the child how to gradually release physical tension in speech

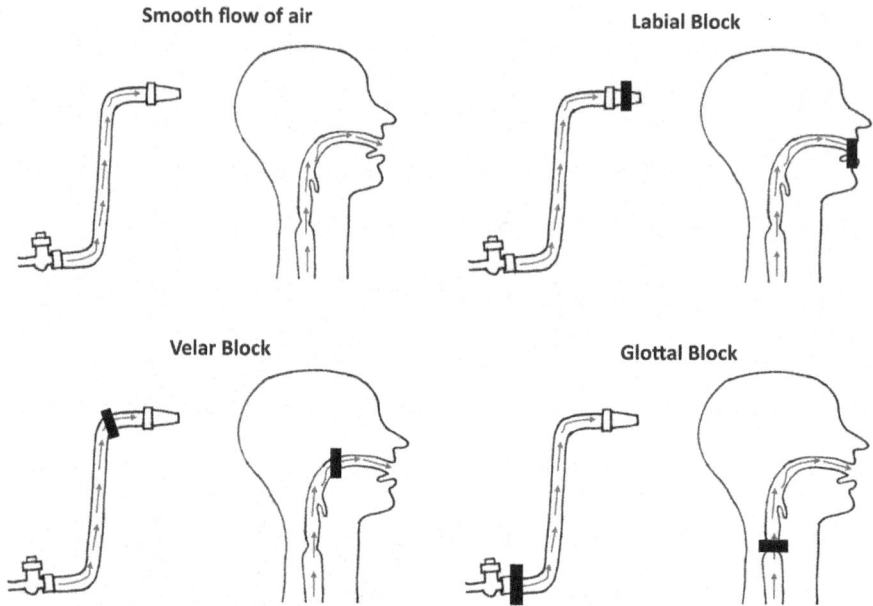

Figure 6.3 The garden hose analogy

Management through the lens of the ICF framework

As discussed in earlier chapters, assessment and intervention of any disorder or condition should include all the components of the International Classification of Functioning, Disability and Health (ICF; WHO, 2001) framework. Within this context, it is reasonable to state that the overall goal of an intervention programme for CWS would be to improve their quality of life by reducing the impact of stuttering. This may be achieved by addressing the three components, body functions and structures; activities and participation; and environmental and personal factors, during evaluation and goal setting. The direct and indirect therapy approaches discussed in earlier sections of this chapter focus on these components of the ICF model. Using direct treatment approaches singly or in combination, clinicians can target body function and work towards establishing and maintaining fluent speech. However, despite a significant reduction in disfluencies in a clinical setting, generalization to natural settings is poor in most CWS. Children might continue to stutter at home, at school, or in any other extra-clinical situation and might continue to experience fear and anxiety. In order to improve activities and participation, it is essential that established fluency is maintained over time and generalized across situations. To achieve this, we recommend that clinicians encourage practice in a variety of situations (such as parent–child interaction, telephonic conversation, speaking with teachers and peers, and interacting with strangers) that are relevant and important for the child. Parents play a major role during this phase of intervention by providing opportunities to communicate, by monitoring their child's performance in natural settings and reporting their observations to the clinician.

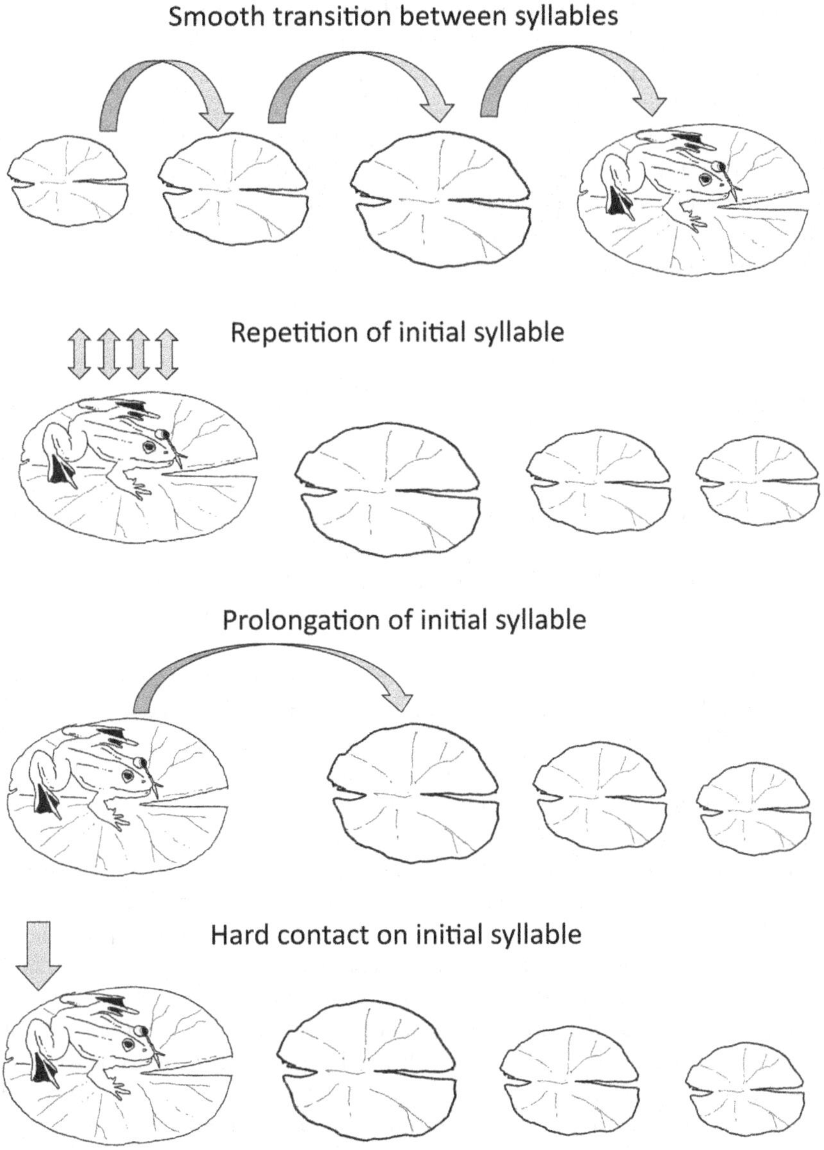

Smooth transition between syllables

Repetition of initial syllable

Prolongation of initial syllable

Hard contact on initial syllable

Figure 6.4 The lily pad analogy

Expected therapy outcomes in school-age children who stutter entail improving self-confidence, achieving independence, and creating a facilitatory environment in addition to the primary goal of reducing stuttering (Cook & Millard, 2018). The ICF model classifies environmental and personal factors as facilitators and barriers, based on whether they aid in the achievement of these outcomes. Indirect approaches explained in earlier sections of the chapter could be helpful in targeting identified barriers through parental counselling, improving awareness and educating parents, peers, teachers, and significant others in the child's milieu, rendering an environment conducive to progress. Establishing fluent speech across situations and providing a facilitatory environment could improve a child's confidence, self-esteem, and attitude towards communication. The result would be a reduced impact of stuttering and an improved quality of life. Thus, a hybrid approach (direct and indirect) and a tailor-made intervention plan are recommended in line with the ICF model. Whether treatment should begin with a direct or indirect approach, when to introduce the said approaches, and whether both may be used simultaneously needs to be decided by the clinician in consultation with the child and the family.

Case example

Child ABC was a 3.5-year-old male who visited the clinic accompanied by his parents who were concerned about his disfluencies. The onset of the disfluencies was reported to be around 3.2 years of age; it coincided with the birth of his younger sister. Case history also revealed a positive family history on the paternal side. The child exhibited initial syllable repetition and occasional blocks; however, blocks were reportedly severe and accompanied by physical tension. The child's overt behaviours were assessed using SSI-4 and overall severity was determined as mild (ICF code *b3300.1*), indicating impaired fluency (under the *body function and structure* domain). The child was primarily unaware of his stuttering and thus no escape or avoidance behaviours were noted. However, a parent perception questionnaire detected a high degree of anxiety in the child's parents. The child's environment was gauged to be supportive (*ICF code e310, e315*) except for a few neighbours who had forbidden their children from playing with him, fearing that their children might develop stuttering (ICF code *e325*). The diagnosis was developmental stuttering.

Based on the current profile, it is essential that the treatment plan for this child follow a hybrid approach. In this case, the immediate and extended family are supportive and could be classified as *facilitators*, while the neighbours serve as *barriers*. Use of direct treatment approaches such as *Lidcombe or response cost* with this child could establish fluent speech involving parents as active participants in therapy. Spreading awareness among the neighbours and others in the child's environment could restore the child's interaction with other children and adults, providing him with ample opportunities to generalize his learnt fluency skills. It might also incidentally help reduce the anxiety experienced by the parents.

The selection of an approach to stuttering intervention in a CWS depends on factors such as the age of the child, duration of stuttering since its onset, the severity of stuttering, the child's awareness of stuttering, comorbid conditions (if any), and the clinician's expertise. Irrespective of the approach chosen, early intervention increases the chances of shorter treatment duration and a greater success rate. The clinician must also educate parents and caregivers about the nature of the problem, treatment options, and what is expected of them in the course of the treatment. Success stories of other people who stutter could be used to motivate parents and gain trust. Clinicians might also need to counsel a child's school teachers or peers to ensure environmental support and acceptance for the CWS. Breaking the dichotomy – *fluent speech is good, disfluent speech is bad* – is extremely essential (Manning, 2009). The clinician must help the child understand that it is okay to stutter and that it can be controlled. Lastly, use of the ICF framework is strongly recommended. As seen in the case vignette above, the ICF framework supports the use of a hybrid approach and guides clinicians to plan intervention with the overall goal of reducing the impact and improving quality of life in CWS.

Summary points to remember

- Treating CWS is different from treating adults with stuttering.
- Several developmental and environmental factors play a crucial role in planning intervention for CWS.
- Treatment decisions significantly depend on the outcomes of a detailed assessment process and the risk factor profile of the given child.
- Treatment approaches are broadly classified into indirect, hybrid and direct approaches.
- Indirect approaches like Parent-child interaction therapy aim at modifying the environment to facilitate fluency in children.
- Hybrid approaches such as RESTART-DCM train parents in a structured manner to reduce demands and enhance a child's capacity across motoric, linguistic, social and emotional domains.
- Direct approaches involve active participation of the child and establish fluent speech using principles of operant conditioning or altering speech production characteristics at the level of different subsystems of speech.
- While selecting a direct treatment approach, a clinician should consider the age of the child who stutters, and the pre-requisite linguistic and cognitive skills.
- Clinicians should appreciate the individuality of each child and plan a custom-made intervention programme. Use of a hybrid approach is encouraged.
- Analogies convey mechanics of fluent speech production to children receiving therapy for stuttering in a simple manner.
- Use of an ICF framework to plan treatment for children who stutter is recommended.

Study questions

1. Outline possible treatment scenarios which can emerge after assessment of CWS.
2. Explain the fluency rules programme and its efficacy for treating CWS.
3. Describe response cost therapy as a treatment option for CWS.
4. With relevant examples, explain the role of analogies in the treatment of CWS.
5. Discuss the protocol followed during the RESTART-DCM programme while treating CWS.

7 Management of stuttering in adults

Vinitha Mary George, Nirmal Sugathan and Preethy Susan Reni

Introduction

Van Riper (1990), a pioneer in the field of stuttering, had professed his inability to find a cause and a cure for stuttering. From the early times, different treatment methods ranging from psychotherapy to surgical approaches have evolved; however, none of these proved to be a persistent solution to stuttering.

The overall quality of life of the person who stutters (PWS) can be significantly compromised by the affective, behavioural, and cognitive correlates of stuttering (Yaruss & Quesal, 2006). According to the International Classification of Functioning, Disability and Health (ICF) (World Health Organization; WHO, 2001) framework, it is important for clinicians to ensure that treatment goals for adults with stuttering should focus on reducing the impact of stuttering on the individual, thereby improving their quality of life. Generally, the approaches of stuttering therapy for adults mainly focus on the body function component of ICF through fluency shaping strategies and stuttering modification approaches. However, according to the ICF model, in addition to the traditional approaches of stuttering therapy, treatment should target all the components of the ICF framework in such a way that improvements in body functions (e.g. enhanced speech fluency) along with modifications of environmental factors (e.g. listener reactions) and improvements in their personal factors (e.g. self-esteem, confidence) would improve activity and participation (e.g. giving a public speech) (George & Bajaj, 2020).

Manning and DiLollo (2018) discussed the four basic principles to bring a positive change in clients with stuttering, which are as follows:

(1) *Move toward rather than away from the problem*: (approach – avoidance continuum). With various activities clients gradually become desensitized to the problem, learn to confront situations and take necessary action (Guitar, 2013).
(2) *Accept responsibility for their actions*: Clients should learn self-monitoring skills and practice speech techniques in all communication situations. Self-confidence develops at this stage which reinforces continued progress in speech (Hubble et al., 1999).
(3) *Cognitive restructuring of the self and the problem*: This refers to clients' desire to improve themselves and their circumstances in a constructive way (Plexico

DOI: 10.4324/9781003367673-7

et al., 2005). This helps them face difficult speaking situations confidently, leading to a better prognosis.

(4) *Take the support of others*: The clinician or a PWS who has succeeded in managing their stuttering can take the role of mentors. Also, involvement in support groups helps clients modify their speaking strategies and recognize indicators of successful change.

Treatment goals

Three primary objectives of therapy when working with a PWS, regardless of age, are (1) to increase their level of fluency, (2) to improve their ability to communicate and (3) to develop greater autonomy. Treatment goals for stuttering depend on the clinician's beliefs and the severity of stuttering. Additionally, PWS have a major role to play in selection of goals important to them. Their desire to achieve these therapeutic goals can be strengthened through ongoing conversations with the therapist (Guitar, 2013).

The American Speech, Language and Hearing Association (1995) has given explicit guidelines for practice in stuttering treatment. These are summarized in Figure 7.1.

The role of the therapist is to select appropriate goals for each PWS based on pre-therapy assessment (Chapter 5), select suitable approaches to achieve these goals, and review these goals through periodic measurement of treatment outcomes.

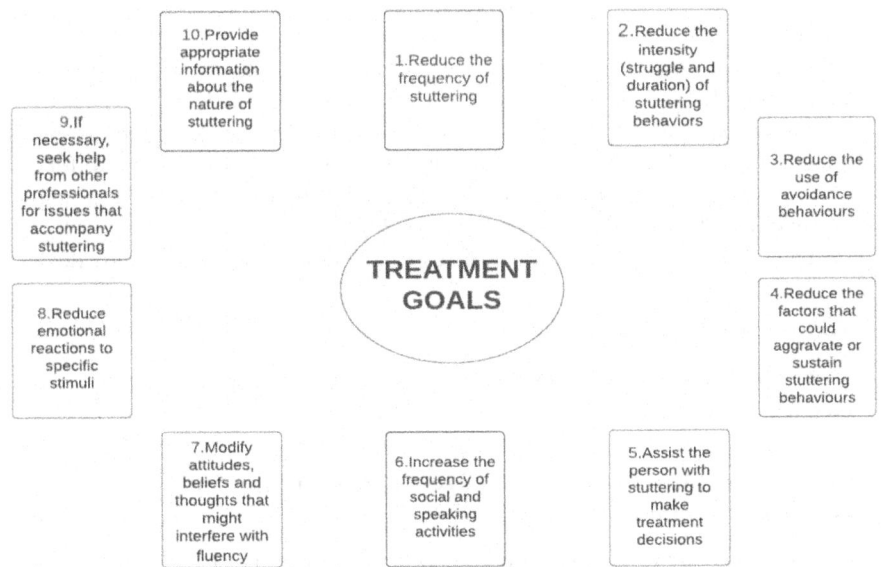

Figure 7.1 Various treatment goals in stuttering treatment

Case example

A male in his early 20s had graduated from a college and was looking for a job. His overt stuttering behaviours (body functions) were blocks (b3300), with intense physical tension (b3301) and occasional prolongations (b3300). He complained that he frequently ran out of breath (b4402) during stuttering moments, and there was slight change in pitch (b3101) when he attempted to speak with reduced breath support. Due to the intense muscle tension during stuttering moments, he perceived his own speech as monotonous and unnatural (b3303). He stuttered more frequently on words with vowels, stops, fricatives and affricates (b320) in the initial position of words. Disfluencies were accompanied by secondary behaviours such as eye blinking, tension around articulators, movement of upper extremities and torso (b3301).

Environmental and personal factors: He was very concerned about his stuttering. His family and friends were very supportive, had accepted his stuttering (e310, e320, e410, e355, e450, e580) and helped him attend speech therapy. However he got rejected in a recent job interview he had attended because the job demanded good interpersonal communication skills. This had severely affected his confidence as a speaker (d8450). Measurement of impact of stuttering using Overall Assessment of Speaker's Experience of Stuttering (OASES; Yaruss & Quesal, 2006) revealed that he had strongly negative affective, behavioural and cognitive reactions to stuttering. He often felt anxious before initiating conversations and angry, ashamed and embarrassed after a stuttering moment. He thought that he could have achieved his life goals more easily without stuttering. He did not have confidence in his abilities as a speaker.

Activities and participation: He had difficulty connecting with people in various social situations due the severity of his stuttering and his reaction to it. He had difficulty engaging in one-on-one conversation (d3503), especially with strangers and on the phone (d3600). He struggled with interpersonal relationships (d730, d750, d760), avoided shopping alone (d6200), had difficulty establishing new friendships (d7200) and avoided social gatherings such as weddings (d910) and sports activities (d920).

The following were the therapy goals in the context of ICF framework:

To improve body function:

Reduce the frequency and severity of disfluencies.
Reduce the tension and effort in communication.

To work on personal factors: (affective, behavioural and cognitive reactions)

Minimize his unpleasant emotional responses (e.g. anxiety, shame, frustration, guilt, and apprehension) to stuttering as well as to communication in general.
Increase self-confidence so that he starts enjoying communication.

Develop self-therapy, self-management and problem-solving skills.
Improve his ability to respond to others' questions about his stuttering.
Improve his ability to cope with teasing/bullying and other listener reactions.

To reduce activity limitations and participation restrictions:

Minimize the impact of stuttering on his ability to interact with others.
Introduce new behaviours to replace old ones
Generalize newly learnt behaviours to facilitate increased speech naturalness
and comfort across a range of communicative situations.

To work on environmental factors:

Bibliotherapy and information giving which could enable him to educate
persons in his environment, making them facilitators.

Treatment approaches

Therapy approaches may vary based on several variables such as the client's age,
severity of stuttering, therapeutic philosophy, treatment goals, and the desired duration and intensity of therapy sessions. Approaches for stuttering intervention can
broadly be classified into fluency shaping approaches and stuttering modification
approaches. According to Manning and DiLollo (2018), the essential difference
between fluency shaping and stuttering modification is the emphasis placed on the
surface and intrinsic features of the disorder by both the approaches. Fluency shaping approaches can be considered as physical therapy for systems involved in speech
production. The primary goal of these approaches is to modify how the speaker uses
respiratory, phonatory, and articulatory systems during speaking. Fluency shaping
assumes that once the person learns a new way to produce fluent speech, the cognitive and affective aspects of stuttering will gradually change.

Stuttering modification approaches, on the other hand, focus on modifying cognitive and affective aspects of stuttering. Unlike fluency shaping approaches, stuttering
modification approaches are less structured. This might make it difficult to have a uniform training module or uniform documentation procedures for these approaches.
It might also take a longer duration to achieve tangible outcomes with stuttering
modification approaches than with fluency shaping methods. The very nature of
these approaches makes it difficult to carry out outcomes research on their efficacy
in the form of large scale randomized controlled trials. However, available evidence
indicates that they have better long-term outcomes (Bernstein Ratner, 2005).

Fluency shaping strategies

The fluency shaping approach is based on two beliefs: First, that stuttering is triggered by stimuli in the environment and can be treated using principles of operant

conditioning. Second, motor control techniques can be used to achieve fluent speech, which can further be shaped into more natural sounding speech.

Fluency shaping usually starts with slow or rhythmic speech on to which other features, such as gentle voicing, are added. The resultant speech will be highly fluent, but might sound very unnatural. It is practised intensely, reinforced and progressively moulded to approximate a natural and typical prosaic pace. Once the client acquires the technique, the session progresses from basic speaking tasks to more challenging speaking situations. Several techniques and programmes have been described under fluency shaping, such as prolonged speech, light articulatory contacts, regulated breathing, flow and slow/passive airflow, Precision Fluency Shaping Program and Camperdown Program.

Prolonged speech

A popular fluency shaping approach, the rationale for prolonged speech (PS) is to modify the existing patterns of three systems, respiration, phonation and resonance, in an individual (Goldiamond, 1965). There is evidence that this brings about a reduction in stuttering. An additional advantage of the approach is a reduced rate of speech due to an increase in vowel duration (Ingham, 1984; Ingham & Andrews, 1973). Even though PS originally refers to the slowing of speech by prolonging vowels, prolonged speech also embraces gentle onset of words, light articulatory movements, smooth transition between sounds, and exaggerated continuity of speech. Some researchers also claim that prolongation serves as a distraction, thus leading to less anticipation of stuttering. It provides more time for the smooth movement of the articulators, enhances coarticulation, and reduces prosodic load (Briley, 2017; Onslow & Ingham, 1987; Packman et al., 2000). The PS treatment approach can be implemented in a programmed or non-programmed manner. Initially, the client is asked to speak at a very slow rate. The rate of prolongation is reduced in a graduated manner in such a way that syllable durations are systematically shortened in order for the speech to get faster. Finally, a controlled normal rate is achieved after having established fluent speech. A *controlled normal rate* is considered to be the rate at which a PWS can speak with reduced or no stuttering. It must be noted that the final rate varies for each individual, though usually a target of 180–200 syllables per minute is aimed at, since this is considered as the normal range (Ingham, 1987).

During *programmed* PS sessions, individuals are instructed to bring down their rate of speech by fixing syllables or words per minute, while the *non-programmed* version of the PS technique does not fix the rate of speech as a basic requirement, and features of prolongation are not delineated (Onslow et al., 1996). Individuals are instructed in a manner that they decrease their speech at a rate that they are comfortable with while maintaining 95% fluency at each level. The various steps of the programmed PS technique are provided in Table 7.1.

PS is the one of the most commonly used and researched techniques for behavioural management of stuttering, and several versions of the technique have emerged in the last few decades (Ingham, 1984; Shames & Florence, 1980). PS-based programmes may produce dramatic results, with subjects experiencing zero to near zero

Table 7.1 Steps to be followed while teaching prolonged speech

Step 1	Prolongation of the initial syllable of a word with a speech rate of around 60 syllables/minute. Speech rate will then be increased to 120 or 160 syllables/minute. It is recommended that individuals with severe stuttering should prolong all syllables in a word.
Step 2	Prolonging the initial syllable of the word only during a stuttering moment when anticipated to have stuttering, while being continuously monitored by the therapist.
Step 3	Same as Step 2; however, the client self-monitors the use of the technique.
Step 4	Generalization of the achieved fluency to speaking situations beyond the clinic. The therapist monitors the client's fluency and use of the technique when stuttering is anticipated.
Step 5	Generalization of fluency to daily speaking situations with less support from the therapist; the client self-monitors their fluency.
Step 6	Monthly follow-ups for six months after the termination of therapy; booster therapy if required.

stuttering instances. However, a major drawback of PS is that the PWS may stutter to some extent despite using the technique. Also, relapse is a common occurrence (Boberg & Kully, 1994a; Onslow et al., 1996). The relapse rate could be high if the rate of speech is not gradually shaped to normal sounding rate at the later stages of the establishment phase.

Light articulatory contacts

The first technique that is often used as a means to reduce muscular tension during speech production is known as light articulatory contacts (Boberg & Kully, 1994a). The rationale behind this technique is that PWS frequently produce consonants with hard articulatory contacts, leading to excessive tension in the articulators, which impedes airflow in the oral cavity. Teaching the client to produce loose articulatory movements helps to reduce articulatory tension and promotes continuity and ease of articulation. Light articulatory contacts are particularly relevant to the production of those consonants which involve complete closure of the vocal tract. The technique helps to prevent development of excessive pressure and tension in the articulators. The steps involved in teaching light articulatory contacts are as given in Table 7.2 below.

This technique is often combined with other fluency shaping techniques such as slow rate, easy onset phonation and continuous airflow blending to achieve better outcomes from therapy (Blomgren, 2010; Ingham, 1984).

Regulated breathing method

Regulated breathing (RB) is another behavioural technique that inhibits stuttering by modifying speech-related breathing patterns to patterns which are incompatible with stuttering (Azrin & Nunn, 1974). The rationale behind the technique is that stuttering is a habitual disorder of the initiation and maintenance of airflow and should be eliminated if the speech behaviours of the individual who stutters are

Table 7.2 Various steps involved in training using light articulatory contacts

Step 1	Teach the client the concept of soft movement of the articulators during articulation. For example, the clinician may ask, "How relaxed does the tongue feel?" and emphasize loose contacts between articulators, as well an uninterrupted airflow while saying a word.
Step 2	Ask the client to pull or stretch the first syllable of words spoken. Emphasize slow approximation of the articulators and prolonged vowel phonation.
Step 3	Teaching contrastive drills to help the client differentiate between hard and soft contacts of articulators. Emphasize kinaesthetic feedback (e.g. producing a word with hard and then again with soft contacts).

incompatible with these airflow anomalies. Teaching regulated breathing involves five stages. These are represented schematically in Figure 7.2. In order to complete these five stages, the PWS is progressively taken through approximately eight steps. These are summarized in Table 7.3 below.

Flow and slow method/modified airflow

The technique, also known as passive airflow, is based on the assumption that stuttering is due to excessive tensing of the vocal folds, called laryngospasm, which is precipitated by a variety of stressors. The feedback receptors within the vocal folds then trigger a learnt set of coping behaviours which are perceived as stuttering (Schwartz, 1976). To eliminate this malfunction, people who stutter are made to relax the vocal folds by maintaining passive airflow. The feedback signals that usually trigger stuttering in the brain are, therefore, curtailed, thus reducing the chances of stuttering. The passive airflow technique has essentially three components as given in Figure 7.3. Initially, the PWS is asked to begin a passive airflow followed by slowing down the first syllable of the utterance they produce. Such practice is then encouraged at increasing levels of linguistic complexity. It is finally generalized across different tasks and situations. The second phase consists of intense home training and group meetings once a week for a year.

Incorporation of passive airflow procedures into conversational speech during the initial phase of therapy demands a greater effort and considerable concentration. Once the technique is established, it may be possible to achieve a success rate of 89% after one week of intensive training. Also, the chances of relapse post one year after the treatment using passive airflow therapy are as low as 17% (Falkowski et al., 1982; Schwartz, 1976).

Precision Fluency Shaping Program

The Precision Fluency Shaping Program is developed based on the notion that articulatory and phonatory gestures are distorted in PWS and speech production requires reconstruction through intensive over learning of appropriate speech targets (Webster, 1980). Adhering to this concept, the goal of the programme is to learn specific phonatory and articulatory behaviours which increase the chances of fluent speech production. The programme revolves around establishing a very slow speech

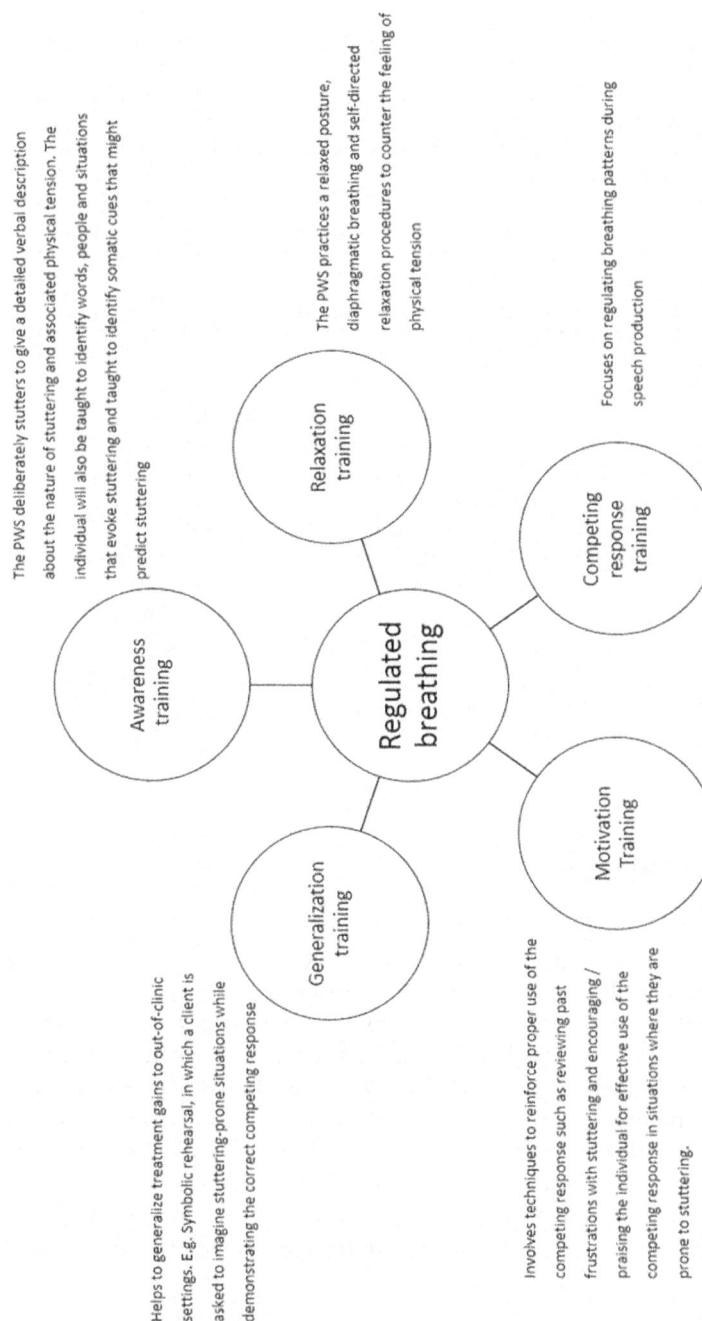

The PWS deliberately stutters to give a detailed verbal description about the nature of stuttering and associated physical tension. The individual will also be taught to identify words, people and situations that evoke stuttering and taught to identify somatic cues that might predict stuttering

The PWS practices a relaxed posture, diaphragmatic breathing and self-directed relaxation procedures to counter the feeling of physical tension

Focuses on regulating breathing patterns during speech production

Helps to generalize treatment gains to out-of-clinic settings. E.g. Symbolic rehearsal, in which a client is asked to imagine stuttering-prone situations while demonstrating the correct competing response

Involves techniques to reinforce proper use of the competing response such as reviewing past frustrations with stuttering and encouraging / praising the individual for effective use of the competing response in situations where they are prone to stuttering.

Awareness training

Relaxation training

Competing response training

Regulated breathing

Motivation Training

Generalization training

Figure 7.2 Stages of regulated breathing

Table 7.3 Steps involved in teaching regulated breathing to someone who stutters

Step 1	Bisyllabic words, prolonging the initial syllable with an audible /h/
Step 2	Words with more than two syllables, prolonging the initial syllable with an audible /h/
Step 3	Sentence production, prolonging the initial syllable with an audible /h/
Step 4	Bisyllabic words, prolonging the initial syllable with an inaudible /h/
Step 5	Words with more than two syllables, prolonging the initial syllable with an inaudible /h/
Step 6	Sentence production, prolonging the initial syllable with an inaudible /h/
Step 7	The client can use passive airflow during or before an approaching stuttering moment. Initially clinician monitored, gradually moving to self-monitored production.
Step 8	Generalization with and without the therapist's support.

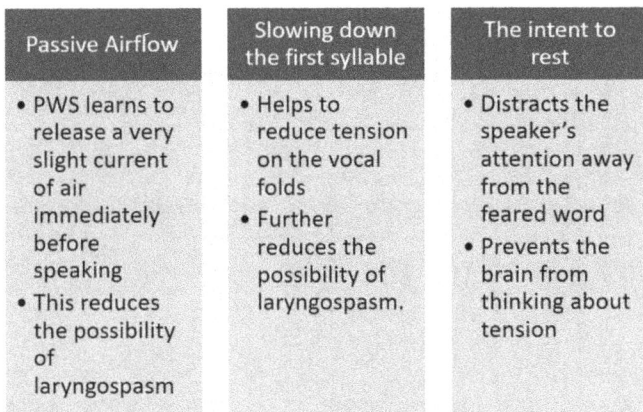

Figure 7.3 The airflow technique

rate. This is achieved by prolonging syllables up to two seconds. The client is then taught a range of skills, depending on the class of speech sounds being practised.

After establishing these skills, the previously taught targets will be practised on words of various syllable length, short, generated sentences and spontaneous speech. The daily practice routine consists of 10 to 20 periods, each period lasting for 20 minutes. The training progresses from one stage to the next after the client attains an accuracy of more than 84% on two successive 20 minute periods. The transfer of the skills achieved involves production of simple messages followed by double and multiple messages over telephone. This is followed by generalization of skills achieved to different communication settings along with intensive home training.

Camperdown Program

This programme involves behavioural treatment, and can be used with PWS who are 12 years of age older (Cocomazzo et al., 2012). The programme is intended to

Table 7.4 Stages of the Camperdown Program

Stage I: Teaching treatment components	The individual learns to use a fluency shaping technique and to use fluency self-rating scales such as Stuttering Severity Scale and the Fluency Technique Scale (O'Brian et al., 2003).
Stage II: Establishing natural sounding stutter-free speech with the clinician	The fluent, though unnatural sounding speech is gradually shaped into speech that sounds natural, while retaining the attained level of fluency.
Stage III: Generalization	The individual develops strategies for controlling their stuttering during everyday speech.
Stage IV: Maintaining stuttering control	The individual develops problem-solving skills for long-term maintenance of the fluency that they have achieved and for self-management of any increase in stuttering.

reduce stuttering in everyday speech. A fluency shaping technique suitable to the client is introduced in order to reduce disfluent episodes. The Camperdown Program lays a lot of emphasis on self-management and enables clients for a possible relapse post-treatment. It consists of four stages. These are summarized in Table 7.4.

One of the major advantages of the Camperdown Program is that it helps PWS to set realistic goals for themselves and to self-evaluate outcomes routinely. It trains PWS to evaluate their fluency in everyday speaking situations and alter the practice activities based on their performance, without the support of a clinician. By the end of the programme, the PWS gains the ability to self-evaluate their level of anxiety related to speaking. The programme also enables clients to identify any variables in their environment that might increase or reduce their disfluencies, and trains them to device strategies for gaining control over their stuttering in the long-term.

Stuttering modification techniques

These are also called traditional approaches or non-avoidance approaches. The major goal of these approaches is to decrease fear, avoidance and struggle that might accompany stuttering. This is achieved through a few steps where the client recognizes their stuttering, gets desensitized to the experience of stuttering, gradually learns new cognitive and behavioural responses to stuttering and changes their stuttering into an easy and smooth form, thereby replacing the old, complex stuttering to easy stuttering. Stuttering modification strategies require assistance from the clinician as well as an effort from the PWS.

Guitar (2013) discussed the suggestions to start therapy using stuttering modification techniques. A stuttering modification technique may be used if the client

1. hides or disguises stuttering,
2. avoids speaking or withdraws from speaking situations,
3. perceives personal punishments as an outcome of stuttering,
4. does not feel confident about himself as a communicator, and/or
5. displays a successful response towards stuttering modification trial therapy.

One of the most prominent and popular stuttering modification approaches was put forth by Van Riper (1982). This approach has six stages: Motivation, identification, desensitization, variation, modification/approximation and stabilization (MIDVAS). Details of each of these can be viewed in Table 7.5 below.

In the MIDVAS approach, the clinician's tasks revolve around how to help the speaker achieve the goals of increased fluency, better communication skills, and most importantly, a more assertive lifestyle. Together, the client and the clinician start the process of understanding and changing the behavioural and cognitive patterns that have dominated the person's communication choices for so long.

When using a stuttering modification approach, the clinician decides how to sequence and combine the various methods and techniques for changing behavioural features of the speech of the PWS by following the client's lead. These treatment approaches help reduce the limiting effects of stuttering, allowing PWS to improve their quality of life regardless of their extent of overt fluency.

Hybrid approaches

There is evidence that social, emotional, and cognitive factors interact with each other and contribute to persistence of stuttering. Intervention for stuttering must, therefore, address these in addition to speech production. Hybrid approaches facilitate such holistic intervention for stuttering through use of a combination of two or more approaches, such as fluency shaping, stuttering modification and/or alternative approaches (which will be discussed in the latter part of this chapter). Some of the hybrid approaches discussed in the literature are the Comprehensive Stuttering Program (CSP), the iGlebe cognitive behaviour therapy (CBT) programme and the Successful Stuttering Management Program (SSMP).

The Comprehensive Stuttering Program (CSP)

The Comprehensive Stuttering Program (CSP) (Boberg & Kully, 1985, 1994b; Kully et al., 2007) is an intervention programme for adolescents and adults that addresses overt stuttering and the attitudinal and emotional consequences of stuttering (Figure 7.4). To assist clients in reducing stuttering and managing persistent stuttering, the approach combines speech restructuring with stuttering modification strategies. Additionally, it employs techniques from cognitive behaviour therapy to assist individuals in reducing learnt avoidance, struggle, and anticipating behaviours and enhancing speech-related attitudes and confidence. This programme is delivered as group or individual therapy at the Institute for Stuttering Treatment and Research (ISTAR), University of Alberta, Canada (Langevin & Kully, 2012).

Langevin et al. (2010) investigated the five-year longitudinal treatment outcomes of the ISTAR Comprehensive Stuttering Program. Results of the study revealed that participants had maintained clinically and statistically substantial decreases in stuttering and increases in speech rates compared to pre-treatment assessments at the five-year follow-up. It was evident that speech improvements made by the end of the treatment programme remained stable over the five-year follow-up period

Table 7.5 The six stages of MIDVAS therapy

Stages	Goals	Description	Activities
Motivation	To motivate and prepare the client to be an active participant in the treatment process	• Clinicians guide and share information about the treatment process. • The clinician gets an idea of the client's expectations from therapy as a rapport is built between the client and the clinician, enabling them to work towards common goals.	1) The clinician shares positive information about stuttering. 2) The client shares feelings and emotions regarding the disorder.
Identification	To identify, analyze and confront the overt and covert cognitive attributes of stuttering	• Supports the client to understand their stuttering, the client has to take the lead. • By understanding the overt and covert features of stuttering, the client achieves his primary step to self-management.	The client can 1) Prepare a list of things that they do when they stutter to identify the overt features of stuttering and 2) Prepare a list of things that they do because of stuttering to identify the covert features of stuttering, such as avoidance behaviour, anxiety, fear, helplessness and the decisions that they take as a consequence of stuttering.
Desensitization	Desensitization to the overt and covert features of stuttering	• Introduction to voluntary stuttering, intentional stuttering or pseudo stuttering, where the client has to try stuttering on purpose.	1) The clinician models a few repetitions and prolongations for the client to imitate. 2) The PWS tries experimenting by adding the struggle that occurs during severe stuttering moments, such as airway blocks and voicing. 3) The PWS tries voluntary stuttering in various speaking situations in clinical and extra-clinical settings.
Variation	To alter the features of stuttering	• Altering the client's responses to stuttering or to listener reactions in a pre-planned or innovative manner. • The clinician can model or give suggestions regarding the change.	1) Self-observation, identifying typical cognitive or behavioural responses the PWS gives to a stuttering moment, and altering them (e.g. Going and waiting outside a hall full of people instead of completely avoiding the situation). 2) Varying responses to listener reactions (e.g. requesting the listener to be patient rather than trying to hurry through an utterance).

(Continued)

Table 7.5 (Continued)

Stages	Goals	Description	Activities
Modification/ Approximation	To alter the reflexive and out of control stuttering to an easy and smooth moment	• Cancellation – It is also called post-event modification as the client changes the features of stuttering after it occurs. The client pauses after a stuttered word, pantomimes his stuttering and analyses the evident physiological aspects of his stuttering. The client is then asked to combine the appropriate features required to produce the stuttered word in a smooth manner. • Pullout or para–event modification. The client will catch the disfluency as soon as it begins and use the appropriate combinations of features to utter the word smoothly. • Preparatory set or the pre–event modification. The client begins the word with a smooth form of stuttering, when that moment of stuttering is anticipated or pre–plans to modify the moment of stuttering.	Cancellation – Asking himself/herself questions like, "What are the articulatory postures that prevent me from producing the next sound or syllable"? Pullout – Improve the airflow and voicing or altering the vocal tract. Pullouts can also be facilitated through a technique called "freezing", which involves staying at the same articulatory posture at which the block occurred, till the muscles gradually relax. Preparatory set – Fluency modification techniques like regulated airflow, gradual onset of constant phonation and light articulatory contacts are essential for an easy preparatory set.
Stabilization	To transfer the new abilities from a clinic setting to daily life situations	• Increasing resilience in speaking situations. • The client continues improving their skills in monitoring and altering stuttering after terminating formal therapy sessions.	1) Taking part in stressful speaking situations 2) Learning various speaking strategies.

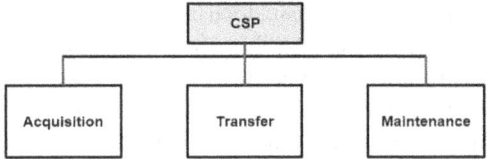

Figure 7.4 The Comprehensive Stuttering Program

because there were no significant changes between immediate post-treatment and follow-up assessments.

iGlebe CBT program

iGlebe is a specially designed cognitive behavior therapy (CBT) programme for adults with stuttering who experience social anxiety due to their stuttering. This programme is a self-directed standalone internet-based treatment developed by the Australian Stuttering Research Centre. It does not require the assistance of a speech pathologist or psychologist. The programme is customized for each individual with stuttering, and it covers seven modules which include an introduction to the programme, the negative thoughts the individual has about stuttering, a psycho-education component, the creation of a social anxiety disorder formulation by the user, behavioural experiments based on responses uploaded by the individual to repair the problematic self-focused attention, and maintenance and prevention of relapse (Menzies, Packman, et al., 2019). Several clinical trials have established that iGlebe is effective in treating social anxiety associated with stuttering in adults, and it is considered as a treatment that is cost-effective, feasible and a promising alternative to in-clinic CBT (Menzies et al., 2019; Helgadóttir et al., 2014).

Successful Stuttering Management Program (SSMP)

The Successful Stuttering Management Program is an integrated approach developed by Breitenfeldt and Lorenz (1989) with an aim to promote acceptance of stuttering, reduce fear and avoidance of stuttering, and reduce the effort that accompanies stuttered speech. The SSMP was developed to provide group intervention for both adolescents and adults who stutter; however, the programme can be adapted to provide individual intervention for stuttering. It has its roots in stuttering modification techniques, but it also incorporates fundamental components of CBT to recognize and address anxiety-inducing beliefs. The Successful Stuttering Management Program consists of three phases: (i) confrontation of stuttering, (ii) modification of stuttering, and (iii) maintenance (Blomgren, 2012).

The confrontation phase which lasts for approximately two weeks is the main component of SSMP. Its aim is to modify attitudes and beliefs of the PWS about stuttering. Desensitization and CBT exercises are used to change attitudes and perception of the PWS. The second phase of SSMP lasts for three days and involves learning specific stuttering modification techniques to reduce the severity of stuttering moments. The third, maintenance phase, focuses on establishing a maintenance plan and motivating the PWS to generalize the newly learnt cognitive and behavioural patterns to situations outside the clinic. Clients are encouraged to join a support group for PWS after discharge from intervention. The major advantage of SSMP is that the programme targets stigma associated with stuttering and encourages self-acceptance through thoughts such as "It is OK to stutter". The major drawback of the programme is that it focuses on modifying stuttering rather than a reduction in stuttering moments, as fluency enhancement is not a goal of the programme.

Group therapy

One of the earliest applications of group treatment in the field of communication disorders was the use of speech in social situations beyond the usual speech production drills (Backus, 1957). According to Luterman (1991), there are two types of groups: Therapy groups and counselling groups. Group therapy for clients with fluency disorders usually serves both purposes, counselling as well as therapy. Group therapy must ideally be used in conjunction with individual therapy. However, in some cases it might be the only service available due to time and cost constraints, especially when the client to clinician ratio is low (Manning & DiLollo, 2018). A group setting allows for bringing about a change in both overt and covert aspects of the disorder and facilitating its maintenance and generalization. Some activities that are possible in a group are a natural extension of an individual treatment session; others encourage application of learnt skills and divergent thinking as members have the opportunity to observe how others have dealt with similar problems (Levy, 1983). The characteristics of group therapy for stuttering are given in Table 7.6 below.

Table 7.6 Characteristics of a typical group session for stuttering intervention

Group characteristics	*Rationale*
Group size should be around seven members with a range of six to ten (Conture, 2001; Van Riper, 1990)	• The size of the group should be small enough that members have the opportunity to get to know and trust one another • Smaller groups of fewer than five participants limit the sense of being in a group and increased speaking demand on the participants • More than ten participants could limit potential participation.
A reasonable time distribution of group members' participation should be announced.	• It is important to avoid situations in which one member dominates the discussion by taking too much talking time.
Clinicians can assume an active or passive role or both.	• The clinician selecting a theme and playing an active role in directing the interaction ensures that quiet members also contribute equally. • The clinician taking a passive role in the group session lets members lead the session and facilitates a free-flowing exchange of thoughts and ideas, leading to an increased camaraderie between group members.

According to St Louis (2006), a typical group therapy session should feature a theme and a lesson, should include something fun, and should involve some real experiences for the participants, not just ideas. Participants in the group can be engaged in specific activities such as relaxation-imagery exercises, which involve progressively relaxing the skeletal muscles. Role-play such as ordering food in a restaurant, public speaking, attending interviews and the like, can be useful in helping the speaker reconsider negative experiences associated with past fluency failure and experiment with various coping responses for future anxiety-provoking situations. Observers can analyze interpersonal aspects of the situation and offer constructive feedback and alternative ways of responding to the situation. Other than preparing participants to deal with anxiety involved in public speaking, group therapy also encompasses basic communications skills such as maintaining eye contact with members of the group, organization and sequencing of ideas, and maintaining an appropriate rate and timing of speech.

Alternative approaches for the treatment of stuttering

Alternative approaches for stuttering treatment work under the premise that stuttering occurs as a result of faulty auditory processing or defective neural processes underlying linguistic function, or psychological distress rather than a faulty speech production mechanism. In contrast to fluency shaping, stuttering modification, or hybrid approaches which are based on interaction between a qualified speech-language pathologist (SLP) and individuals who stutter, alternative approaches rely on feedback-altering devices or psychological and pharmacological intervention methods which require minimal or no input from an SLP.

Cognitive behaviour therapy

Cognitive behaviour therapy (CBT), as the name suggests, uses cognitive and behavioural methods to enable individuals to cope with unfavourable external circumstances. The unhelpful thoughts and distressing feelings that arise as a result of such circumstances might adversely affect persons who stutter. For instance, many individuals who stutter might be afraid of other people judging their speech fluency in social and/or occupational situations. Providing treatment for stuttering in adults using solely speech restructuring programmes could lead to psychosocial aspects of stuttering, such as anxiety, frustration, negative attitudes towards speaking situations, social anxiety and phobia in these individuals not getting addressed. This might serve as a barrier to long-term improvement (Menzies et al., 2009; Cream et al., 2003; Messenger et al., 2004). CBT helps PWS modify their patterns of thought and behaviour to constructively cope with difficult or challenging speaking situations.

A CBT programme specially designed for PWS by Menzies et al. (2008) focuses on reducing the anxiety related to speaking and the duration of treatment usually lasts for 15 hours. The programme includes procedures from three domains of CBT such as cognitive restructuring, graded exposure, and behavioural experiments. During cognitive restructuring, a PWS is trained to identify unhelpful thoughts that might create speech-related anxiety. Gradual exposure involves individuals gradually confronting anxiety-provoking circumstances and repeating that exposure until anxiety levels are no longer considered overly unpleasant. Behavioural experiments are carried out in conjunction with graded exposure and are aimed to assess the negative outcomes expected by participants and compare them with the actual outcomes of the exposure exercises. Providing CBT for PWS combined with speech restructuring has been clinically proven to have a significant influence on the individuals' capacity to engage in everyday speaking tasks with less psychological distress, anxiety and avoidance.

Rational emotive behavioural therapy for stuttering

One of the original forms of CBT is Rational Emotive Behavioural Therapy (REBT) developed by Albert Ellis (1974), a psychologist. This is a form of psychotherapy and a principle of life that can be applied well to stuttering treatment along with the other treatments, such as stuttering modification and avoidance reduction approaches. REBT is based on the fundamental principle that our emotions are not a direct result of the things that happen to us. Instead, it is the belief we have about these things that make us upset and worried (Dryden & Branch, 2008). Individuals with stuttering tend to lay a lot of value on fluency, and consequently develop the fear of speaking which further worsens their struggles and avoidance behaviour. REBT works towards helping individuals with stuttering to restructure their beliefs by identifying and modifying the irrational beliefs and negative thoughts in order to enable them to accept themselves the way they are regardless of their stutter (Neiders, 2011; Neiders & Ross, 2013).

Altered feedback therapies

Altered feedback systems that provide delayed auditory feedback (DAF) and frequency altered feedback (FAF) act as artificial exogenous speech signals and thus enhance fluency. In addition, these devices mask the speaker's speech signal as a result of which fluency typically improves.

Delayed auditory feedback

Delayed auditory feedback (DAF) implies that individuals hear their own speech with a pre-defined time delay. It has been used for intervention since the 1960s (Goldiamond, 1965; Perkins, 1973; Ryan & Van Kirk, 1974; Shames & Florence, 1980). In conventional therapy, a DAF time delay is introduced at an optimal setting that induces fluent speech, and then gradually reduced to a zero delay. The DAF is then faded out steadily as the individual learns to maintain fluency outside the clinic and without the aid of DAF. DAF also helps the PWS focus on more stable proprioceptive feedback while ignoring auditory feedback systems that may be presumed to be faulty in those who stutter (Guitar, 2013).

The procedure requires the user to first set a delay time on the device. The time delay is set to either 50 or 75 milliseconds, with a maximum delay up to 220 milliseconds (Antipova et al., 2008). Van Borsel, Reunes, et al. (2003) who tested the effect of DAF on nine adults who stutter found that DAF reduced the number of stuttered words significantly across different speaking situations such as face-to-face and telephonic conversation, monologue, and oral reading. Although DAF consistently reduces stuttering for most speakers across these situations, the effects of feedback do not eliminate stuttering. Although there is evidence that DAF provides increased levels of fluency even under no auditory feedback conditions; the major question of whether DAF continues to work in the long-term remains unanswered (Van Borsel, Reunes, et al., 2003).

Frequency altered feedback

Frequency altered feedback (FAF) involves giving the PWS the feedback of their own speech output with a shift in pitch. Similar to DAF, FAF replicates the effect of having another speaker at the same time (Armson & Stuart, 1998; Rastatter et al., 1998; Stuart et al., 1996). In FAF, instead of altering the feedback timing of the speech signal, the pitch of the feedback altered to varying notes is used to enhance speech fluency. As with DAF, the extent of change in signal needed for FAF to be effective varies from person to person (Ward, 2006). Obtaining optimum results using an FAF device is usually through trial and error. A study that explored the effectiveness of FAF revealed that the condition demonstrated a reduction in stuttering only in 50% of a group of PWS. In contrast all of the participants showed a reduction in stuttering under DAF (Natke, 2000). However, FAF has been found to be more effective when used together with DAF, with a reported efficacy of up to 80% on clinical trials (Zimmerman et al., 1997).

A study by Stuart et al. (1997) on the effect of monaural and binaural alterations in DAF and FAF among adults with stuttering revealed a 60% to 75% reduction in the frequency of stuttering as compared to the non-altered feedback condition, with a greater decrease in stuttering frequency in the binaural as compared to the monaural AAF condition. Andrade and Juste (2011) conducted a systematic review of the efficacy of DAF in adults with stuttering by collecting data from various resources, such as research articles, letters to the editor, case studies, studies on fluent speakers as well as persons with neurogenic stuttering. Interestingly, in contrast to the findings of the earlier studies, the systematic review indicated that effectiveness of AAF devices in reducing the frequency of stuttering is not yet well established as the results of most of the studies in the review were found to be inconclusive.

Computerized feedback devices

Computerized feedback devices are different from altered feedback. They use computer technology that helps PWS improve the regulation of the physiological aspects underlying speech generation. They provide feedback on the control of respiratory and phonatory functions. They are particularly useful for implementation of techniques for fluency enhancement, such as soft glottal onsets and soft articulatory contacts for consonants that require precise coordination between breathing and phonation. For instance, a computerized feedback device might monitor vocal intensity through a microphone, thus providing feedback in the use of a gentle voice onset. Feedback devices such as Dr. Fluency differentiate diaphragmatic breathing from clavicular breathing and give information about patterns of exhalation, such as gradual exhalation, pre-voice exhalation, uncontrolled exhalation or attempting to speak on residual air. By providing accurate visual feedback regarding the physiological aspects of speech, these devices free the clinician to concentrate on treating the attitudinal, affective and cognitive aspects of stuttering (Keyhoe, 1998).

App-based intervention for stuttering

The advent of apps which can run on computers or smartphones has increased the feasibility of self-therapy for stuttering. These apps can also serve as adjuncts to therapy when frequent follow-ups might not be possible, or when the client is in the generalization and maintenance phases of therapy. Some of the popular apps are described below.

FluencyCoach

FluencyCoach is a free software application that simulates the effects of "Choral Speech" using altered auditory feedback (AAF) technology (speaking simultaneously with another person). FluencyCoach provides either delayed (DAF) or frequency altered (FAF) feedback. DAF offered by FluencyCoach ranges from 25 to 225 milliseconds with increments of 10 milliseconds, allowing the client to gradually transition from slow speech targets to a normal speech rate. The FAF provided by the application ranges from one-half octave below to one-half octave above the actual pitch. The FAF functionality is useful to improve fluency without affecting the naturalness of speech. The application also provides additional recording and playback functionality for self-evaluation purposes in order to identify particular words, syllables or sounds on which the person stutters consistently.

Speech4Good

The Speech4Good stuttering and speech therapy with DAF app is developed for iPhone operating system devices and offers delayed auditory feedback (DAF) at adjustable levels 20–300ms. The application also provides additional features such as a visual dashboard which helps the PWS practice, view speech graph (oscilloscope) displays in real-time, add notes, or record and playback speech samples. The custom-built library which is a part of the app helps saving and organizing files as well.

Stamurai

Stamurai is a mobile app developed in India to help learn and practice speech therapy for those who struggle with stuttering. Its co-founders Anshul Agarwal, Meet Singhal and Harsh Tyagi are IIT-Delhi graduates with the vision to make speech therapy affordable and accessible for individuals who stutter. Stamurai offers features such as video tutorials on understanding stuttering and its causes, cancellations, preparatory sets, and voluntary stuttering. The app also provides self tutorials on fluency shaping techniques such as light contacts, proprioception, easy onset, pausing, and speech rate modification. Additional features offered by Stamurai include breathing and relaxation practice; practicing feared sounds in isolation; daily self-assessment of speech fluency, meditation packages that improve confidence and focus and help identify anxiety, fear, muscle tension and a negative self-image; daily support groups (including a support group exclusively for Hindi speakers); group video calls and practice sessions; and individual stuttering therapy by a trained speech-language pathologist. The app is currently in use in over 150 countries by more than 50,000 people.

Drug therapy

It is postulated that people stutter due to increased dopamine levels and decreased activity of the striatum. Dopamine blocking drugs such as olanzapine and risperidone have demonstrated some reduction in core behaviours and secondary behaviours. Some studies suggest that this category of drugs can lead to increased activity of the striatum and a reduction in stuttering behaviour by about 40% to 60% (Wu et al., 1997; Maguire et al., 2020). Another group of drugs includes serotonin-specific reuptake inhibitors which are commonly used in the treatment of obsessive-compulsive disorders and depression. There is evidence that these medicines can induce stuttering in persons who do not stutter. However, mixed findings have been seen among some people who stutter (Brady, 1998). When found effective, these drugs significantly reduce the severity of moments of stuttering and increase the percentage of fluent speaking time, together with a significant decrease in speech-related anxiety.

Among all the categories of drugs with which clinical trials were conducted to reduce stuttering behaviours, dopamine blocking medications were found to be most effective (Maguire et al., 2000). However, adaptation to these drugs over a certain period of time and the damaging effects of these drugs on the nervous system such as tardive dyskinesia, prolactin elevation, sexual dysfunction, and dysphoria in the long-term are issues that still need resolution.

Botox therapy

Botox treatment could be administered to those PWS who experience laryngeal spasms as the core feature of their stuttering. Attempts have also been made to use Botox to control tremors of the articulators and unnecessary movements of lips. However, the outcomes of treatment of stuttering using Botox are not unambiguously positive. In this treatment, Botox is injected into the thyroarytenoid muscles of the larynx on both sides (Brin et al., 1994) in order to reduce the laryngospasm and thereby increase fluency. Its effectiveness varies across individuals, and the procedure needs to be repeated every few months to maintain any effect. The reported outcomes are an increase in speech rate due to reduction in laryngeal blocks and a decrease in frequency of stuttering. However, benefits of the Botox treatment do not overweigh its drawbacks such as the need to undergo painful injections repeatedly on an ongoing basis, a resultant breathy voice and occasionally a lower pitch (Ward, 2006).

Issues of speech naturalness in stuttering

It has been noticed that treatment techniques targeting speech fluency might result in outcomes affecting the speech naturalness of those who stutter (Novelli, 2018). Although speech naturalness can improve with stuttering treatment, it may not necessarily be perceived as normal (Martin et al., 1984; Hausman, 2019). In a study by Onslow et al. (1992), the speech of persons who had very severe stuttering prior to treatment was perceived as unnatural after treatment compared to those who had less severe stuttering. The aim of stuttering treatment in adults should not be limited to reducing the core behaviours of stuttering, but should also focus on the speech naturalness in order to maintain the quality of the post-therapy speech (Franken et al., 1995).

In addition, the modality of the speech sample assessed (Martin & Haroldson, 1992), the length of the speech sample (Onslow et al., 1992), stuttering frequency and pause duration may also influence speech naturalness ratings (Hausman, 2019). In addition, Teshima et al. (2010) reported that speech was rated to be more natural after five years post-treatment as compared to ratings given immediately after treatment.

Research has demonstrated that regular feedback through the use of speech naturalness ratings facilitates an improvement in the speech naturalness of stutter-free and spontaneously fluent speech (Ingham et al., 2001; Novelli, 2018). Such feedback can be given either through ratings by the clinician or through self-ratings by the client. The clinician can also provide a model to the client on appropriate prosodic features that need to be applied along with stutter-free speech (Ingham & Onslow, 1985; Ingham et al., 2001).

Relapse of stuttering

Most adults who stutter remain with residual stuttering related behaviours even after treatment, and it is unlikely that there will be no stuttering. Various authors have identified relapse as a regular event following treatment for adults with stuttering (Bloodstein & Bernstein Ratner, 2008; Craig, 1998; Kuhr & Rustin, 1985; Perkins et al., 1979; Silverman, 1981; Van Riper, 1990). Martin and Haroldson (1981) reported an estimated relapse at around 30% while Craig and Hancock (1995) found that 71.7% of 152 adults experienced relapse, although a majority of them regained their fluency subsequently.

Yairi and Ambrose (2005) in their longitudinal studies, have supported the assertion that genetic elements contribute to stuttering persistence and recovery (Sheehan & Martyn, 1966). Some adults with stuttering are genetically predisposed to relapse of stuttering (Cooper, 1972; Neaves, 1970). The presence of overt stuttering could serve as a measure of relapse. Relapse criteria of 2% syllables stuttered (SS) (Craig et al., 1984; Evesham & Fransella, 1985) or 4% SS (Boberg, 1981) may be applied, according to some researchers. For example, after therapy is terminated, if a PWS reports to the clinic with a gradual increase in the number of stuttering moments and assessment reveals the % SS to be greater than 4%, it can be considered as relapse of stuttering.

There are various factors such as changes in the attitudinal and cognitive variables, often in the form of negative self-talk, which can trigger a relapse. For example, Craig and Hancock (1995) reported that PWS with increased levels of trait anxiety were three times more likely to experience a relapse. Geetha (2007) discussed 20 factors that might influence a relapse of stuttering (Figure 7.5).

Relapse can range from short periods to long episodes. It can range from mildly interfering episodes to episodes that are vastly handicapping. Based on affective, behavioural and cognitive aspects of the problem, a clinician should be able to identify the threshold of relapse for each PWS. However, PWS themselves are the best persons to determine the presence and degree of relapse. When, for instance, a PWS is no longer confident in managing their own speech and when their decisions are based on the possibility of stuttering, it is essential to seek professional help for the relapse of stuttering.

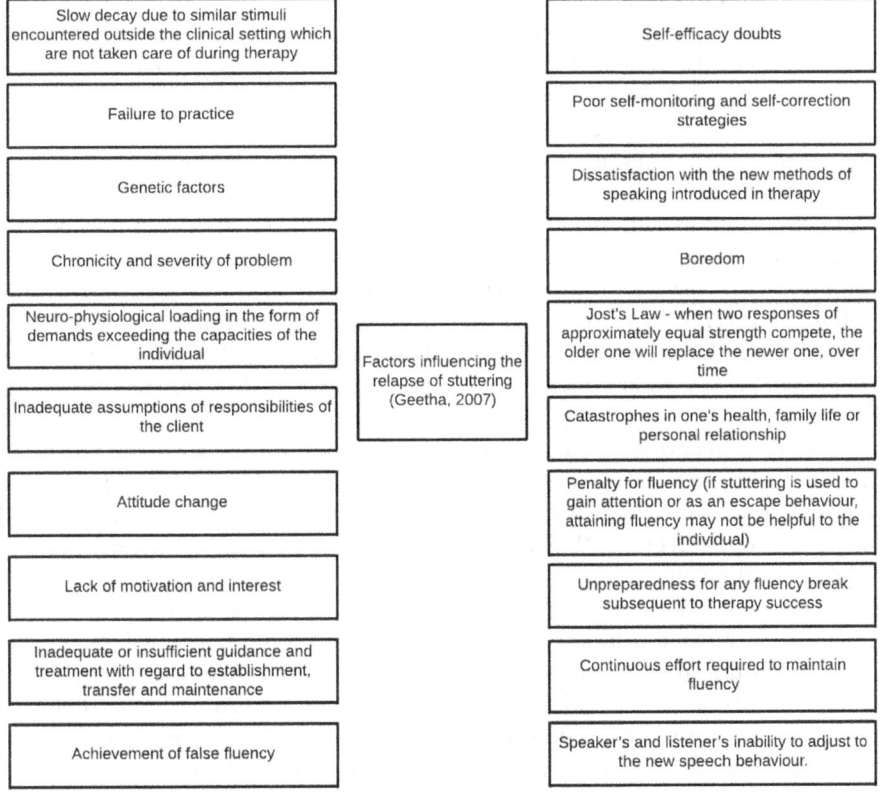

Figure 7.5 Factors influencing relapse

According to Van Riper (1990), relapses and remissions on a regular basis can be observed among a majority of adults who stutter if long-term follow-up investigations are conducted, and these are not exceptional cases. For all clients, a follow-up in some form is mandatory. Literature suggests that regular follow-ups for at least two to five years are essential following formal treatment for adults who stutter (Bloodstein & Bernstein Ratner, 2008; Conture & Guitar, 1993)

An option of continuing therapy for stuttering in some form is necessary for as long as clients feel the need for professional support. Coming back to the clinic for follow-ups should not be viewed as an indication of failure by the clinician or the client. In fact, successfully managing stuttering should be viewed as a long-term process. It should be considered as a natural part of the process of change. However, most PWS do not require intensive individual sessions for relapse. Group sessions or support group meetings occasionally can help them reacquire their fluency skills and maintain continued progress.

Recovery from stuttering

Stuttering reportedly affects between 5% (Mansson, 2000) and 11% (Reilly et al., 2013) of preschool-aged children. However, the prevalence of stuttering in school-going children has been estimated to be around 1.3% to 1.4% (Craig & Tran, 2005; Craig et al., 2002). Stuttering persists into adulthood for about 0.2% of females and 0.8% of males (Bloodstein & Bernstein Ratner, 2008; Craig & Tran, 2005). This reduction in the occurrence of stuttering is related to its recovery rate.

In 70% to 80% of children before puberty, a significant reduction or disappearance of stuttering symptoms occurs naturally without known triggers or without any clinical intervention. Yairi and Ambrose (1999) reported that 75% to 80% of young children with stuttering recover spontaneously. Girls have been seen to recover at a higher rate than boys. If spontaneous recovery is seen in a child, it is usually seen within the first few years after onset, and at the most by 7 years of age (Mansson, 2000). However, recovery may occur in adolescence or adulthood in some instances (Finn, 2004; Martyn & Sheehan, 1968; Neumann et al., 2019). Recovery figures might vary across studies due to variations in criteria used by different researchers (Table 7.7).

The term "recovery" can be interpreted as (a) a positive change in their speech or (b) learning to live with the disorder (Anderson & Felsenfeld, 2003). Spontaneous recovery from stuttering before or after puberty has also been called "non-assisted" or "unassisted" recovery (Ingham, 1984; Ingham et al., 2005), "self-recovery" (Shearer & Williams, 1965) or "spontaneous late recovery" (Neumann et al., 2019), although it could be a result of a former treatment or self-management.

Recovery rate is usually assessed using behavioural measures such as frequency and severity of stuttering behaviours observed or experienced. Arya and Geetha (2013) studied factors associated with recovery and relapse of stuttering in adults following treatment and reported that domains contributing to the treatment outcomes were individual-related, therapy-related, environment-related, behaviour-related and personality-related factors.

Table 7.7 Criteria to assess the recovery of stuttering

Authors	Criteria to assess recovery
Bloodstein & Bernstein Ratner (2008); Chang et al. (2018); Yairi and Ambrose (1999).	The percentage of stuttering-like disfluencies should be less than 3%.
Iverach, O'Brian, et al. (2009)	The core behaviours or overt symptoms of stuttering, as well as covert symptoms in the form of negative emotions or avoidance of speaking situations, should not be present in the speech of a person with stuttering.
Finn (1997)	The speech of a PWS should be no different from that of a person without stuttering, and the fluent speech should not be restricted to any familiar speaking situations.
Yairi and Ambrose (1999)	Fluent speech should persist for at least 12 months.
Wingate (1964a)	Recovery was attributed to a change in attitudes towards stuttering and was indicated by acceptance, desensitization, or an increasing awareness of their own capabilities in the PWS.
Finn (1996)	Improved motivation, self-confidence, and self-awareness, and speech management strategies were common elements that helped those people who consider themselves as recovered from stuttering.

Webster (1998) asserted that systematic use of stuttering modification or fluency shaping techniques bring speech motor control processes under voluntary control and the activation of the brain is focused more on the motor systems in the left hemisphere, particularly the supplementary motor areas. Additionally, the use of cognitive or behavioural techniques brings emotional reactions such as fear under control, consequently controlling right hemisphere activation. Fluency skills become more involuntary and require less focus as clients practice these skills and become more proficient in all speaking situations. The altered state of the brain would also become automatic as the fluency skills are maintained.

Evidence-based practice in stuttering treatment

The term evidence-based practice (EBP) is defined as "the explicit and unbiased use of current best research in making clinical and health policy decisions" (Sackett et al., 1996; p. 71). EBP allows clinicians to offer the best possible research-based, customized treatment (Schlosser & Raghavendra, 2004). This entire process can be summarized in a framework of three key elements, namely, external scientific evidence, clinical expertise and client/patient/caregiver perspective. The implementation of EBP involves five steps (Bothe, 2004) as depicted in Figure 7.6 below.

In stuttering treatment research, meta-analyses, systematic reviews and randomized controlled trials are considered as good quality evidence (Bothe, 2004). However, very few studies in the realm of stuttering are randomized controlled trials (RCTs). Nonetheless, literature reviews related to stuttering intervention since the 1980s point to many aspects of stuttering treatment which tend to be beneficial for

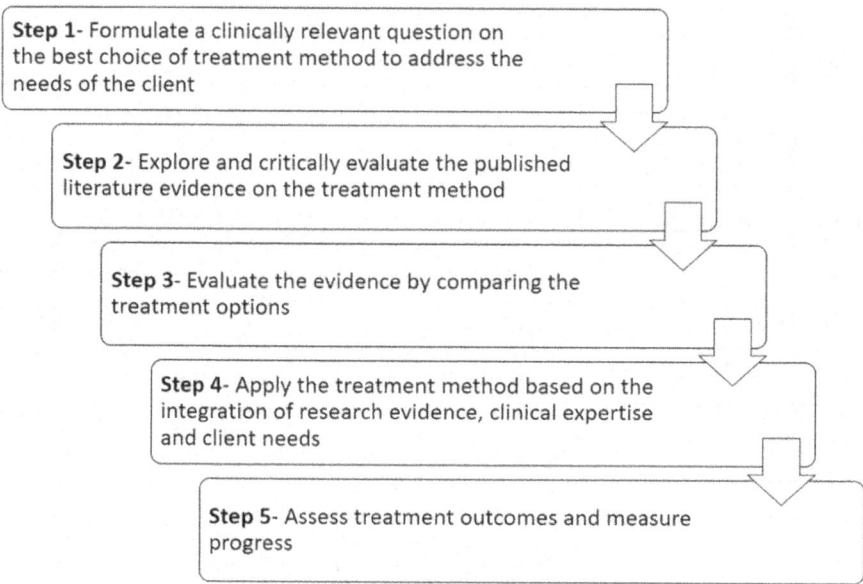

Figure 7.6 The five steps in evidence-based practice

achieving positive treatment outcomes. Providing at least 100 hours of treatment specifically for adults with stuttering, structured and planned transfer of fluency skills, reporting data on maintenance or long-term follow-up, beginning therapy with the use of shorter utterances, modifying phonatory and respiratory control, and most importantly, the use of prolonged speech, have been demonstrated as effective for the reduction of stuttering behaviour (Andrews et al., 1980; Ingham & Cordes, 1998; Ingham, 2003). Prolonged speech is also reported to be effective in the cross-linguistic generalization of the gained fluency to languages which are untreated among bilingual adults with stuttering (Priyanka & Maruthy, 2019).

Recently, Brignell et al. (2020) conducted a systematic review of stuttering treatment for adults. Electronic databases and clinical trials were searched, from which the researchers reviewed five RCTs, four clinical trials and three systematic reviews. Speech restructuring or fluency shaping techniques such as the Camperdown Program were found to be effective treatment methods since on average, they could reduce stuttering frequency by 50 to 57%. In addition, there is also evidence of the benefits of intervention using modified phonation intervals in adults who stutter (Ingham et al., 2015).

Multiple studies have shown evidence of the efficacy of combined approaches, such as the Comprehensive Stuttering Program (Langevin et al., 2010; Langevin & Boberg, 1996; Boberg & Kully, 1994a). These are based on the ICF framework given by the World Health Organization (WHO, 2001).

It is important to put together the most relevant research evidence in order to facilitate the best possible evidence-based decisions in the treatment of stuttering in adults.

It is essential that the clinician and client together identify the desirable outcomes and use evidence-based treatment methods which demonstrate these outcomes.

It is evident from this chapter that there is a wide variety of approaches and their combinations available for intervention of stuttering in the adult population. Beginning clinicians might either make the mistake of adhering to a single approach that they think works or feel lost among the multiple approaches. The solution we would like to offer them is to stay abreast of current evidence related to stuttering intervention in adults, view this information in the light of each patient's profile to shortlist approaches that they feel would help that particular PWS, and finally, include the PWS as an active contributor to therapy-related decisions. Such careful and individualized decision-making before implementation of intervention could certainly bring about a positive change in the lives of those who stutter.

Summary points to remember

- The three objectives of stuttering therapy are to increase the level of fluency, improve the communication ability and develop greater autonomy.
- Fluency shaping approaches modify the way a speaker uses the various systems involved in speech production, resulting in stutter-free speech.
- Stuttering modification approaches focus on desensitizing the individual to their stuttering and to external variables that might serve as barriers and addresses the struggle, fear, and avoidance during stuttering moments.
- Group therapy helps the individual achieve maintenance and generalization of fluency to various speaking situations.
- Alternative approaches for stuttering therapy use instruments such as DAF and FAF, psychological approaches, various computer-based programmes and pharmacological drugs to improve speech fluency.
- Improving speech naturalness should be one of the goals in fluency therapy. This is because stuttering behaviours as well as techniques used to improve fluency result in compromising the naturalness of a person's speech.
- Chances of relapse after the treatment ranges from 30% to 71.7% as indicated by various studies.
- Recovery from stuttering without treatment depends on many factors such as a genetic predisposition to stutter, age and gender of the individual, etc.

Study questions

1. Write a short note on voluntary stuttering.
2. How can we treat laryngospasm in adults who stutter?
3. Describe any two evidence-based treatments for adults with stuttering.
4. Explain relapse and recovery of stuttering in adults.
5. What are the various alternative approaches to stuttering therapy?

8 Acquired neurogenic stuttering

Rakesh Chowkalli Veerabhadrappa
and Santosh Maruthy

Introduction

As discussed in Chapter 3, stuttering can broadly be classified into two types – developmental and acquired stuttering (non-developmental). Unlike developmental stuttering, which is more commonly seen in children, acquired forms of stuttering are more commonly seen in adulthood. Among the two types of acquired stuttering, psychogenic stuttering results from emotionally distressing events. The other type of acquired stuttering, acquired neurogenic stuttering (ANS), is caused by an insult or injury to the nervous system in the form of a stroke, traumatic brain injury, encephalitis, drug abuse, etc. Guitar (2019) defines ANS as "stuttering that appears to be caused or exacerbated by neurological disease or damage". In contrast to developmental stuttering, where stuttering is the first and only/predominant presenting feature, ANS is relatively less discussed, probably because the underlying neurological condition overwhelms the patient and caretakers in most instances. Also, there is relatively limited research data available on acquired forms of stuttering compared to developmental stuttering. However, stuttering due to neurological trauma forms the largest sub-group among the different types of acquired stuttering.

Apart from the term ANS, a few authors use the term "neurogenic disfluency" as they don't consider acquired neurogenic stuttering as a true form of stuttering. However, the usage of such a phrase might create some confusion between two different phenomena that might occur with neurological damage: A speech disorder presenting as stuttering-like disfluencies (blocks, single-syllable repetitions, and prolongations) along with avoidance, struggle, tension, and escape behaviours; and an increase in typical disfluencies (revisions, pauses, interjections, whole-word, and phrase repetitions) followed by a neurological insult. ANS is also known as *stuttering associated with acquired neurological damage* (SAAND). The term was coined by Helm-Estabrooks (1999). Other terms for ANS include neurological stuttering, stuttering of sudden onset, cortical stuttering (Rosenbek et al., 1978), organic stuttering (Van Riper, 1982), and neurogenic acquired stuttering (Guitar, 2019). Nonetheless, ANS and SAAND are the two most commonly used terminologies in research and clinical setup. Due to its simplicity and frequent usage in speech-language pathology, we prefer using the term ANS coined by Canter (1971) in this chapter over SAAND. This chapter discusses possible etiologies, types of ANS, the speech characteristics of ANS, evaluation and

DOI: 10.4324/9781003367673-8

differential diagnosis of ANS from other fluency disorders and treatment approaches for the reduction of symptoms of ANS.

The most common causes of ANS include cerebrovascular accident (CVA)/ stroke, traumatic brain injury, drug abuse and misuse, and degenerative diseases such as progressive supranuclear palsy, Alzheimer's disease, Parkinson's disease, and tumours (Helm-Estabrooks, 1999). In rare instances, uncontrollable seizures, cryo-surgery, renal dialysis, anoxia, thalamic stimulation, or bilateral thalamotomy could lead to ANS (Duffy, 2005). Recent case reports indicate that ANS might also be one of the sequelae of long term COVID-19 (Furlanis et al., 2023). Most clinicians and researchers agree that ANS is an independent fluency disorder. However, some authors in the past have argued that it is a part of speech and language disorders such as apraxia, dysarthria, and aphasia. This could be due to the frequent co-occurrence of ANS with these speech and language disorders.

Theys et al. (2011) reported an incidence of ANS as 5.3% following stroke, and males were more affected than females, with a gender ratio ranging from 2:1 to 10:1. The incidence and prevalence of ANS are not well established due to the lack of availability of adequate data (Theys et al., 2011). A majority of the studies on ANS are single case studies, case reports, or studies with a smaller sample size (Tani & Sakai, 2011). A few authors, in contrast, question the lack of incidence data given the frequent occurrence of ANS in clinical practice, mainly in the hospital setup (Lundie et al., 2014).

Subtypes of ANS

As most of the literature on ANS is based on single case studies, we will attempt to describe the disorder based on multiple cases. Canter (1971) wrote an entire article that categorized ANS into three subtypes based on the foci of neural damage. The first, *dysarthric stuttering*, is when the site of damage would be in the cerebellar region or Parkinson's disease, which causes a lack of neuromotor control that leads to stuttering. It is frequently characterized by imprecise articulation and slurred speech with disfluency. The second is *apraxic stuttering*, which occurs due to poor motor planning that can cause disturbances in sequential organization, transitionalization, selection, and initiation of motor speech movements. Repetitions and silent blocks, along with articulatory groping behaviour, are the most common characteristics of this sub-group. *Dysnomic stuttering* forms the third sub-group with predominant disturbances in word retrieval, which is associated with the aphasic population. Persons with dysnomic stuttering often exhibit disruption in the forward flow of speech with inappropriate halts. These are accompanied by articulatory groping behaviour, pauses, interjections, and word or phrase repetitions. One should be vigilant in the differential diagnosis between ANS and other behaviours associated with neurological disorders such as palilalia (phrase and word repetitions produced with decreasing loudness and increasing rate). It must be noted that ANS is characterized by involuntary repetitions of the correct sound/syllables and not sounds that are incorrectly produced as a result of aphasia (Rosenbek, 1984).

Speech deficits are usually some of the earliest signs of neurological deficits. Any subtle changes in the nervous system due to lesions may result in a speech deficit, which may vary from very mild to severe speech impairment. ANS may be an early diagnostic sign of neurological problems in patients. Helm-Estabrooks (1999) explained this persuasively as:

Fluent speaking is, perhaps, the most refined motor act performed by humans, requiring complex coordination of many different muscle groups. Therefore, it can be sensitive to even small changes in neurological status, which may be why stuttering occurs in a wide range of neurological disorders, from Parkinson's disease to closed head injury. If this fact is ignored, clinicians may be overlooking an important early indicator of neurological disease.

(p. 265).

Nature of lesions

Stuttering followed by CVA may be accompanied by heterogeneous lesions on both hemispheres. Except for the occipital lobe, most cortical and subcortical structures are implicated in ANS, unlike developmental stuttering (DS), where a limited number of sites are identified. Stuttering associated with right hemisphere lesions has been reported in the literature (Harrison, 2004), including lesions in the right-sided subcortical areas (Soroker et al., 1990). Multiple sites in the left hemisphere are observed to be associated with ANS, including the putamen and internal capsule, the striatum, and the left supplementary motor area (Ciabarra et al., 2000; Harrison, 2004).

ANS has also been associated with bilateral lesions. Stuttering that results from unilateral damage is transient in nature, lasting for a week, whereas in the case of bilateral lesions, it is usually of a persistent nature (Helm-Estabrooks, 1999). Furthermore, some researchers have reported instances of different stuttering linked to lesions in the left subcortical area, basal ganglia, and pontine nucleus (Ciabarra et al., 2000).

There are some shreds of evidence in the literature where lesions have led to the recovery of developmental stuttering and, in contrast, the re-emergence of stuttering where the patient had recovered from developmental stuttering many years ago (Andy & Bhatnagar, 1992; Mouradian et al., 2000). Some authors hypothesize that knowledge of the site of lesion associated with neurogenic stuttering may have a significant potential contribution to understanding developmental stuttering (Guitar, 2019). However, a few authors contradict this as they see developmental and neurogenic stuttering as two separate entities. Watson and Freeman (1997) believe that neurological conditions do not contribute to understanding developmental stuttering reliably. In contrast to the wide variability in the site and nature of lesions associated with ANS, relatively specific brain centres are known to be affected in developmental stuttering. Also, speech characteristics of developmental stuttering are heterogenous in nature unlike in ANS, in which they are restricted to a set of motor speech disruptions.

Literature also reports that a variety of drugs can cause stuttering. Journal of Psychopharmacology and a French journal, Prescrire International, published a review article in 1998 constituting 24 cases related to stuttering and drugs. Findings revealed that drugs such as antipsychotics, mood stabilizers, tranquilizers, antidepressants, and antiepileptics are directly linked with stuttering (Ward, 2006). The link between these drugs and stuttering was confirmed when there was a cessation of stuttering on withdrawal of the drugs in all 24 cases. Medical practitioners frequently prescribe these drugs; however, there is a poor understanding of the interaction between these drugs and stuttering. Many contradicting studies have been reported in the literature. Guillaume et al. (1957) reported a significant reduction in stuttering followed by administering anticonvulsive drugs in two out of three epileptic patients. Contrasting results were observed by Supprian et al. (1999), who reported an increase in epileptic brain activity and stuttering followed by the administration of clozapine. There is no clear explanation of the effect of drugs on stuttering. A look into the literature might confuse the reader further as some of the drugs such as Prozac (antidepressants), propranolol (beta-blockers) as well as benzodiazepine tranquilizers reduce stuttering in some people who stutter (PWS); in contrast some non-prescription drugs such as alcohol, nicotine, and caffeine reportedly increase stuttering. Brady (1998), in his review of literature on drugs and stuttering, stated that the involvement of numerous neurotransmitters and their complex relationship may lead to the variability in the effect of drugs on stuttering. Also, given the heterogeneity of stuttering, finding out what variables contribute to the effect of drugs on stuttering is challenging. Most of the findings in the literature are based on a single case report or a small sample size, where the generalization of the results is highly questionable. Most of the observations are individualistic. These lacunae demand randomized clinical trial studies with a large sample size to better understand the relationship between drugs and stuttering.

Characteristics of ANS

The speech characteristics and type of disfluencies in ANS vary across patients based on the etiology. In individuals with PD, the disfluencies consist of frequent attempts to produce rapid movements (repetitions), articulatory freezing (pauses), and frequent prolongations or silent blocks. Among the core behaviours, repetitions are the most frequently observed disfluency in ANS (Penttilä & Korpijaakko-Huuhka, 2015), especially in head injury patients. Ludlow et al. (1987) compared repetitions to a gunshot, where they are fast, uncontrollable, intermittent, unpredictable bursts with poor intelligibility. Along with repetitions, prolongations and longer pause duration without struggle were also observed. In stroke patients, the nature of repetitions varies, where repetitions of short segments of sounds were observed in syllables and shorter words as well as in longer words and phrases (Van Borsel, van der Made, et al., 2003). Ellis and Rittman (2009) analyzed the speech of six individuals with subcortical stroke, and the results showed an increase in the frequency of disfluencies and disfluency rate compared to the control group. Some characteristics are striking and more evident in ANS, compared to developmental stuttering. These characteristics are given in Table 8.1.

Table 8.1 Features of acquired neurogenic stuttering

Domain	Characteristics
Loci of Disfluencies	Disfluencies are observed on both grammatical and functional (substantive) words. Disfluencies are not limited to the initial position; they are also observed in the medial and final positions.
Adaptation Effect	Reduced or lack of adaptation effect in reading task
Secondary Behaviours	Rare association of secondary symptoms (fist-clenching, eye blinking, facial grimacing, escape, and avoidance) with stuttering behaviour
Emotional Reactions	Reduced anxiety, fear, and concern about stuttering
Consistency Effect	Consistency is seen in stuttering behaviour across speech tasks (spontaneous speech and reading).

ANS need not be associated with any specific site of lesion (Lebrun et al., 1987). As ANS may result from damage to almost any part of the brain, there is no strong rationale that could justify localizing the site of the lesion (Rosenbek, 1984). However, symptomatology varies with the lesion site. The possible etiology/site-specific disfluency characteristics of ANS are given in Table 8.2.

Loci of disfluencies within sentences or words

In ANS caused due to stroke, disfluencies are observed in the initial position of words. However, unlike developmental stuttering, disfluencies are also observed in the medial and final positions of words (Bloodstein, 1995), such as "barrist-er-er-er", "school-b-b-boy", and "tourna-me-me-me-ment" (Canter, 1971; Helm-Estabrooks, 1999). Canter (1971) also observed that the loci of stuttering in his patients tended to increase in /l/, /h/, and /r/ sounds. A recent case report based on five ANS patients reported similar loci of stuttering in adults with ANS and persistent developmental stuttering (Max et al., 2019). However, replicated studies with a larger sample size are required to confirm these findings.

Adaptation effect

The reduction of disfluencies with successive readings of the same text is referred to as the adaptation effect (Johnson & Knott, 1937). The adaptation effect and its assessment have been addressed in detail in Chapter 3. The presumed absence of an adaptation effect during reading is often thought to be associated with acquired neurogenic stuttering, as reported by several single case studies (Guitar, 2019; Tani & Sakai, 2011). However, this is not an obligatory characteristic of ANS because the adaptation effect varies based on the cause and site of the lesions. Recent studies have reported the absence of an adaptation effect in ANS (Balasubramanian et al., 2010; Krishnan & Tiwari, 2011). Hence, during differential diagnosis between ANS and other fluency disorders, speech-language pathologists (SLPs) should rely more on other variables, such as case history, to make a clinical decision.

Table 8.2 Etiology-specific disfluency characteristics of ANS

Sr. No.	Study	Structure	Etiology	ANS disfluency characteristics
1.	Lebrun and Leleux (1985)	Cortical	Right hemisphere lesion	Repetitions mostly on the initial position of words and only a few in medial and final positions
2.	Ludlow et al. (1987)		Traumatic brain injury	Rapid and frequent repetitions likened to guns firing
3.	Van Borsel et al. (2009)		Bilateral frontal dysfunction with a right preponderance	Frequent interjections followed by whole–word repetitions Functional words are stuttered on more than content words
4.	Ardila and Lopez (1986)		Right brain damage	Repetitions, blocks, and prolongations in the initial position. Only a few are in the medial position Iterations in all positions within the word
5.	Van Borsel and Taillieu (2001a)	Subcortical	Subarachnoid bleeding in the interhemispheric fissure	Part–word repetitions and frowning
6.	Van Borsel, van der Made, et al. (2003) Van Borsel and Taillieu (2001)		Left ventrolateral thalamus infarct Parietal intracerebral hematoma on the left Left parieto-occipital epidural hematoma	Whole–word, part–word, phrase repetitions Interjections
7.	Tani and Sakai (2011)		Basal ganglia lesions	Initial position consonant prolongations. Most frequent disfluencies are syllable and part–word repetitions, followed by blocks.
8.	Ellis and Rittman (2009)		Subcortical stroke (left basal ganglia) Head injury secondary to epileptic attack. Extensive cortico-subcortical lesion (fronto-temporo-parietal cortex and basal ganglia) in the left hemisphere.	The percentage of disfluencies ranges from 3–5% Filled pauses, syllable, and word repetitions Majority of disfluencies on the medial position of the sentence
9.	Van Borsel et al. (2010)			Lexical words stuttered more often than grammatical words
10.	Leder (1996)		Parkinson's Disease	Rapid repetitions, articulatory freezing, frequent prolongations, or silent blocks

Secondary behaviours

Developmental stuttering, especially in older children and adults, is not only characterized by speech disfluencies but often also by a complex set of secondary behaviours. A detailed account of these secondary behaviours can be found in Chapter 3. In contrast, it has been suggested that the absence of secondary behaviours in people with ANS is one of the criteria that could be used for differential diagnostic purposes (Canter, 1971; Helm-Estabrooks, 1999). There is a difference of opinion regarding this finding among various researchers. In many carefully reported clinical studies, investigators have commented on the lack of secondary behaviours in people with ANS (Dworkin et al., 2002). However, a few researches also suggest the presence of secondary behaviours in people with ANS (Rosenbek et al., 1978). The presence or absence of secondary behaviours needs to be interpreted in the light of the onset of stuttering relative to the onset of the neurological lesion/disease and the timing of the speech assessment relative to stuttering onset. The time elapsed between the onset of stuttering and the fluency assessment on which the published report is based may not have been sufficiently long for learnt secondary behaviours to develop fully in some adults with ANS. Even though secondary behaviours are very rare in ANS, they do not imply their complete absence. Some patients do exhibit secondary behaviours with stuttering; however, they may be very mild in nature and might usually go unnoticed.

Attitudes and emotional reactions

Evidence-based research highlights that children and adults with developmental stuttering often show significantly elevated speech–related negative attitudes (Veerabhadrappa, Krishnakumar, et al., 2021; Veerabhadrappa, Vanryckeghem, et al., 2021a) and other negative emotional reactions towards their communication ability (Vanryckeghem et al., 2001; Veerabhadrappa, Vanryckeghem, et al., 2021b). Further, potential differences in terms of temperament in developmental stuttering have been confirmed by research (Anderson et al., 2003). In contrast, very little systematic research has been conducted regarding speech–associated attitudes and emotional reactions in people with neurogenic stuttering. Based on clinical observation, Helm-Estabrooks (1999) and Canter (1971) proposed that adults with ANS may be annoyed due to their stutter but seldom develop marked anxiety as a result of their speech disfluencies. In order to rule out speech-related attitudes, anxiety, or any other behavioural issues, it is advisable to include test batteries in the assessment protocol, such as the Behavioural Assessment Battery (BAB) (Vanryckeghem & Brutten, 2018).

Consistency in stuttering behaviour

Usually, the disfluencies seen in ANS are not specific to speech tasks (Helm-Estabrooks, 1999; Van Borsel & Taillieu, 2001). However, in some patients, repetitions were observed to be speech task specific. Abe et al. (1993) observed repetitions only during spontaneous speech but not during reading or repetition tasks in a male patient with brain stem infarct and bilateral medial thalamic stroke. In the context of complexity of the speech task, the proportion of the repetitions in TBI patients stayed the same with an increase in the complexity (paragraphs, sentences, and words) (Jokel et al., 2007). Also, the frequency of stuttering in spontaneous speech increased in monologue compared to conversation tasks. However, these results cannot be reliably generalized as these studies are based on single cases. Until studies with larger samples are reported, it is safer to believe that stuttering behaviour is consistent in neurogenic stuttering across speech tasks.

Other speech or language problems accompanying neurogenic stuttering

Although neurogenic stuttering may occur as the patient's only speech disorder, concomitant speech or language problems will often occur. Speech problems such as dysarthria, apraxia, language problems such as paraphasias, anomia, transient expressive aphasia, and memory problems have been reported in individuals with ANS (Mazzucchi et al., 1981).

Assessment and diagnosis of acquired neurogenic stuttering

ANS can manifest itself in many different ways depending on several factors, including the nature of the associated disorder, the underlying etiology, and the time since onset. As mentioned before, often it is not the only communication disorder the patient is experiencing. It may include aphasia, dysarthria, motor or cognitive problems, or chronic pain that affects their performance. All of these conditions might influence the nature and severity of ANS. Assessment of ANS must, therefore, be a highly individualized process, with information gathered along several different dimensions and synthesized into a coherent clinical picture. Ringo and Dietrich (1995), and Helm-Estabrooks (1999) developed a set of guidelines to assess and differentially diagnose ANS. They recommended these guidelines not only as an aid to accurate diagnosis but also to build substantial evidence for further literature support on the subject of ANS.

Step 1: A detailed case history

This is the first step in the assessment process and is of utmost importance in the differential diagnosis of ANS. The following information could be obtained from the patient or caregiver at the initial meeting or through the patient medical file, and supplementing information can be obtained during the interview. It includes

1. Stuttering onset and its association with neurological damage
2. Pre-morbid handedness of the individual
3. Education and employment history
4. Extent to which stuttering affects verbal communication
5. Health history with the date including the following:
       History of neurologic diseases, head trauma, period of unconsciousness, seizures, substance abuse (prescriptive and non-prescriptive medications), surgery and hospitalization, psychiatric problems, and treatments
6. Patient's level of concern, fear, and anxiety related to stuttering
7. Progression of the disorder (improving or deteriorating)

8. Patient's past and family history of treatment for speech-language or learning problems
9. History of developmental stuttering; if yes, age of onset of stuttering

Case history taking is both an art and a science. A detailed case history is crucial for making an accurate diagnosis. The case history plays a vital role in the differential diagnosis of neurogenic, developmental, and psychogenic stuttering. It is challenging for a trained SLP to identify or label a fluency disorder only on the basis of a recorded spontaneous speech sample. This could be due to the similarities in the perception of disfluencies observed during advanced developmental and acquired neurogenic stuttering. Hence, the case history plays a pivotal role in making an accurate diagnosis.

Step 2: Direct evaluation of speech

1. Formal tests should be administered to assess stuttering severity, such as Stuttering Severity Instrument 4th edition (SSI-4) (Riley, 2009).
2. Speech samples should be audio-video recorded for an approximate total duration of 10 minutes, including spontaneous speech and reading samples.
3. Speech samples should be analyzed for stuttering-like disfluencies (part-word, single-syllable and monosyllabic whole-word repetitions, blocks, and prolongations). Also, note secondary behaviours associated with stuttering, if any. Suvi and Leipakka (2012) gave new guidelines to analyze disfluencies and to count syllables in ANS speech samples. During syllable count, interrupted words, discourse particles, and interjections are omitted. Also, syllable count does not include repetitions due to word searching behaviour in ANS. Suvi and Leipakka suggested using Yairi's (2007) stuttering-like disfluencies (SLDs) and other disfluencies (OD's) classification to analyze stuttering speech samples. A detailed account of SLDs and ODs can be found in Chapter 2.
4. Check for the position of disfluencies, adaptation effect, and proportion of stuttering moments on function versus content words using standard passages.
5. Patients should be asked to speak under fluency-inducing conditions and their speech pattern evaluated in terms of speech rate and fluency, such as delayed auditory feedback, choral reading, and auditory masking. Generally, unlike developmental stuttering, speech fluency does not improve under these conditions for neurogenic stuttering.
6. Check for the number of disfluencies during automated speech tasks such as counting numbers, singing, and reciting the months of the year. Usually, the number of disfluencies will not reduce during automated speech tasks, in contrast with developmental stuttering.

Step 3: Assessment of other components, including language and cognition

1. The possible existence of underlying language problems should be assessed. Helm-Estabrooks (1999) recommended using standard diagnostic tools for

aphasia to exclude the possibility of a language disorder (palilalia, word-finding difficulties) expressing itself as stuttering.

2. ANS can coexist with other neurological conditions such as apraxia or dysarthria. It is essential to administer neuropsychological tests to determine the patient's capabilities for accurate diagnosis and treatment plans.

3. Also ANS is seldom accompanied by negative emotional reactions as noted in the section on characteristics of ANS; it is essential to rule out their presence. Assessment of speech-related negative attitudes, anxiety, disruptions, and behavioural changes using BAB (Vanryckeghem & Brutten, 2018) can aid holistic assessment, preparation of an individualistic treatment plan and estimation of the prognosis.

Differential diagnosis

It is crucial to distinguish neurogenic stuttering from other forms of fluency disorders such as developmental and psychogenic stuttering (see Table 8.3). Differential diagnosis assists in planning intervention.

Treatment of neurogenic stuttering

Following CVA or TBI, standalone ANS is very rare, and it presents itself with other communication disorders such as aphasia, dysarthria, and apraxia. Hence, with the help of a detailed case history and interview, the clinician should try to identify the possible existence of pre-morbid developmental stuttering or any other speech and language disorders.

The interference of other neurological disorders in the intervention programme, such as dementia and Parkinson's disease, must be considered before making a treatment plan. Not all patients with neurogenic stuttering require therapeutic intervention because immediately after brain injury, stuttering may appear and may gradually resolve independently without any formal intervention (De Nil et al., 2007).

Helm-Estabrooks (1999) recommended a few guidelines to select patients who could potentially benefit from treatment. As per guidelines given by Helm-Estabrooks, not all patients who present with disfluencies followed by brain damage require or warrant treatment. For example, a patient presenting with mild stuttering may be exempted from therapy if it does not interfere significantly with their communication ability. In other cases, although neurogenic stuttering may significantly hinder communication, these patients do not warrant treatment for stuttering due to the presence of severe comorbid conditions such as fatal or progressive neurological disorders. Similarly, therapy may not be warranted in conditions such as single-sided cortical lesions regardless of the presence or absence of aphasia. In the presence of aphasia, the aphasia acts as a greater barrier to communication than the stutter. Also, the patient might be more concerned about aphasia than stuttering. Even in the absence of aphasia or other speech and language disorders, it is appropriate to wait for spontaneous recovery and reassure the patient that there would be recovery resulting in near normal speech (De Nil et al., 2007). If the patient has persistent stuttering and is concerned and motivated for therapy, then the SLP may decide to

Table 8.3 Differential diagnosis between neurogenic, psychogenic, and developmental stuttering

Sr. No	Neurogenic stuttering	Developmental stuttering	Psychogenic stuttering
1	Disfluencies are generally not restricted to the initial position of a word	Disfluencies are typically observed in the initial position	Disfluencies are usually observed in initial and middle positions and on stressed syllables
2	Sudden onset, usually seen in adulthood, followed by brain damage	Gradual onset, generally during preschool age (2–5 years)	Sudden, coincides with traumatic events in life and is usually seen in teenage and adulthood
3	Caused due to neurological disease or damage	No specific cause, multiple predisposing factors	Chronic stress and traumatic event
4	No changes with altered feedback	Usually vulnerable to altered feedback	No changes with altered feedback
5	The proportionality of disfluencies is not directly related to grammatical function	Disfluencies are seen more often on content words than functional words	Grammatical errors are observed; however, the proportionality is unknown
6	Absence of stuttering related anxiety and secondary behaviours	Presence of stuttering related anxiety and secondary behaviours	Rare; however, situation avoidance is exhibited with bizarre or unusual struggle behaviours
7	Conversational partner and speaking situation independent	Stuttering behaviour may vary depending upon the conversational partner and speaking situation.	Conversational partner and speaking situation independent
8	Absence of adaptation effect	Presence of adaptation effect	Absence of adaptation effect
9	No changes with fluency-inducing/ enhancing conditions	Stuttering reduces with fluency-inducing/ enhancing conditions	The patient may stutter more or severely in these conditions
10	Prognosis varies with the nature and extent of brain damage. Lesions involving both hemispheres lead to persistent stuttering.	There is no cure for adult chronic stuttering; nonetheless, the severity can be reduced drastically with therapy. Prognosis is better in children with early identification and intervention.	The prognosis depends on the underlying psychological trauma. It may improve significantly with resolving the psychological trauma but not always. Dramatic improvement with trial therapy is a hallmark of psychogenic stuttering.

start with the intervention programme. However, the patient's adequate linguistic and cognitive abilities are essential for the behavioural management of stuttering.

Treatment approaches

Unlike developmental stuttering, neurogenic stuttering treatment is entirely behavioural due to a lack of emotional and cognitive components. However, for a few patients where neurological causes have been identified, the treatment proceeds in the form of neurosurgery or medications.

Broadly speaking, there are three options available to treat neurogenic stuttering: Behavioural management, surgical management and medications. These may be employed singly or in combination.

Behavioural management

The behavioural management of ANS includes therapeutic techniques used to treat developmental stuttering. These include pacing, stuttering modification, fluency shaping, auditory masking, altered auditory feedback, and biofeedback techniques such as electromyographic biofeedback (EMG).

Auditory masking and altered feedback

Masking and delayed auditory feedback (DAF) have been suggested for treatment of neurogenic stuttering (Helm-Estabrooks, 1999; Marshall & Starch, 1984). However, the prognosis and the generalization of induced fluency using these methods is questionable. Rentschler et al. (1984) described a 41-year-old adult male with neurogenic stuttering due to an overdose of the drug chlorazepate dipotassium. Auditory masking using binaural white noise at 90 decibels resulted in a noticeable reduction of stuttering behaviour. Nevertheless, with a lower intensity masking noise, stuttering relapsed. Downie et al. (1981) reported that DAF was effective with two Parkinson's patients with stuttering. Krishnan and Tiwari (2011) observed a marked reduction in disfluencies in a patient with ANS under a masked auditory feedback (MAF) condition.

Pacing or rhythmic speech

A few patients with ANS may respond to the pacing technique. In this speech technique, the patient is asked to utter one syllable at a time, reducing the speech rate and eliminating the coarticulation across syllables. This results in staccato rhythmic speech. This treatment technique was invented by Helm (1979) for the treatment of palilalia (fast repetition of words and phrases) and, due to its effectiveness, was implemented in the treatment of neurogenic stuttering by Helm-Estabrooks (1999). The pacing technique can be used for patients who have difficulty reducing their speech rate. Pacing boards (Helm-Estabrooks & Kaplan, 1989) or moulds

(Rentschler et al., 1984) that fit over the patient's finger are used, and patients are instructed to move their finger from one place to another while enunciating each syllable. Once patients reduce their speech rate, portable pocket-sized pacing boards can be used to facilitate generalization. Patients can gradually progress from using a pacing instrument to tapping a table, tapping their thighs or fingers, eliminating the need for an overt device. Generally, patients achieve fluent speech. However, generalization and progression to non-staccato speech are challenging. Krishnan and Tiwari (2011) employed the pacing technique to reduce disfluencies in a 56-year-old patient with ANS. At the end of seven therapy sessions, there was a significant reduction in disfluencies, and the subject and the caregiver were satisfied with the therapy outcomes.

Stuttering modification and fluency shaping techniques

Market et al. (1990) conducted a survey and found that a few clinicians employed fluency shaping techniques (easy onset and slower speech rate) to treat acquired neurogenic stuttering and found it to be successful. Clinically, SLPs have used stuttering modification tools such as preparatory sets, cancellations and pullouts to treat ANS with modest therapeutic outcomes (Market et al., 1990).

EMG biofeedback

Biofeedback techniques similar to those employed with developmental stuttering have been used for ANS. EMG biofeedback aids in the reduction of stuttering related excessive muscle tension during speech. Patients are trained to use biofeedback to reduce masseter muscle tension to a maximum of 5 milli volt electrical activity. A baseline skin conduction will be established before training. Steps for muscle relaxation training might include deep breathing, a relaxed body posture, and relaxation of specific muscles such as the neck, jaw, and shoulders. Acquisition of 95% fluency is essential at each step before progress is permitted. The hierarchy is completed first with direct EMG feedback followed by indirect feedback from the clinician (i.e., with instrument feedback, followed by without instrument clinician feedback, and lastly, self-monitoring from the patient). Training patients to relax the masseter muscle during speech with the help of EMG biofeedback resulted in a considerable reduction in neurogenic stuttering (Rubow et al., 1986).

Surgical management

In some cases, stuttering may reduce or resolve after neurosurgery. Donnan (1979) described a female patient with neurogenic stuttering following cerebral ischemia. Patients exhibited fast repetitions of syllables with word-finding difficulties. A carotid angiogram revealed stenosis of the left carotid artery with plaques due to hemorrhage. An endarterectomy was performed, and the patient started speaking fluently by the time he was shifted to the ward after two weeks. A post-surgical angiogram revealed an uninterrupted blood flow in the left carotid artery. The surgery for the neurological problem thus led to an incidental resolution of stuttering. A few patients have also experienced stutter-free speech after thalamic stimulation. Andy and Bhatnagar (1992) stimulated the thalamus of four patients by placing electrodes in order to treat mesothalamic damage in these patients. The thalamic stimulation resulted in stutter-free fluent speech in all four patients. Thus, surgical correction of the underlying neurological dysfunction might resolve stuttering.

Medications

As discussed earlier in this chapter, drugs have various effects on fluency. There is reported evidence that suggests varying degrees of success in treating developmental stuttering using pagoclone, olanzapine, and haloperidol (Guitar, 2019). However, these drugs are not meant for the treatment of ANS. There is evidence to suggest that these drugs could either induce fluency or result in stuttering. Drugs adminis-tered for asthma, depression, schizophrenia, Parkinson's disease, anxiety, and seizure disorders can cause stuttering in patients with no history of developmental stuttering (Duffy, 2005). In most of these cases, stuttering has either reduced or disappeared upon withdrawal or reduction in the dosage of these pharmaceutical agents. Elliott and Thomas (1985) described a 22-year-old female developing stuttering after the administration of Alprazolam for anxiety and depression. A double placebo con-trol study confirmed the negative side effects of Alprazolam on speech fluency. In contrast, a few studies reported stuttering reduction when drugs were administered to reduce the other concomitant symptoms (Turgut et al., 2002). Quader (1977) reported two patients with neurogenic stuttering who were administered Amitripty-line (an antidepressant), resulting in a reduction of stuttering. Together these reports indicate that ANS might either result from or be eliminated by the administration of various pharmacological agents. In such cases, the SLP should consult with the neuro-physician to achieve optimal management of the stuttering in relation to other medical or psychological disorders.

Irrespective of the treatment approach, prognosis depends on the site and extent of the neurological lesion, the presence of comorbidities, and the general health status of the patient. There is limited data available on neurogenic stuttering pro-jecting the long-term benefits of the above-mentioned treatment approaches. One possible reason for this could be that the causes of ANS are many and varied. As a result, acquiring data from a homogenous sample becomes difficult. Another reason could be the frequent occurrence of severe comorbid conditions (paralysis, dysarthria, dysphagia), where the patient and caregiver's primary concerns would be treatment of these comorbidities to enable the patient to carry out day-to-day activities and reduce the impact of the neurological insult on their quality of life. As a result, most of the evidence related to intervention for ANS is based on case reports.

Case example

History – medical and neurological findings:

A 54-year-old man was referred to the Department of Speech and Hearing from the Department of Neurology, Kasturba Hospital, Manipal, with a complaint of speech difficulties. He had suffered from a stroke two months ago, which was followed by right-sided weakness and no speech output. During the period of spontaneous recovery, he complained of speech abnormalities in the form of disfluencies. Other reported problems were difficulty recognizing familiar faces, difficulties in reading and writing, and poor arithmetic skills. Pre-morbid history revealed that the patient worked as a life insurance officer and was a native speaker of the Kannada language. He could read and write Kannada language and was right-handed pre-morbidly.

Medical history indicated dilated cardiomyopathy (DCM) with severe left ventricular dysfunction (LVD) for which the patient was under medication. A magnetic resonance imaging (MRI) scan was carried out at Manipal. The findings revealed a chronic neurological insult with hemosiderin deposition bilaterally in the postcentral gyri (the deposition on the left was more significant than that on the right). The present scan did not indicate any evidence of an acute infarct.

Assessment and management of communication skills:

His language evaluation was carried out using the Kannada version (Chengappa & Kumar, 2008) of the Western Aphasic Battery (WAB) (Kertesz, 1982), which revealed moderate conduction aphasia (Aphasia Quotient = 66.2). His cognition seemed to be intact, as he was alert, oriented, attentive, and could follow commands. Upon administration of the Kannada articulation test (KAT), inconsistent substitution and distortion errors were observed. Speech assessment using the Frenchay Dysarthria Assessment – Second Edition (FDA-2) (Enderby & Palmer, 2008) did not reveal any dysarthric characteristics. The patient's speech sample was rated as 4 on the AYJNIHH (1984, as cited in Sebastian et al., 2000) speech intelligibility rating scale (a scale of 0 to 6 where 0 = normal speech intelligibility and 6 = speech cannot be understood even when context is known), indicating fairly intelligible speech after careful listening, although some words are unintelligible.

Fluency assessment was carried out using the Stuttering Severity Instrument (SSI-3)[1] (Riley, 1994). The speech sample consisted of a Kannada monologue as the patient could not read. The frequency, duration, and physical concomitants scores were 16, 10, and 2, respectively, indicating moderate stuttering (percentile 61–77). Core behaviours consisted of blocks and repetitions, with repetitions being more frequent. Disfluencies were observed in the initial, medial, and final positions of words. Secondary behaviours included occasional fidgeting with the hands and poor eye contact. When the patient was subjected to fluency-inducing conditions, results revealed no difference or improvement in speech on using MAF. A temporary improvement in fluency was seen with delayed auditory feedback (DAF) given at a 50ms and 75ms delay, but disfluencies soon reappeared. Singing did not affect stuttering behaviours. The patient was diagnosed as a case of conduction aphasia with neurogenic stuttering and was recommended a follow-up for speech and language therapy. Demonstration therapy was conducted for a day, after which online therapy was recommended in order to make follow-ups feasible and avoid a long commute for the patient.

In the demonstration session, the pacing or rhythmic speech technique was used with the help of a metronome to reduce stuttering, and the semantic feature analysis (SFA) technique was used for aphasia intervention. The metronome was set to 140 beats per minute, the patient was asked to produce one syllable per beat. A slight reduction in speech rate was observed while using the metronome. The patient would have benefitted from speech and language therapy, but did not continue with the therapy programme, probably because he prioritized his comorbid condition (DCM with LVD and right-side paresis) over a compromised speech and language output.

If the patient in the above case example did follow-up for therapy, an ideal therapy plan should be centred on the individual as a whole, rather than the speech symptoms in isolation. The framework given by the International Classification of Functioning, Disability and Health (ICF; WHO, 2001) is best suited to plan therapy along these lines.

The ICF framework for neurogenic stuttering

As described in many of the previous chapters of this book, the ICF provides a unified, standard, and systematic framework for intervention, using a biopsychosocial model. It ensures simultaneous focus on the individual, family, and community levels (George & Bajaj, 2020). The practice of applying the biopsychosocial model of functioning and disability to understand the characteristics, assessment, and management of stuttering was initiated by Yaruss (1998). Yaruss and Quesal (2004) superimposed the ICF model on developmental stuttering, describing it in terms of body structures and functions, activity limitations, participation restrictions, and contextual factors. However, in contrast to developmental stuttering where a single structural anomaly cannot be stated under "body structures", an individual with ANS would receive an ICF code indicating only a structural impairment of the nervous system (s110 Structure of brain). Similar to developmental stuttering, they may face difficulties with respect to body functions, participating in daily living activities, receiving support from caregivers, etc. Figure 8.1 depicts the characteristics of neurogenic stuttering in the ICF framework.

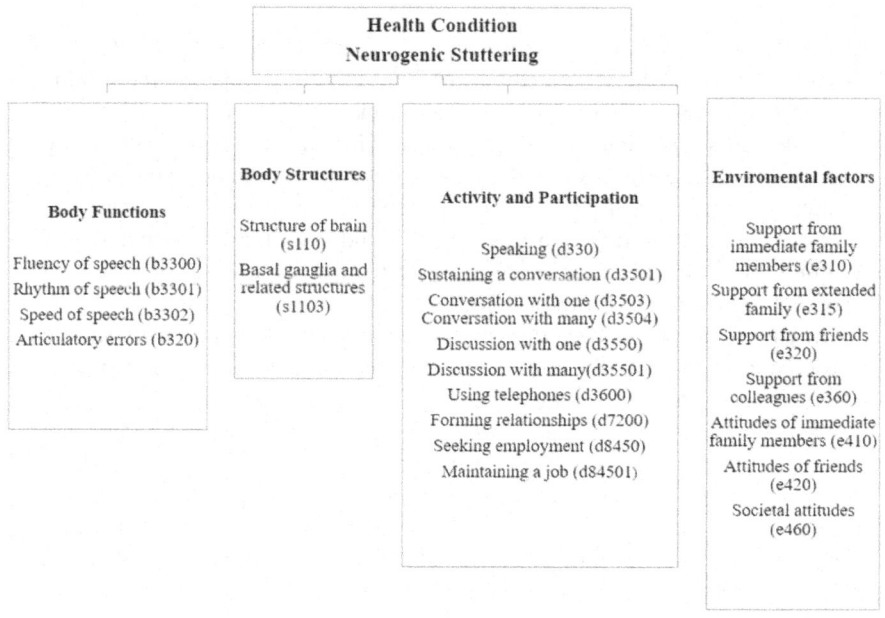

Figure 8.1 Characteristics of neurogenic stuttering in the ICF framework

Body structure

A neurological insult is the most common cause of ANS (Craig-McQuaide et al., 2014; Helm-Estabrooks, 1999; Tani & Sakai, 2011). ANS has been reported after lesions to almost all areas of the brain except the occipital lobe (Tani & Sakai, 2011). The codes for body structures would thus pertain to the structure of the brain (s110 structure of the brain). Specifically, a lesion in the basal ganglia and related structures (s1103) is the most common impairment noticed in neurogenic stuttering (Craig-McQuaide et al., 2014; Tani & Sakai, 2011).

Body functions

Similar to developmental stuttering, a person with ANS has difficulties in speech and voice functions, specifically the fluency (b3300), rhythm (b3301), and speed of speech (b3302). Unlike developmental stuttering, there may not be any consistent loci of disfluencies. For instance, repetitions, prolongations, and blocks may not occur only on initial syllables of words. The frequency of disfluencies on function words might not be lower than content words. Also, articulatory errors (b320) might co-occur with disfluencies (Tani & Sakai, 2011). A study revealed that accessory characteristics of eye blinking and facial grimaces were observed in neurogenic stuttering, but these were not associated with speech-related anxiety (Tani & Sakai, 2011).

Activity limitations and participation restrictions

Specific aspects of communication such as speaking face to face (d330), speaking through a telephone (d3600), and sustaining a conversation (d3501) might be affected in those with ANS. In addition, conversations with one or many persons (d3504, d3503), or a discussion with an individual or group of people (d3550, d35501) could be equally impaired because unlike developmental stuttering, variability with respect to person, place, and situation may not be seen in neurogenic stuttering. The codes for an individual with ANS would also include codes pertaining to difficulties participating in social settings (d7202), forming relationships (d7200), or continuing employment (d845, d8450, d84501). These difficulties in social participation and quality of life might also be a result of the stroke or any brain injury.

Environmental factors

Environmental factors play a significant role in the lives of persons with neurogenic stuttering. To overcome barriers faced by a person with neurogenic stuttering in the form of social isolation, stigmatization, low self-esteem, poor quality of life and communication breakdown, positive and enriching support from people in the patient's environment is essential. The support and attitudes of a spouse or any immediate family member (e310, e410), friends (e320, e420) and colleagues (e360), as well as societal attitudes (e460) have the potential to serve as facilitators as the therapist works towards improving the person's quality of life.

Case example

Mr. Y, a 32-year-old right-handed male reported that he suddenly became restless with rigid leg and hand movements (b735) on the right side on April 16, 2012. He was an auto rickshaw driver by profession. After the symptoms appeared, his family members immediately took him to a nearby hospital. Magnetic resonance imaging (MRI) revealed mild cerebral infarctions in the left basal ganglia (s1103) and pons. He returned home after seven days of hospitalization. He resumed walking as before, and resumed activities of daily living. After discharge from the hospital, his family members noticed that he was speaking faster than his usual rate of speech (b3302). In addition, they identified unclear speech (b320) and repetitions of sounds (b3300) while he spoke. As his family depended solely on his income, he needed to continue working. But his communication with people was affected (d3501, d3503, d3504) as his speech was unintelligible. In addition, he experienced giddiness (b755) while driving and had to discontinue his work soon after (d84501). Speech and language assessment ruled out the presence of aphasia (Aphasia Quotient of WAB 94/100). Also, he was found to have normal intelligence upon psychological assessment. His oral peripheral mechanism examination revealed normal structures and functions, although distortions were observed while speaking occasionally. He exhibited sound and syllable repetitions without any facial grimaces or struggle during conversation and reading tasks. He was aware of the difference in his speech but not self- conscious of it. He seemed to be confident about going to work and conversing with his friends. He showed a willingness to engage in telephonic conversations (d3600). Despite being self-motivated to overcome his difficulties, societal attitudes (e460) such as poor social acceptance and stigmatization of the disorder by the society acted as a barrier to his progress.

This example of holistic assessment and documentation along the lines of the ICF model demonstrates how the assessment process itself aids the clinician in planning goals for therapy. These goals, then, are directed at rehabilitation in terms of reducing the presenting symptoms as well as resuming activities, participation and a quality of life as close to pre-morbid status as possible, within the limits of the impairment.

To conclude, ANS was earlier perceived to be a part of speech and language disorders due to brain damage. Although this scenario has gradually changed with more objective assessment and treatment of ANS, research related to ANS is still in the cradle, so to speak. Consequently, there has been a dearth of evidence-based data regarding treatment approaches and prognosis for the disorder. Therefore, ANS requires the attention of clinicians and researchers who can contribute to existing literature with additional evidence-based research.

Summary points to remember

- ANS, also known as SAAND, is frequently seen in adulthood with a sudden onset.
- Neurogenic stuttering is a sub-group of acquired stuttering caused due to neurological trauma such as stroke, traumatic brain injury, drug abuse and misuse, infections such as meningitis and encephalitis, brain tumour, and degenerative disorders.
- A detailed case history is a very crucial component of the assessment process.
- Disfluencies in ANS are present on both content and functional words and are not restricted to initial syllables.
- ANS is rarely associated with secondary behaviours and is not characterized by anxiety or fear related to stuttering.
- Fluency-inducing conditions do not affect neurogenic stuttering; an adaptation effect is usually absent.
- Not all patients with ANS warrant treatment.
- Treatment approaches include medications, surgical management, and behavioural therapy such as pacing, biofeedback, and stuttering modification therapy.
- Long-term benefits of intervention approaches for ANS are not well documented.

Study questions

1. Write a short note on the pharmaceutical management of ANS.
2. What questions would you include in case history taking for an adult male with suspected ANS?
3. Do all patients with ANS warrant treatment? Justify your answer.
4. Write a treatment plan for an adult male with ANS.
5. Write a note on the speech characteristics of ANS.

Note

1   The SSI-3 was used because of the unavailability of the SSI-4 in the clinic when this case study was documented. We recommend the use of SSI-4 or the latest version of any assessment instrument whenever possible.

9   Cluttering

Pallavi Kelkar

Introduction

Fluency has been defined and redefined over the past few decades (Bloodstein et al., 2021; Van Riper, 1984; Guitar, 2019), popular definitions often encompassing cohesion, coherence and prosodic aspects of speech. Despite this clarity in the definition of fluency, the primary focus of public education, assessment, intervention and research has been stuttering (Ward, 2018). The other fluency disorder, cluttering, hitherto called an orphan (Van Riper, 1971) in the field of speech-language pathology, is the focus of this chapter.

The presence of cluttering has been detected as early as the ancient Greek period. As Ward (2018) states, "Demosthenes, originally thought to have had a stutter, more likely suffered from cluttering" (p. 143). The period from 1964 to 1970 saw cluttering receive recognition as a separate disorder, as well as an increased interest in defining and describing cluttered speech (Myers, 1996). This period was followed by a relative lull in academic and research interest in cluttering. In the 1990s, however, therapists and researchers took to studying cluttering with renewed vigour. This period also saw the inception of the International Cluttering Association (ICA)[1] with representatives from countries the world over. This gave an added impetus to discussion and collaborative research on cluttering (Reichel et al., 2014; Reichel et al., 2019). The last two decades have witnessed what La Salle (2010) called a renaissance in the area of cluttering research and practice, with new guidelines for assessment (van Zaalen et al., 2011) and structured approaches to cluttering intervention (Myers, 2011). One of the factors stimulating these advances in assessment and intervention is the present definition of cluttering that focuses purely on core speech symptoms accompanying the disorder.

Definition and characteristics

Evolution of the definition

The earliest description of cluttering can be found in Track II among the four developmental tracks of stuttering (Van Riper, 1971). Weiss (1964) first described cluttering as the verbal manifestation of a central language imbalance. The central language imbalance manifested itself symptomatically as problems in speech,

DOI: 10.4324/9781003367673-9

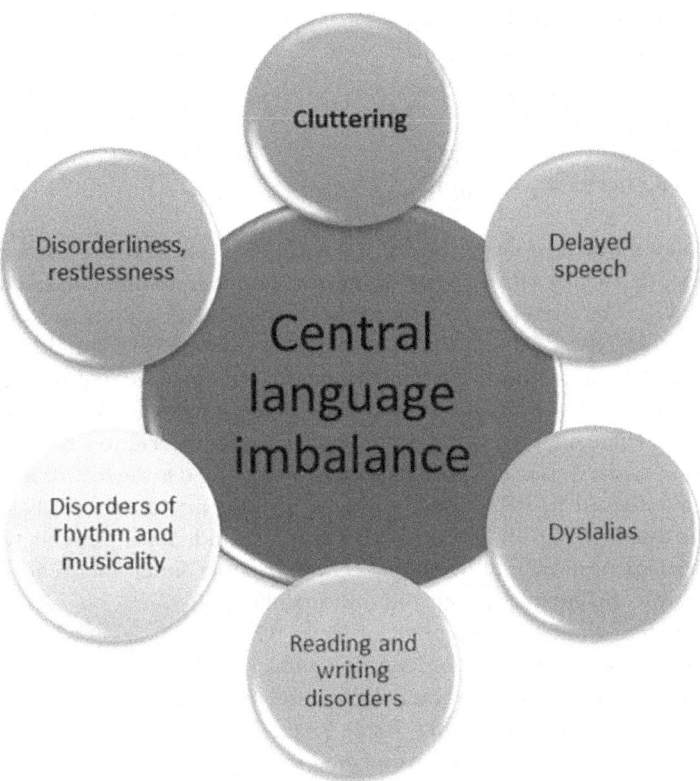

Figure 9.1 Weiss's view on cluttering

language, reading, writing, attention, rhythm and musicality, etc. Weiss's description can be pictorially represented as the cluttering iceberg (Figure 9.1). According to Weiss (1964), among all the possible features seen in people who clutter (PWC), three symptoms were essential to arrive at a diagnosis of cluttering. These were labelled as "obligatory symptoms" and were as follows:

1. Excessive number of repetitions
2. Short attention span and concentration
3. Lack of awareness of the problem

Other than the three obligatory symptoms, Weiss put forth a list of "facultative symptoms" which might or might not be present in a PWC. The facultative symptoms were

1. Tachylalia (fast bursts of speech or festinating speech)
2. Dysrhythmic breathing
3. Dysphonia
4. Articulatory errors

5. Monotony and lack of rhythm
6. Poor fine motor abilities
7. Disorganized thought processes
8. Language difficulties
9. Reading or writing deficits
10. A strong hereditary component

St Louis (1992) defined cluttering as "a speech/language disorder" characterized by "abnormal disfluency which is not stuttering, and a rapid and/or irregular speech rate" (p. 49). The presence of a language component in cluttering was reiterated by Daly (1993), who defined cluttering as "a disorder of speech and language processing resulting in rapid, dysrhythmic, sporadic, unorganized and frequently unintelligible speech. Accelerated speech is not always present, but an impairment in formulating language almost always is" (p. 107). His description of cluttering was also in line with Weiss's (1964) perspective, when he described five areas that are necessarily affected in PWC. In his linguistic disfluency model (Daly & Burnett, 1999), he asserted that "Cluttering exists when an individual presents with one or more impairment in each of five broad communicative dimensions reflecting cognitive, linguistic, pragmatic, speech and motor abilities" (p. 226).

Similar to St Louis's (1992) point of view, Ward (2006) acknowledged the possible presence of either speech or language problems when he described two strands of the disorder, one in which motor deficits are prominent and the other characterized primarily by language deficits (Table 9.1).

Although all of these definitions seemed to focus on both, the underlying processes as well as the manifestations of cluttering, the focus subsequently shifted to a definition that focused primarily on the core identifiable symptoms of cluttering necessary for a reliable and valid diagnosis. The first such working definition of cluttering was given by St Louis et al. (2003) and updated four years hence (St Louis,

Table 9.1 Subtypes of cluttering

Author	Subtypes	Description
Ward (2006)	Motoric cluttering	Tachylalia, excessive coarticulation, articulation errors, lack of speech rhythm, monotonous speech, festinant speech, fluency disruptions
	Linguistic cluttering	Syntactic errors, problems in lexical access, semantic paraphasia, maze behaviours (pauses, hesitations and revisions due to linguistic dead ends), deficits in language organization, sequencing or cohesion
van Zaalen (2009)	Phonological cluttering	Problems in phonological encoding precipitated in word structure errors, coarticulation (especially at a fast speech rate, in multisyllabic words, or linguistically complex situations)
	Syntactical cluttering	Problems in grammatical encoding, word retrieval precipitated as normal disfluencies (especially at a fast speech rate or linguistically complex situations)

Myers, et al., 2007). A refined version of this revised working definition is the lowest common denominator (LCD) definition of cluttering (St Louis & Schulte, 2011) that is presently in use:

> Cluttering is a fluency disorder wherein segments of conversation in the speaker's native language typically are perceived as too fast overall, too irregular, or both. The segments of rapid and/or irregular speech rate must be further accompanied by one or more of the following: (a) excessive 'normal disfluencies'; (b) excessive collapsing or deletion of syllables; and/or (c) abnormal pauses, syllable stress or speech rhythm.
>
> (p. 241–242)

The definition is followed by a few clarifications that might be useful for beginning clinicians during assessment of cluttering. Firstly, it allows for cluttering to be present in a non-native language sample if the speaker is multilingual and has gained mastery over that language. This is especially applicable to the Indian scenario where almost every child understands and/or speaks a minimum of two languages. Secondly, the definition allows for symptoms to be present even in a few communicative situations for a person to be diagnosed with cluttering. Thirdly, it clarifies that the rate of speech might not necessarily be faster than typical speakers, but is fast for that individual and leads to intelligibility being compromised. The definition thus effectively distinguishes cluttering from a mere fast rate of speech. Being a symptom-based definition, the LCD definition allows a uniform conceptualization of cluttering across researchers and clinicians. It facilitates more efficient management by distinguishing the core areas to be worked on from associated problems or co-occurring disorders. The speech characteristics contained within the bold lines in Figure 9.2 are the features included in the current definition of cluttering. Those outside the bold lines but within dotted lines represent features that were included in previous definitions but have been excluded from the current (LCD) definition. The characteristics listed in dotted lines deserve a mention because although their presence is not currently of diagnostic significance, they might be present in persons who clutter as reported by several authors. This will be clearer to the reader in subsequent sections of this chapter. Some of the characteristics such as problems in reading and writing or inattention might be present in some PWC but would warrant a separate diagnosis, such as specific learning disabilities or attention-deficit hyperactivity disorder. The LCD definition thus prevents over-diagnosis or under-diagnosis of cluttering and ensures that the concomitant (non-speech) problems get a separate diagnosis and appropriate intervention.

The LCD definition does have a few limitations. One of these (Figure 9.2) is the exclusion of the linguistic component of cluttering (Kaul et al., 2022; Logan, 2020; Ward, 2018). Kaul et al. (2022) asked naïve listeners from Pune, India to opine on a speech sample of a PWC and a typical speech sample. The themes that emerged were coded with +1 for every positive comment and -1 for a negative comment for each of the two samples. A large difference in the total scores obtained would indicate that a particular trait effectively differentiated typical speech from cluttered speech.

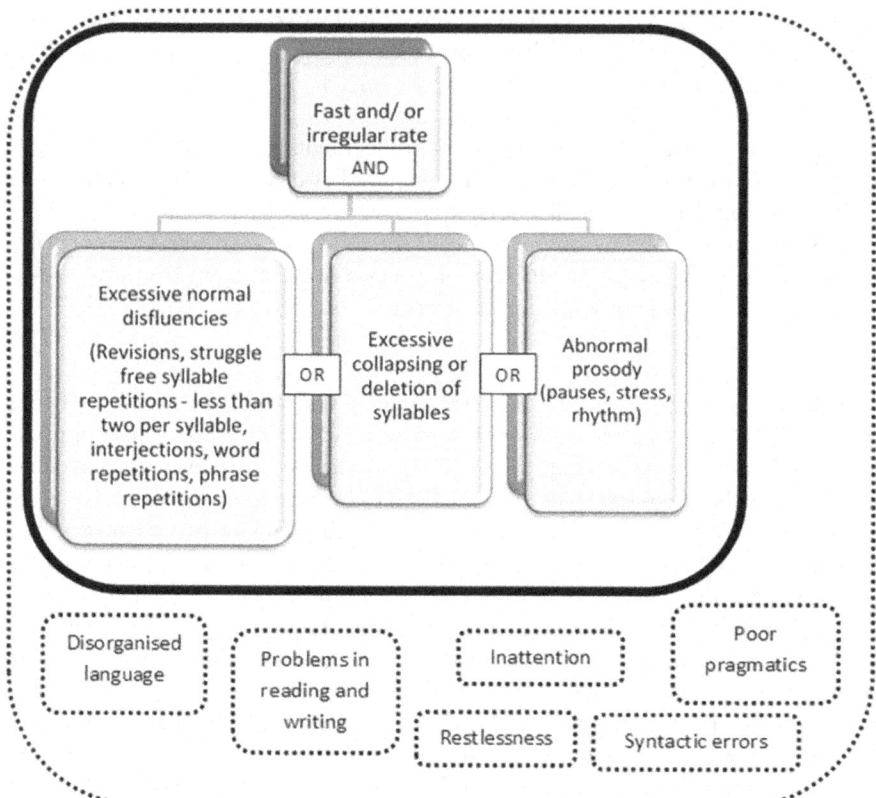

Figure 9.2 Characteristics of cluttering included in and excluded from the current definition

Interestingly, rate of speech, prosody, clarity, fluency as well as content of speech (indicating a linguistic component) stood out as differentiating features between typical and cluttered speech for naïve listeners. The World Health Organization (WHO, 2016) tries to be slightly more inclusive of language related symptoms in its recent definition of cluttering by mentioning faulty phrasing patterns:

> A rapid rate of speech with breakdown in fluency, but no repetitions or hesitations, of a severity to give rise to diminished speech intelligibility. Speech is erratic and dysrhythmic, with rapid jerky spurts that usually involve faulty phrasing patterns.

> (2016, ICD-10 F98.6, p. 345)

Another limitation is the acknowledgement that even typical speakers might exhibit the disfluencies that PWC exhibit, though at a lower frequency. The decision about the threshold at which these disfluencies might be considered reflective of cluttering is not specified. This still leaves a lot of scope for subjectivity in the diagnosis of cluttering.

The co-existence of cluttering and other disorders

Since the earliest description of cluttering as being a result of a central language imbalance (Weiss, 1964), cluttering has been known to frequently coexist with stuttering. Some researchers described cases where cluttering evolved into stuttering (Weiss, 1964), while some put forth cases where cluttering was missed initially but noticed later, once the symptoms of stuttering abated after therapy (St Louis & Myers, 1998). It was earlier estimated that around 32% to 40% of people who stutter also show symptoms of cluttering (Daly, 1993; Preus, 1981). However, recent epidemiological studies demonstrate this proportion to be about 17.6% (Howell & Davis, 2011). After applying the LCD definition, Ward (2018) estimated cluttering to be present in 25% of the cases that reported with stuttering. In such cases, the resultant speech problem could either be termed as stuttering-cluttering or cluttering-stuttering, depending on which of the two fluency disorders is relatively more prominent.

Cluttering also reportedly co-occurs with a number of other disorders, such as attention deficit-hyperactivity disorder (AD/HD) (Molt, 1996; St Louis, Myers, et al., 2007), specific learning disorders (SLD) (Ward, 2018), autism spectrum disorder (ASD) (Scaler Scott, 2011) and Down syndrome (Van Borsel, 2011; Van Borsel & Vandermeulen, 2008). Ward (2018) argued that in fact, cluttering in most cases manifests as a result of the influence of these disorders. This was put forth by Ward in the form of a multifactorial model of cluttering. Figure 9.3 presents a simplified version of the model for conceptual clarity. Ward (2018) asserted that each of these disorders has some features that culminate in a fast or irregular rate of speech. For

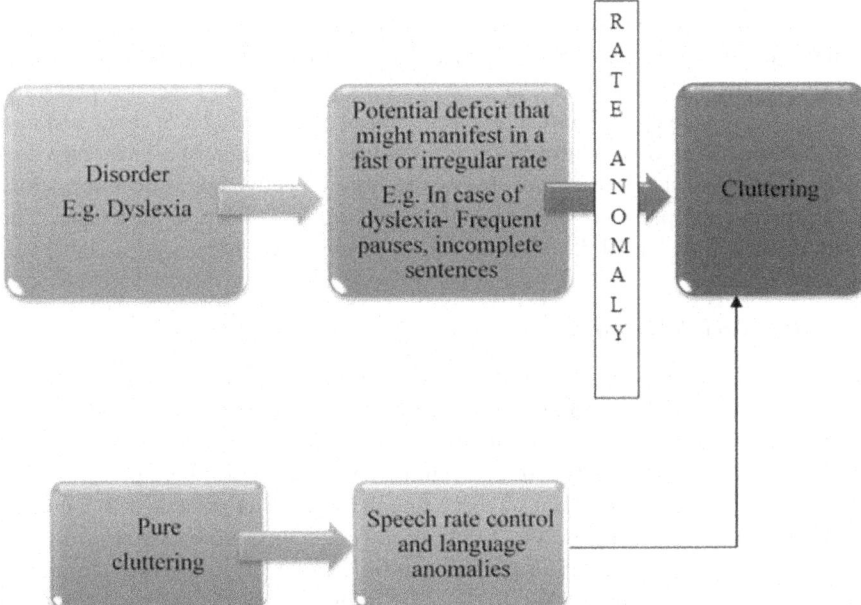

Figure 9.3 A simplified version of the multifactorial model of cluttering

example, disrupted speech rhythm in ASD or disinhibition in AD/HD might manifest in rate abnormalities and consequently cluttering. According to Ward (2018), "Those who clutter without any concomitants must (to meet criteria for the LCD definition) in some way activate the rate component of the model" (p. 166).

Ward's model, however, does not seem to be watertight in its explanation. For instance, a child with a learning disability (LD) who might have disorganized language output, but none of the features of cluttering from the LCD definition, would not be diagnosed with cluttering. Based on a study of 103 Dutch speaking children, van Zaalen (2011) outlined similarities and differences in children with LD and children with cluttering. It might just be, then, that these disorders have some neurophysiological underpinnings in common with cluttering and might, therefore, tend to co-occur frequently with cluttering. This might not necessarily mean that "external influences play a significant part" (p. 166) in its manifestation, as Ward (2018) asserts. The model also does not explain why pure cluttering exists, with no external influences to manifest it. In fact, as per recent evidence, the prevalence of pure cluttering may not be as low as it has been reported so far (St Louis et al., 2010) and needs to be ascertained with more data. Until then, cluttering could just be considered as a separate entity that may or may not co-occur with any other disorder. The LCD definition can, in fact, help identify if cluttering coexists with these disorders and reduce the risk of over-diagnosis or under-diagnosis of cluttering in the presence of these disorders. This is elaborated on in the subsection on differential diagnosis.

Subtypes of cluttering

As is apparent from the evolving definition of cluttering, there have been varied opinions about whether it is speech inaccuracy or language organization that culminates in cluttered speech. Along the way, some researchers have also presented case-based evidence of different subtypes of cluttering. Ward (2006) described two such subtypes – motoric cluttering and linguistic cluttering. More recently, van Zaalen (2009) postulated that cluttering results from defective linguistic automation. The resultant subtypes were phonological cluttering or syntactical cluttering. The predominant symptomatology of each of these subtypes is summarized in Table 9.1.

Cluttering spectrum behaviour

Recall that one of the limitations of the LCD definition is a lack of a specific threshold to differentiate typical from cluttered speech disfluencies. In fact, one of the possible reasons for a reported low prevalence of cluttering might be that some cases are either masked by a concomitant disorder and consequently miss being diagnosed as cluttering. Another reason might be that some persons either present with a limited breadth of symptoms from the LCD definition or the entire breadth of symptoms at a lower severity. This might deter clinicians from giving a diagnosis of cluttering. Ward (2006) attempted to address this issue by using the term "cluttering spectrum

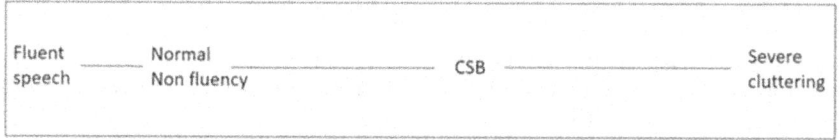

Figure 9.4 Schematic representation of the concept of cluttering spectrum behaviour (CSB)

behaviour" (CSB), as "a speech/language output that is disrupted in a manner consistent with cluttering, but where there is a) insufficient severity; b) insufficient breadth of difficulties; or c) both, to warrant a diagnosis of cluttering" (Ward, 2010b, p. 258).

CSB (Figure 9.4) thus lies on a continuum ranging from completely fluent speech at one end and severe cluttering at the other (Ward, 2011b). The term can also be used with cases that predominantly present as language or other speech disorders, with some elements of cluttering. A child with ASD, for instance, might have a monotonous speech output which lacks rhythm. This might not be combined with or result in a fast and/or irregular rate of speech. The said child would, thus, not satisfy the LCD definition. A diagnosis of ASD accompanied by CSB can be given to this child. The benefit of this would be that the intervening therapist would take a note of the symptom associated with cluttering and ensure that appropriate goals and activities are directed towards improving prosody. The term thus facilitates greater awareness of the presence of a few symptoms of cluttering which might otherwise go unnoticed, as well as their timely amelioration.

Onset and development

Most parents bring a child who exhibits cluttered speech for assessment around the age range of 6–8 years. This is not to say that cluttering might not surface before this age. Howell and Davis (2011) found the average age of detection of cluttering or cluttering-stuttering to be around 4.5 years of age. Ward (2018) cites an exception of a 3.5-year-old who fit into the LCD definition, though no similar cases seem to have been cited till date. The speech and language related symptoms of cluttering might be more noticeable in continuous discourse, which is more likely to emerge during primary school years. An excessive number of typical disfluencies, coarticulation or language disorganization might easily be dismissed by parents as a normal variation in a young child. The chances of this happening are even higher in countries such as India with multiple languages and dialects being spoken across states, where listeners might make allowances for errors in speech production (Reichel et al., 2019). This is perhaps why the average age of first reporting cluttering is pushed further to middle school years as per anecdotal evidence from India. The above reasons, coupled with relatively lower amount of self-awareness and perceived impact as compared to stuttering (Kelkar & Mukundan, 2016), might prevent preschool children from being brought to a speech clinic.

Prevalence and sex ratio

Very few studies have reported the incidence and prevalence of cluttering till date. The proportion of persons with disfluencies that manifest with pure cluttering has been estimated to lie between 5% and 16% (Bakker et al., 2005; St Louis & McCaffrey, 2005). Becker and Grundman (1970) reported a 1.5% incidence in school-going children with cluttering in the age range of 7–8 years. More recently, van Zaalen and Reichel (2017) found the prevalence of pure cluttering to be around 1.1% in Dutch children and 1.2% in German children in the age range of 10–12 years. Arnold (1960, as cited in Op't Hof & Uys, 1974) reported a male to female of 4:1. Howell and Davis (2011) shared an even more skewed gender ratio on the basis of their study of 17 PWC out of which 15 were males (about 88%). Self-reports of cluttering, however, reveal much higher prevalence figures of 11% to 16% and an almost equal male to female ratio (Fagnani et al., 2009) with males showing only a slightly higher prevalence than females (Sommer et al., 2021). Findings from India are closer to those of Howell and Davis (2011) with reference to gender distribution. A study by Kelkar and Mukundan (2016) on impact of fluency disorders included nine PWC (in a purposive sample of persons with fluency disorders who visited the fluency clinic), all of whom were males. Prevalence of cluttering has been seen to peak around four to six years of age (Sommer et al., 2021).

Etiology

Neurophysiologic basis of cluttering

Neuroanatomical correlates of cluttered speech can be found in the medial frontal cortex, specifically the anterior cingulate cortex, the putamen and the supplementary motor area (Alm, 2011; van Zaalen et al., 2009). The anterior cingulate cortex is responsible for volitional movements, error correction and monitoring, while the supplementary motor area helps in assembling and sequencing words and phrases.

The disinhibition that is characteristic of cluttering has been correlated with low occurrence of alpha waves in EEG recordings, indicative of a high activation of the medial frontal cortex (Alm, 2011). Cluttering has also been postulated to result from a hyper-dopaminergic state, which might explain the EEG abnormalities as well. The neurotransmitter dopamine controls flow of signals through the basal ganglia and as a result affects the excitation of the frontal cortex. An increased release of dopamine results in overexpression of dopamine receptors, resulting in a poor ability to estimate timing and rate of speech, which is one of the defining features of cluttering.

Brain imaging studies (van Zaalen et al., 2009) have reported high levels of activation in the ventrolateral thalamic nucleus, which might be associated with disinhibition of the supplementary motor area. The hyper-dopaminergic state might be a result of excessive synaptic release of dopamine, poor reuptake of dopamine from the synaptic cleft, or an overexpression of dopamine receptors (Alm, 2011).

Cluttered speech has also been seen to be associated with functional magnetic resonance imaging scans showing a reduced activity in the anterior lobe of the cerebellum bilaterally (Ward et al., 2015). As the anterior lobe is involved in the process of articulation (Fiez & Raichle, 1997), its under-activation correlates with the symptomatology of cluttering.

Central auditory processing

One of the causal explanations of cluttering might lie in central auditory processing deficits. Children who clutter have been seen to perform poorly as compared to age matched controls on right and left competing conditions in the Staggered Spondaic Word Test (Blood et al., 2000). Ward (2018) reported preliminary findings of a study investigating temporal processing tasks in 5 PWC and age matched controls, where significantly higher thresholds were obtained for PWC in an interval detection task.

Motor speech control

According to Ward (2011a), cluttering involves a breakdown in motor speech control at the planning, programming as well as execution levels of motor speech processing. Studies on voice onset times (VOT) and vowel duration time (VDT) in PWC have produced variable results, probably as a function of the task employed. However, the conclusion obtained from these studies as well as studies on speech kinematics is that an increase in linguistic complexity results in motor speech breakdowns in PWC (Ward, 2011a).

Effects of drugs

Effects of inhibitor and stimulant drugs on cluttered speech are in agreement with neurophysiologic findings on cluttering. Chlorpromazine, which blocks dopamine receptors, has been known to improve speech in PWC (Langova & Moravek, 1964). On the other hand, dopamine stimulant phenmetrazine worsens cluttered speech.

Genetic predisposition

The heritability of cluttering is not completely known at this point. This is because of the lack of feasibility of family, twin or adoption studies on a large scale, owing to insufficient number of cases with pure cluttering. Preliminary conclusions, however, can be drawn from genetic studies related to stuttering. For example, St Louis (1996) reported a family history in 39% of their participants who cluttered, while Howell and Davis (2011) reported it to be 47%. Their conclusions, however, were based on sample sizes smaller than 20. Lan et al. (2009) found some alleles of a gene for dopamine receptors influenced the risk of stuttering. As cluttering often co-occurs with stuttering (Daly, 1999), there is a possibility that the same gene might be related to the occurrence of cluttering as well. In a single case study by Op't Hof and Uys (1974), cluttering was seen to follow an autosomal dominant pattern of inheritance. The researchers also observed that symptoms specific to cluttering were inherited as opposed to a general language deficit.

The microgenetic model of cluttering

The various factors discussed above could work individually or in combination to manifest cluttering. The factors that might serve as potential contributors to the emergence of cluttered speech have been well summarized in the form of a micro-genetic model (Goral-Polrola et al., 2016). The model describes a complex interaction of four distinct components: (1) Main interactive factors, (2) Distal interactive factors, (3) Modelling factors and (4) Behaviour. Main interactive factors, according to the model are the motoric, linguistic and neuropsychological subcomponents of cluttering. Distal interactive factors comprise of both, genes as well as the pre-natal and peri-natal environment. Modelling factors constitute low levels of self-awareness or awareness of one's surroundings, which tend to affect the processes of attention and perception and consequently result in a higher tolerance for speech errors. The fourth component, behaviour, addresses the complex presentation of cluttering, involving a range of speech and language components, such as fluency, phonology, syntax and semantics.

The complex presentation of cluttering as described in the LCD definition as well as the microgenetic model makes cluttering assessment a challenging task. A systematic assessment protocol is described in the following subsection.

Assessment

Drawing from the various perspectives on cluttering and the LCD definition presented in the earlier part of this chapter, it follows that the assessment protocol for cluttering needs to be comprehensive enough to cover the necessary and sufficient symptoms of cluttering. Two rules of thumb for the assessment of cluttering that might be of use to the beginning clinician are as follows:

Rule 1. The lesser the attention to speech, the greater the cluttering
Rule 2. The more the complexity of the utterance, the greater the cluttering

The assessment protocol

With the above criteria as a backdrop, the assessment protocol for cluttering is described below.

Case history

In line with the characteristic features of cluttering, the case history should delve into the age of onset of the problem, as well as the nature of onset (sudden or gradual). The clinician should probe for any history of neurological injury or a family history of dis-fluency, so as to differentially diagnose developmental from neurogenic cluttering. Eliciting a developmental, academic and social history at this point would be helpful, not from a diagnostic point of view but as a clue to the presence of concomitant deficits.

This should be followed by the description of the problem in the patient's or caregiver's own words. This would reveal valuable information about the presence or absence of symptoms listed in the LCD definition as well as types of disfluencies. For instance, a parent may describe their adolescent's speech as "too fast sometimes", or "difficult to understand". Parental descriptions, in some cases, might also give leads about the concomitant presence of stuttering.

The initial interview should also probe for the presence of feared sounds or words, the patient's awareness of the problem, as well as conditions that improve or worsen fluency. This could serve as important information in the process of unambiguously ruling out concomitant stuttering. Towards the end of the interview, the clinician might attempt asking the patient about their feelings about their speech difficulty. This would in turn help in gauging their level of motivation for therapy.

Oral reading

Similar to the assessment protocol for stuttering, cluttering assessment, too, must include a reading sample. However, the cluttering assessment protocol should include more than one reading sample. Reading samples with varying levels of linguistic difficulty (van Zaalen et al., 2011) as well as reading of prepared and unprepared passages (van Zaalen, Wijnen, et al., 2009b) is recommended so as to investigate if speech worsens with an increase in linguistic complexity of the task or a reduction in attention to the task. Reading might also alert the therapist to the presence of covert or interiorized stuttering (Ward, 2018) because the client can no longer substitute or avoid words (see Chapter 3).

Narration

A narration sample in the cluttering assessment protocol must be on a topic that the PWC knows well or is interested in, so as to elicit a relaxed speech sample, as cluttering worsens in relaxed or informal speaking conditions (Table 9.2). The clinician must ask the client to narrate on a topic that requires them to think and organize the content of their speech. Tasks that involve listing out of events are not recommended (van Zaalen et al., 2008; Ward, 2006). van Zaalen et al. (2011) recommend a sample duration of at least 10 minutes in order to elicit sufficient information on the presence of any syntactic, semantic or pragmatic deficits in language.

A video recording of the above tasks is essential. Ward (2018) recommends that the therapist pretend to stop recording while actually continuing to record, to elicit a sample where the PWC is less self-conscious (remember rule 1 above). This should, of course be followed by informing the PWC about what was done once the sample is elicited, in line with ethical practice.

Conversation

A conversation task is a great way to elicit unguarded speech (rule 1), increase the linguistic demands (rule 2). It helps the clinician look for difficulties in sentence formulation, word finding, transpositions, and articulatory clustering (Ward, 2018). Prosodic difficulties which are included in the LCD definition, as well as other

Table 9.2 Key differences between stuttering and cluttering

Feature	Stuttering	Cluttering
Age when detected	2 years to 5 years of age	4.5 to 10 years of age
Subtypes	Developmental, neurogenic, psychogenic	Developmental, neurogenic
Core behaviours	Syllable repetitions, prolongations, hard blocks, silent pauses	Syllable, word and phrase repetitions, revisions, interjections
Language	Syntax, semantics and pragmatics are unaffected unless accompanied by a concomitant language delay	Syntactic errors, word retrieval problems, problems in language organization, lack of cohesion in a narrative and inappropriate turn-taking in conversation might be present
Articulation	Unaffected unless accompanied by a concomitant articulation disorder	Coarticulation, collapsing of syllables and syllable deletion errors seen
Feared sounds or words	Usually present, especially in moderate to severe stuttering	Absent
Consistency effect	High. The presence of feared sounds and words predisposes a person to stutter on the same sound or word on repeated readings.	Low. The loci of both, disfluencies and syllable collapsing might vary from one reading to the other.
Secondary behaviours	Present as visible tenseness of lips, jaw tremors, audible sounds or movements of extremities	Absent. No visible signs of struggle
Feelings and attitudes	Helplessness, anxiety, frustration, low self-esteem, anger	Anxiety, sadness, low self-confidence (to a lesser extent than stuttering)
Fluency enhancing conditions	Over-learnt speech, informal interactions, delayed auditory feedback, reading a well-prepared text	Difficult speaking situations, formal interactions, delayed auditory feedback, reading an unknown text
Therapy goal	Drawing attention away from speech	Drawing attention towards speech

features not in the definition, such as difficulties with turn-taking, topic maintenance, conversational repair, etc. can be elicited using a conversation task.

Phonological tasks

These include word and sentence repetition tasks, backward counting, etc. Repeated repetitions of the same word would give information about the consistency of articulation errors in speech. Repeating words with varying stress patterns gives information about prosodic abilities, while repeating sentences of varying complexity increases the demands on the language mechanism as well as on auditory memory (van Zaalen et al., 2011).

Story retelling

This task simultaneously assesses the ability of the PWC to paraphrase a narrative while retaining its key points; linguistic cohesion and coherence; syntax; articulation; as well as prosodic patterns in speech.

Self-awareness

The client can be asked to listen to his own recorded speech and rate various speech parameters (e.g. clarity, speed, etc.) on a scale of 1 to 5. The clinician or the caregiver can simultaneously rate the same aspects. A comparison of these ratings can provide information about how accurately the PWC can describe their problem, or in other words, the degree of self-awareness. In cases with poor self-awareness, this assessment would serve as a baseline for increasing self-monitoring skills in the PWC.

Ratio disfluencies

Subsequent to the analysis of the reading and narration samples, a ratio of the non-stuttering-like disfluencies (NSLD) to the stuttering-like disfluencies (SLD) can be calculated. A ratio of 1.7 or more has been seen to indicate possible cluttering (van Zaalen et al., 2011).

Formal assessment tools

In order to ascertain a diagnosis of cluttering or cluttering-stuttering and to quantify the amount of cluttering (and stuttering, if any), it is essential to administer the following battery of formal tests.

PREDICTIVE CLUTTERING INVENTORY (PCI; DALY, 2006) AND PCI-REVISED (VAN ZAALEN, WIJNEN, ET AL., 2009A)

The PCI, a clinician-administered tool, consists of 33 items distributed between the domains of pragmatics, speech motor, language-cognition and motor coordination-writing problems. The clinician rates each item on a 7-point Likert type scale, where "0" indicates "Never" and "7" indicates "Always". The checklist was initially created as a diagnostic tool, a score of more than 120 indicating pure cluttering, and a score ranging from 80 to 120 indicating mild cluttering or cluttering-stuttering. The checklist was revised by van Zaalen, Wijnen, et al. (2009a). The revised PCI contains 33 items of which the ones in line with the LCD definition are italicized. With a 6-point Likert type scale for every item, if the total score of the italicized items in section one exceeds 24, cluttering is indicated. The second section includes items that give information about the linguistic component of cluttering, and the third and fourth sections give information about communication skills. Ward (2018), however, expressed concern over the use of the above checklists as diagnostic tools for lack of adequate evidence to validate the scoring system and recommends using them as outcome measures rather than diagnostic tools.

MODIFIED CHECKLIST OF CLUTTERING AND ASSOCIATED BEHAVIOURS (COCAF; WARD, 2018)

This checklist includes features related to speech rate, fluency, articulation, language, and other features that might be related to cognition, attention, writing, etc. These are rated by the therapist on a 3-point scale, where 1 indicates that the feature is within normal limits, 2 indicates that it appears more commonly than in typical speakers, and 3 indicates that it is a strong feature. There are two additional columns to indicate whether the feature was observed during assessment or whether it is seen in extra-clinical situations. This automatically ropes in the caregiver in the assessment process, while simultaneously alerting the PWC to features they might not have been aware of.

CLUTTERING SEVERITY INSTRUMENT (CSI; BAKKER & MYERS, 2011)

A value addition to cluttering assessment, the CSI is a software that facilitates quantification of cluttering. The clinician must listen to the speech sample a minimum of three times in the CSI, during which the cluttering moments are selected by the clinician. Based on this assessment, the software calculates the percentage of the sample cluttered. In addition, the clinician also rates eight different aspects of speech on visual analogue scales – overall intelligibility, speech rate regularity, speech rate, articulation precision, typical disfluency, language disorganization, discourse management, and prosody. On each scale, the clinician can provide both a point estimate and a range estimate to account for variability across tasks and situations. To increase inter-rater reliability, each scale also has five descriptive anchors ranging from "normal" to "extremely deviant". A combination of the visual analogue scale ratings and the percentage sample cluttered gives a weighted CSI score (based on expert opinions of 31 fluency specialists). The CSI can thus be used to tailor therapy to the needs of the PWC as well as to measure the outcomes of therapy.

STUTTERING SEVERITY INSTRUMENT-4 (RILEY, 2009)

Administration of the SSI-4 is an inseparable part of cluttering assessment. This is to ensure that stuttering is ruled out before arriving at a diagnosis of pure cluttering. In cases of cluttering-stuttering, it helps to quantify the stuttering and guide treatment. In combination with the LCD definition, the PCI and the CSI, the SSI-4 enables an accurate diagnosis of cluttering.

THE MOUNT WILGA HIGH LEVEL LANGUAGE TEST (SIMPSON, 2006)

Ward (2018) recommends using this test for picking up subtle language difficulties that might be missed by formal language assessment tools. This is a freely downloadable tool. However, language proficiency in English might vary across populations even though English might be the primary language of communication. If items in the above tool seem difficult for most typical speakers in a region, an informal assessment of language through tasks such as narration and conversation is recommended.

In the context of comprehensive assessment of cluttering, a recently developed Fluency Assessment Battery (FAB; van Zaalen & Reichel, 2015) deserves a mention. The battery includes the Predictive Cluttering Inventory-Revised (van Zaalen, Wijnen, et al., 2009a), followed by an analysis of rate of speech, grammatical encoding, phonological accuracy and fluency through various speech tasks, such as reading, story retelling and spontaneous speech. One of the unique aspects of the FAB is measurement of mean articulatory rate (MAR) and articulatory rate variation (ARV) in addition to speech rate and articulatory rate. For measuring MAR, articulatory rate over five consecutive sequences of 10–20 syllables is measured. The mean of these five values is the MAR. ARV is measured both within a speech task and between two speech tasks, such as reading and story retelling. According to van Zaalen and Reichel (2015), MAR values in typical speakers range from 4.5 to 5.5 syllables per second and ARV values range from 1 to 3.3 syllables per second. ARV values greater than 3.3 within tasks or less than 1.0 between tasks are considered abnormal values. Fluency assessment involves the use of the SSI-4. Grammatical encoding is checked through retelling of the Wallet story. Assessment involves noting the down the number of main issues and side issues in the story that the client was able to retell, noting down errors in syntax, etc. Phonological encoding is evaluated using the Screening Phonological Accuracy Test (SPA; van Zaalen, Wijnen, et al., 2009b). These assessments reportedly help differentially diagnose phonological from syntactic cluttering. Finally, the FAB also includes assessment of speech motor control using the Oral Motor Assessment Scale (OMAS). Although more empirical evidence is required to provide robust evidence of the differential diagnostic characteristics of the FAB, it does enable comprehensive assessment and documentation of core speech behaviours in those who clutter.

A fundamental difficulty in all the above assessments (except the SSI-4) is that they rely heavily on the clinician's judgement and are, therefore, susceptible to large inter-judge variability. Beginning clinicians might often find themselves in a dilemma over scoring a behaviour as within normal limits or beyond. A guiding rule for them would be to decide based on whether (and how much) the feature compromises on the intelligibility and coherence of the speech output and consequently on the ease of communication.

Assessment of language and articulation

If the above assessment protocol indicates the presence of a language delay or speech sound errors, these need to be assessed and quantified through formal testing. In India, the MISHA Test of Communication Development in Marathi (Sanghi et al., 2021) the Assessment of Language Development (ALD; Lakkanna et al., 2021), or the Linguistic Profile Test (LPT; Ali Yavar Jung National Institute for the Hearing Handicapped, 1988a) are tools with an indigenous normative for children, while adolescents can be tested using the Manipal Manual of Adolescent Language Assessment (MMALA; Karuppalli & Bhat, 2016). Articulation can be assessed formally using the Photo Articulation Test (PAT; Ali Yavar Jung National Institute for the Hearing Handicapped, 1988b) available in multiple Indian languages. If presence of a language delay or speech sound disorder is detected, these will be considered concomitant disorders and not included under the diagnosis of cluttering. This is further touched upon in the next subsection.

Differential diagnosis

Since stuttering and cluttering often coexist, it is of primary importance especially for beginning clinicians to be able to distinguish one from the other. Table 9.2 summarizes the key differences in the two fluency disorders.

Cluttering might have some features in common with disorders such as learning disabilities, AD/HD or childhood apraxia of speech. Cluttering has also been known to co-occur with several disorders like SLD, AD/HD, ASD, etc. In such cases, clinicians might tend to clump all the features under one diagnosis, either that of cluttering or the co-occurring disorder. It is, however, important to understand similarities and differences between cluttering and these disorders to steer away from an incorrect or, more often, an incomplete diagnosis. The LCD definition has helped this along to some extent. A few salient differential diagnostic indicators are summarized in Table 9.3.

Assessing attitudes and feelings

A feature of PWC that has been stressed on since its earliest definitions (Daly, 1993; Weiss, 1964) is the unawareness of the problem. It is, however, important to interpret this phrase with caution and examine its various implications. Unlike persons who stutter, PWC do not exhibit anxiety specific to sounds or words (Ward, 2006). While some PWC might be completely unaware of their speech disorder unless it is pointed out by significant others, some might be well aware, though they might not be aware of precise moments of cluttering or might underestimate the severity of their cluttering. In fact, recent reports of PWC reveal that they might, in fact, have negative attitudes towards speaking situations which might be triggered when they are unable to express their thoughts as cohesively as they would like to or when listeners frequently ask them to repeat what they said (Daly & Burnett, 1999; Ward, 2018). As a result, they might often experience anxiety, frustration, sadness, and poor self-confidence (Daly, 1993; Reichel, 2010).

Till date, there are no standardized instruments to assess attitudes of PWC. Modifications of tools for assessing stuttering related attitudes, however, are presently being used to assess attitudes related to cluttered speech. One such tool is the Perceptions of Speech Communication (PSC; Daly, 1993) which is created by substituting stuttering in the Perceptions of Stuttering Inventory (PSI; Woolf, 1967) by the word "communication".

Similarly, the St Louis Inventory of Life Perspectives and Speech/Language difficulty (SL. ILP-SL) (St Louis, 2005) has been adapted for use with persons with cluttering, from the St Louis Inventory of Life Perspectives and Stuttering (St Louis, 2001). The questions investigate different aspects like the degree of handicap felt, the desire to get help, the severity of the problem, the importance given to the problem,

Table 9.3 Similarities and differences between cluttering and other disorders

Disorder	Similarities	Differences
Learning disabilities (LD)	Reading and writing deficits, problems in handedness, poor language organization	Rate of speech might not always be affected in children with LD. Reading and writing deficits are relatively milder in children who clutter as compared to children with LD. Children with LD have poor mathematics and reasoning abilities while these are usually unaffected in children who clutter.
Attention-deficit hyperactivity disorder (AD/HD)	Short attention span, poor self-inhibition, language deficits	A fast or irregular rate of speech may not always be present in AD/HD. Language deficits in AD/HD might be reflective of language delay, while those in cluttered speech reflect language disorganization.
Childhood apraxia of speech (CAS)	Inconsistent articulatory errors, poor prosody	CAS exhibit a slow rate of speech while PWC show a fast or irregular rate. There are more substitution errors in CAS, while more coarticulation errors in cluttering. The struggle and frustration seen in CAS is not seen in cluttered speech.
Delayed language development	Difficulties in language organization and sentence formulation; pragmatic difficulties	A discrepancy in chronological and language age may not be seen in PWC.
Speech sound disorder	Coarticulation, especially for long and complex words, sound transpositions	Errors in a speech sound disorder are consistently seen for specific sounds, while those in cluttered speech are inconsistent and might display no particular pattern. Errors in cluttered speech are not a result of an organic deficit, as might be seen in speech sound disorders as a result of conditions such as tongue tie.

etc. High scores on many items in the ISL indicate that the person experiences severe suffering, disability and handicap as a result of their cluttering. The Communication Attitude Test (CAT; Brutten & Vanryckeghem, 2006) might also be used for self-assessment of attitudes towards communication in a PWC.

Assessing impact of cluttering

Although the impact of stuttering can be successfully quantified using a variety of tools (Ayre & Wright, 2009; Yaruss, Coleman, et al., 2010; Yaruss & Quesal, 2006; Yaruss, Quesal, et al., 2010), no standardized tool for assessing impact of cluttering is presently in use. Kelkar and Mukundan (2015) constructed the Impact Scale for Assessment of Cluttering and Stuttering (ISACS). The tool then underwent preliminary validation using data from 52 persons with fluency disorders and their significant others (Kelkar et al., 2018). A significant feature of the tool is that it assesses impact of fluency disorders from two perspectives – that of the person with the fluency disorder and that of their significant other. However, owing to the relatively small proportion of PWC in the sample, the scale is currently in the process of standardization. Given the large number of persons exhibiting stuttering-cluttering or cluttering-stuttering, the common neurological underpinnings for both fluency disorders and similar communicative barriers faced by persons who stutter (PWS) and PWC, the tool seems to be a promising addition to assessment of cluttering. Both parallel forms of the ISACS, the ISACS(A) and (B) are reproduced in Appendix B so as to be useful to clinicians for holistic assessment of cluttering (and stuttering). The case examples below reflect the need for assessment of impact of cluttering. The relationship between impact and severity of cluttering symptoms might not necessarily be a linear one. Delving further into the nature of this relationship could be an interesting direction for future research.

Case examples

A 52-year-old male reported to the clinic with a speech problem that he described as "speaking at a very fast speed. . .. My thoughts run faster than my speech". The complaints were reportedly seen in both languages that he spoke, Hindi and English, but it was seen more frequently in Hindi, his native language. He was a businessman by profession and felt that his speech impacted his growth opportunities to some extent. Based on his symptomatology in line with the LCD definition, he was diagnosed as exhibiting cluttering spectrum behaviour. His total score in the CSI was 22.3%. Impact score on ISACS (A) was 33.6%.

Another male, a college student, was diagnosed with cluttering, his symptoms being of a much higher severity than the previous case example. His score on the CSI was 51.6% and that on the ISACS(A) was 57.6%.

Another male with a diagnosis of cluttering was embarrassed to reveal to anyone in his extended family that he was seeking therapy for his speech disorder.

These case examples highlight the fact that irrespective of the severity of the presenting features of cluttering, PWC are not only aware of the fact that they have atypical speech, but are also functionally and emotionally affected by it.

Management

A comprehensive assessment protocol as described in the previous subsection facilitates effective and efficient management of the various subcomponents of cluttering. Many of the popular approaches to cluttering management recommend a synergistic mode of intervention. Synergism refers to the coordinated and synchronous movements of the various components of the speech mechanism. A synergistic mode of intervention thus follows the rationale that working on one aspect of communication would also affect others. Three such approaches are discussed below.

Profile analysis and synergistic treatment (Daly, 1993)

In line with the five key areas listed in the linguistic disfluency model, Daly (1993) recommended a profile analysis of features associated with cluttering. Subsequent to the analysis, each of the five dimensions should be targeted in each therapy session. This is feasible only if a synergistic approach to therapy is used, where more than one goal is addressed simultaneously.

The cognitive-behavioural approach and the A-frame model (Myers, 2011)

The model depicts the intervention of stuttering as a triangle shaped home set on a foundation of meta-awareness, which represents the cognitive part of the approach. It involves familiarizing the PWC with the nature of cluttering and increasing their awareness of their own cluttering related behaviours and their frequency of occurrence. The central beam of the triangle or the "A-frame home" is rate control. The three walls of the triangle (or the insulation of the A-frame home) depict three essential components of intervention, namely, monitoring, modulation and moderation of cluttering related behaviours. Myers (2011) advocates the use of several auditory, visual and movement analogies for increasing meta-awareness of the various aspects of cluttering, primarily rate and coordination of speech movements. Strategies for improving self-monitoring as well as monitoring of the feedback received from the listener; moderation of rate and control over compulsive, impulsive and propulsive moments during speech; and modulation (voluntary variation) of clarity, intelligibility, prosody and rate of speech are encouraged. In this manner, the model targets both, motoric and linguistic aspects of cluttering through a systematic and structured approach.

Ward's synergistic treatment protocol (Ward, 2006)

Ward (2006) strongly recommended gathering of information about the PWC from multiple sources like parents, teachers, and other professionals, if any, to formulate an individualized treatment plan. This is followed by a four-step protocol, which starts with identification of cluttering. This step involves working on the client's knowledge of his own cluttering and helping them set realistic and tangible goals. The second step, monitoring and self-awareness, builds further on the first step by training the client to detect and self-monitor errors made. The third step involves modification or gaining control over the various affected aspects of speech. The final step helps the client maintain the acquired fluency and make the client self-reliant.

Numerous other models have been advocated for use with PWC. For instance, van Zaalen and Reichel (2014) stress on the use of a four-component model, targeting thoughts, feelings, verbal-motor and communicative components of cluttering.

Bennett Lanouette (2011) incorporates therapy for language disorders to improve language organization and thus reduce cluttering in a cognitive-linguistic approach.

A closer look at each of the above approaches reveals some common speech-related goals that may be targeted for a majority of PWC. Various techniques and activities can be employed to work towards realizing these goals. Myers (2011) put forth an exhaustive list of techniques to facilitate monitoring, modulation and moderation of various aspects of speech output. Reichel et al. (2019) proposed the use of mirror reading, which involved reading a short phrase silently followed by articulating it while looking at a mirror. The process is repeated throughout a reading passage to facilitate a habitual slow rate through short phrases and frequent pauses. Kelkar (2022) proposed the use of two finger feedback, that is, placement of two fingers below the lower jaw to facilitate kinesthetic feedback while jaw opening. This initiates a cycle of self-monitoring and self-correction through engagement of an additional sensory channel. Broad goals that may be targeted in therapy for most adolescents and adults who clutter along with corresponding techniques or activities are summarized in Table 9.4.

Instruments such as delayed auditory feedback (DAF) and metronome may also be employed. However, reports of their use have usually revealed mixed results (St Louis et al., 1996). It might also be a short-term change that might be hard for the PWC to maintain without the use of these appliances.

For school-going children, however, the approach might not be as straightforward. Features of cluttered speech in a school-going child might be noticed by parents and teachers as different or something that needs urgent attention. For the child, although speaking might become a mildly unpleasant experience for often being asked to repeat, the features of cluttering cannot be easily singled out by parents, teachers or the child. As a result, the motivation of the child for self-monitoring and following up for therapy would most likely be poor. To overcome this problem, Scaler Scott and Ward (2013, as cited in Ward, 2018) suggested a backdoor approach. This involves increasing the child's awareness of speech and features related to cluttered speech through alerting them to errors in other people's speech or through demonstration of different types of speech by the therapist through games, where the child detects a certain feature (e.g. coarticulation in speech).

Management of negative thoughts and feelings related to cluttering

A large number of researchers have proposed the use of cognitive approaches to the abatement of negative thoughts and feelings in PWC. The approaches advocated include relaxation, positive self-talk, affirmation training, etc. (Daly, 1993). Reichel (2010) advocated the use of five emotional intelligence skills, namely, emotional self-awareness, impulse control, reality resting, empathy and interpersonal relationships to work on cognitive and affective aspects of cluttering.

Prognosis and recovery

In their longitudinal study of 17 children who cluttered, Howell and Davis (2011) found that 5 children persisted with cluttering while the remaining 12 continued

Table 9.4 Common goals and activities for PWC

Goal	Activity/technique
Self-monitoring	• Negative practice • Evaluating one's own recordings • Focusing on valving of articulators
Speech rate control	• Syllabification (dividing words into syllables) • Over coarticulation • Block design • Prolongation • Alternating between a slow and fast rate of speech • Pausing and phrasing
Language organization	• Retelling a story • Correcting a story • Using index cards for storytelling • Describing similarities and differences
Semantics/word retrieval	• Unscrambling words • Vocabulary building • Word association • Cloze activities (sentence completion)
Pragmatics	• Role reversals in a discourse • Noting listener reactions • Awareness of pragmatic violations • Training in appropriate ways of requesting clarification • Turn-taking in role-play
Prosody	• Emphasis on stressed syllables • Varying syllable and word stress • Using emphatic stress in sentences • Differentiating levels of pitch • Pitch modulation exercises
Oral motor coordination	• Negative practice • Exaggerated articulation • Attending to word endings
Maintenance of fluency	• Discussing relapse • Discussing prognosis • Discussing factors which might contribute to prognosis and relapse

to have cluttered speech. Cluttering that does not receive intervention in childhood and persists into adulthood, however, is unlikely to completely recover (Ward, 2018). Even if intervention is obtained in early years, prognosis with therapy depends on a number of factors like the severity of cluttering, knowledge and expertise of the therapist, and most importantly, the level of self-awareness, persistence and motivation of the PWC. Other variables within and outside the PWC might also contribute to the prognosis to some extent. These can be better understood by familiarizing oneself with the biopsychosocial model (World Health Organization (WHO; 2001).

Superimposing the biopsychosocial model on cluttering

The section on assessment of cluttering and the case examples given above might have made it clear to the readers that the phenomenon of cluttering encompasses many aspects beyond just core speech (and language) symptoms. It includes the thoughts, feelings and behaviours of the PWC, and the resultant effect of these on their daily functioning and quality of life. The environment plays an additional role in influencing all the above variables.

The International Classification of Functioning, Disability and Health (ICF; WHO, 2001) was a big step towards summarizing and quantification of these variables uniquely for every individual. Yaruss (2007) defined these variables in the context of fluency disorders. The impairment, the resultant limitations in function, the environmental and personal variables that might improve or further limit functioning, and the consequent quality of life, together constitute the impact of cluttering. Measuring impact, therefore, is the most crucial to accurate outcome measurement. Assessment and management along the lines of the biopsychosocial model gives the therapist a complete picture of the person rather than the disorder (Fanning, 2018). For instance, therapy using any of the approaches mentioned under management might reduce the impairment. However, if the person's thoughts and feelings about their cluttering or environmental support systems are not addressed in therapy, the reduction in overall impact might not be commensurate with the reduction in core speech symptoms. More importantly, the PWC might still feel dissatisfied with therapy. Tools such as ISACS (see Appendix B) prove to be useful for comprehensively quantifying the different facets of cluttering. Unlike other tools structured along the ICF, the form (B) of the ISACS quantifies the perspective of significant others, which might be a variable that requires intervention.

Expanding the circle of environment a little further then, public attitudes towards cluttering might also have an influence on the degree of impact of the disorder experienced by PWC.

Public attitudes towards cluttering

As opposed to stuttering, the struggle faced by a PWC in the production of fluent speech is not apparent to a listener (Ward, 2010a). As a result, the resultant disorganized output may not be attributed by the listener to a chronic speech disorder, resulting in the PWC being perceived as "stressed, insecure, scared or stupid" (Kvenseth, 2007). The impact of cluttering is perceived as significantly lower than that of stuttering (Kelkar & Mukundan, 2016), which might partly be related to the lower visibility of struggle experienced by a PWC. The reader may recall from the section on the LCD definition of cluttering, that listeners from Pune, India heard two recorded samples, one each of typical and cluttered speech, and rated cluttered speech as less natural, justifying their ratings with reasons such as poorer clarity, fluency, prosody and language organization (Kaul et al., 2022). A follow-up study then investigated acceptability of speech of the PWC in different social roles (as compared to the typical speaker). There was no significant difference in acceptability of speech of the PWC and the typical speaker in any of the social roles studied. This indicates that while the population studied considered cluttered speech to be different, they did not perceive it as unacceptable.

A study comparing attitudes towards stuttering with those towards cluttering was carried out in four countries – USA, Russia, Turkey and Bulgaria – in their native languages (St Louis, Coskun, et al., 2007; St Louis et al., 2011). A convenience sample of a total of 302 respondents from the four countries responded to an adapted version of the POSHA-E (Public Opinion Survey of Human Attributes; St Louis et al., 2009). Mean ages ranged from 26 to 33 years. The POSHA-E was adapted for the study (POSHA-Cl) by adding cluttering to the general section and adding a detailed section on cluttering to the existing detailed section on stuttering. Cluttering was viewed as negatively as mental illness. People seemed to be slightly less tolerant and patient with a PWC than a PWS and slightly more concerned if someone close to them had cluttering than stuttering, though the differences were not significant. They considered that persons with cluttering would be able to socialize, make friends, do well in school, raise a family or lead normal lives. However, ratings for being able to do any job they wanted to were low. The mean ratings for good judgement, earning people's trust or being described as influential were below neutral for cluttering and significantly lower than for stuttering. Although respondents' ratings were relatively neutral across all the four countries, they still rated "wanting to have cluttering" lower than "mental illness" or "using a wheelchair". Furthermore, they could not completely dismiss the possibility of cluttering being caused by viruses or an act of God.

The above findings indicate an urgent need for public education about cluttering so as to facilitate its early identification and intervention, as well as to improve the quality of life of PWC. Recent research has revealed that a large proportion of the general public, when given a description of cluttering, seem to be acquainted with at least one PWC (Blanchet et al., 2015; St Louis et al., 2010). Public education about cluttering and speech therapy might, then, increase footfalls of PWC in speech clinics (Reichel et al., 2019; St Louis et al., 2010). This is likely to stimulate further research, bringing us closer to a data-based definition of cluttering, which in turn could translate to increased efficacy in management of this elusive disorder.

Summary points to remember

- Cluttering can exist alone or along with stuttering.
- The definition of cluttering has evolved over many decades into a symptom-based definition.
- The term cluttering spectrum behaviour ensures identification of subtle features of cluttering.
- The etiology of cluttering has been attributed to multiple factors like auditory processing, motor speech programming, neurophysiological differences related to the basal ganglia and cerebellum, and genes as well.
- Assessment of cluttering must be comprehensive and must account for all the necessary symptoms for its diagnosis.
- Management of cluttering must be structured so as to be efficient, yet individualized enough to account for variations in the symptomatology of every PWC.
- Public education about cluttering and speech therapy is the need of the hour.

Study questions

1. List the essential areas of assessment in a PWC.
2. Explain Weiss's perspective on cluttering.
3. Differentiate between stuttering and cluttering.
4. Explain the concept of cluttering spectrum behaviour.
5. Elaborate on the Cluttering Severity Instrument. Explain how it is a value addition to cluttering assessment.

References

Abe, K., Yokoyama, R., & Yorifuji, S. (1993). Repetitive speech disorder resulting from infarcts in the paramedian thalami and midbrain. *Journal of Neurology, Neurosurgery, and Psychiatry, 56*(9), 1024–1026. https://doi.org/10.1136/jnnp.56.9.1024

Adams, M.R. (1974). A physiologic and aerodynamic interpretation of fluent and stuttered speech. *Journal of Fluency Disorders, 1*, 35–47.

Ahmed, H.H., & Mohammad, H. O. (2018). Social anxiety disorders among stutterers: Effects of different variants. *Egyptian Journal of Otolaryngology, 34*, 155–164.

Ali Yavar Jung National Institute for the Hearing Handicapped (AYJNIHH). (1988a). *Linguistic profile test*. AYJNIHH.

Ali Yavar Jung National Institute for the Hearing Handicapped (AYJNIHH). (1988b). *Photo articulation test*. AYJNIHH.

Al-Khaledi, M., Lincoln, M., McCabe, P., & Alshatti, T. (2018). The Lidcombe program: A series of case studies with Kuwaiti preschool children who stutter. *Speech, Language, and Hearing, 21*(4), 224–235.

Alm, P.A. (2014). Stuttering in relation to anxiety, temperament, and personality: Review and analysis with focus on causality *Journal of Fluency Disorders, 40*, 5–21.

Alm, P.A. (2011). Cluttering: A neurological perspective. In D. Ward & K. Scaler Scott (Eds.), *Cluttering: A handbook of research, intervention and education* (pp. 3–28). Psychology Press.

Ambrose, N.G., & Yairi, E. (1995). The role of repetition units in the differential diagnosis of early childhood incipient stuttering. *American Journal of Speech-Language Pathology, 4*, 82–88.

Ambrose, N.G., & Yairi, E. (1999). Normative disfluency data for early childhood stuttering. *Journal of Speech, Language, and Hearing Research, 42*(4), 895–909.

Ambrose, N.G., Yairi, E., Loucks, T.M., Seery, C.H., & Throneburg, R. (2015). Relation of motor, linguistic and temperament factors in epidemiologic subtypes of persistent and recovered stuttering: Initial findings. *Journal of Fluency Disorders, 45*, 12–26.

American Speech-Language-Hearing Association. (1995). Guidelines for practice in stuttering treatment. *ASHA, 37*(14), 26–35.

Anderson, J.D., & Conture, E.G. (2000). Language abilities of children who stutter: A preliminary study. *Journal of Fluency Disorders, 25*(4), 283–304.

Anderson, J.D., & Conture, E.G. (2004). Sentence structure priming in young children who stutter. *Journal of Speech and Hearing Research, 47*, 552–571.

Anderson, J.D., Pellowski, M.W., Conture, E.G., & Kelly, E.M. (2003). Temperamental characteristics of young children who stutter. *Journal of Speech, Language, and Hearing Research, 46*, 1221–1233.

Anderson, J.D., Wagovich, S.A., & Brown, B.T. (2019). Phonological and semantic contributions to verbal short-term memory in young children with developmental stuttering. *Journal of Speech, Language, and Hearing Research, 62*(3), 644–667.

Anderson, J.D., Wagovich, S.A., & Hall, N.E. (2006). Nonword repetition skills in young children who do and do not stutter. *Journal of Fluency Disorders, 31*(3), 177–199.

Anderson, J.M., Hood, S.B., & Sellers, D.E. (1988). Central auditory processing abilities of adolescent and preadolescent stuttering and nonstuttering children. *Journal of Fluency Disorders, 13*, 199–214.

Anderson, T.K., & Felsenfeld, S. (2003). A thematic analysis of late recovery from stuttering. *American Journal of Speech-Language Pathology, 12*(2), 243–253.

Andrade, C.R., & Juste, F.S. (2011). Systematic review of delayed auditory feedback effectiveness for stuttering reduction. *Journal Da Sociedade Brasileira Fonoaudiologia, 23*(2), 187–191.

Andrews, C., O'Brian, S., Onslow, M., Packman, A., Menzies, R., & Lowe, R. (2016). Phase II trial of syllable-timed speech treatment for school-age children who stutter. *Journal of Fluency Disorders, 48*, 44–55.

Andrews, G., & Craig, A. (1988). Prediction of outcome after treatment for stuttering. *The British Journal of Psychiatry, 153*(2), 236–240.

Andrews, G., Craig, A., Feyer, A., Hoddinott, S., Howie, P., & Neilson, M. (1983). Stuttering: A review of research findings and theories circa 1982. *Journal of Speech and Hearing Disorders, 48*, 226–246.

Andrews, G., & Cutler, J. (1974). Stuttering therapy: The relation between changes in symptom level and attitudes. *Journal of Speech and Hearing Disorders, 39*(3), 312–319.

Andrews, G., Guitar, B., & Howie, P. (1980). Meta-analysis of the effects of stuttering treatment. *Journal of Speech and Hearing Disorders, 45*(3), 287–307.

Andrews, G., & Harris, M. (1964). The syndrome of stuttering. In *Clinics in developmental medicine no. 17.* Spastics Society Medical Education and Information Unit, in association with W. Heinemann Medical Books.

Andrews, G., & Ingham, R. J. (1971). Stuttering: Considerations in the evaluation of treatment. *British Journal of Disorders of Communication, 6*(2), 129–138.

Andrews, G., & Ingham, R.J. (1972). An approach to the evaluation of stuttering therapy. *Journal of Speech and Hearing Research, 15*(2), 296–302.

Andrews, G., Morris-Yates, A., Howie, P., & Martin, N.G. (1991). Genetic factors in stuttering confirmed. *Archives of General Psychiatry, 48*(11), 1034–1035.

Andy, O.J., & Bhatnagar, S.C. (1992). Stuttering acquired from subcortical pathologies and its alleviation from thalamic perturbation. *Brain and Language, 42*(4), 385–401.

Anjana, B.R. (2015). *Disfluencies in two point one to 6 year old Kannada speaking children* [Unpublished thesis submitted to University of Mysore].

Anjana, R., & Savithri, S.R. (2013). *Disfluencies in 2.1 to 6 year old Kannada speaking children* [Unpublished doctoral thesis submitted to the University of Mysore].

Antipova, E.A., Purdy, S.C., Blakeley, M., & Williams, S. (2008). Effects of altered auditory feedback (AAF) on stuttering frequency during monologue speech production. *Journal of Fluency Disorders, 33*(4), 274–290.

Ardila, A., & Lopez, M.V. (1986). Severe stuttering associated with right hemisphere lesion. *Brain and Language, 27*(2), 239–246.

Armson, J., & Stuart, A. (1998). Effect of extended exposure to frequency-altered feedback on stuttering during reading and monologue. *Journal of Speech, Language, and Hearing Research, 41*(3), 479–490.

Arnott, S., Onslow, M., O'Brian, S., Packman, A., Jones, M., & Block, S. (2014). Group Lidcombe program treatment for early stuttering: A randomized controlled trial. *Journal of Speech, Language, and Hearing Research, 57*(5), 1606–1618.

Arya, P., & Geetha, Y.V. (2013). Factors related to recovery and relapse in persons with stuttering following treatment: A preliminary study. *Disability, CBR & Inclusive Development, 24*(1), 82–98.

Aryal, D., & Maruthy, S. (2022). Linguistic factors and stuttering in Nepali speaking adults who stutter. *Clinical Linguistics & Phonetics*, 1–14. https://doi.org/10.1080/02699206.2022.2049880.

Au-Yeung, J., Howell, P., & Pilgrim, L. (1998). Phonological words and stuttering on function words. *Journal of Speech, Language and Hearing Research, 41*(5), 1019–1030.

Ayre, A., & Wright, L. (2009). WASSP: An international review of its clinical application. *International Journal of Speech-Language Pathology, 11*(1), 83–90.

Azrin, N.H., & Nunn, R.G. (1974). A rapid method of eliminating stuttering by a regulated breathing approach. *Behaviour Research and Therapy, 12*(4), 279–286.

Backus, O. (1957). Group structure in speech therapy. In L.E. Travis (Ed.), *Handbook of speech pathology* (pp. 1025–1064). Appleton-Century-Crofts, Inc.

Bajaj, A. (2007). Analysis of oral narratives of children who stutter and their fluent peers: Kindergarten through second grade. *Clinical Linguistics & Phonetics, 21*(3), 227–245.

Bakhtiar, M., Abad Ali, D.A., & Sadegh, S.P.M. (2007). Nonword repetition ability of children who do and do not stutter and covert repair hypothesis. *Indian Journal of Medical Sciences, 61*, 462–470.

Bakhtiar, M., & Packman, A. (2009). Intervention with the Lidcombe Program for a bilingual school-age child who stutters in Iran. *Folia Phoniatrica et Logopaedica, 61*, 300–304.

Bakker, K., & Myers, F. (2011). *Instructional manual for the cluttering severity instrument.* Retrieved May 15, 2016, from https://associations.missouristate.edu/ica/Resources/Resources%20and%20Links%20pages/CSI%20software%20ALL/CSI%20Manual_EN.pdf.

Bakker, K., & Riley, G.D. (2009). *Computerized scoring of stuttering severity (CSSS-2.0).* Pro-Ed Inc.

Bakker, K., St Louis, K.O., Myers, F.L., & Raphael, L.J. (2005). Computer aided assessment of cluttering severity. In *Paper presented at the 8th international stuttering awareness day online conference.* Retrieved March 14, 2021, from www.mnsu.edu/comdis/isad8/papers/bakker8/bakker8.html.

Balasubramanian, T. (1980). Timing in Tamil. *Journal of Phonetics, 8*, 449–468.

Balasubramanian, V., Cronin, K.L., & Max, L. (2010). Dysfluency levels during repeated readings, choral readings, and readings with altered auditory feedback in two cases of acquired neurogenic stuttering. *Journal of Neurolinguistics, 23*(5), 488–500.

Bancroft, S. (2011). *Does changing parent verbal interaction styles increase fluency in children who stutter?* www.uwo.ca/fhs/lwm/teaching/EBP/2011_12/Bancroft.pdf

Barasch, C.T., Guitar, B., McCauley, R.J., & Absher, R.G. (2000). Disfluency and time perception. *Journal of Speech, Language, and Hearing Disorders, 43*, 1429–1439.

Barbara, D.A. (1965). *New directions in stuttering: Theory and practice.* Charles C. Thomas.

Baumgartner, J. (1999). Acquired psychogenic stuttering. In R. F. Curlee (Ed.), *Stuttering and related disorders of fluency* (pp. 269–288). Thieme Medical Publishers.

Becker, K.P., & Grundman, K. (1970). Investigations on incidence and symptomatology of cluttering. *Folia Phoniatrica, 22*(4), 261–271.

Bennett Lanouette, E. (2011). Intervention strategies for cluttering disorders. In D. Ward & K. Scaler Scott (Eds.), *Cluttering: A handbook of research, intervention and education* (pp. 175–197). Psychology Press.

Bernstein Ratner, N. (2005). Evidence-based practice in stuttering: Some questions to consider. *Journal of Fluency Disorders, 30*(3), 163–188.

Bernstein Ratner, N. (2018). Selecting treatments and monitoring outcomes: The circle of evidence-based practice and client-centered care in treating a preschool child who stutters. *Language, Speech, and Hearing Services in Schools, 49*(1), 13–22.

Bertinetto, P.M. (1980). Perception of stress by Italian speakers. *Journal of Phonetics, 8,* 385–395.

Blanchet, P., Farrell, L., Ambrosino, G., & Paler, K. (2015). Survey of students' identification of cluttering and stuttering. *Procedia- Social and Behavioral Sciences, 193,* 44–50.

Blomgren, M. (2010). Stuttering treatment for adults: An update on contemporary approaches. *Seminars in Speech and Language, 31*(4), 272–282.

Blomgren, M. (2012). Review of the successful stuttering management program. In S. Jelčić Jakšić & M. Onslow (Eds.), *The science and practice of stuttering treatment: A symposium* (pp. 99–113). Wiley-Blackwell. https://doi.org/10.1002/9781118702796.ch8

Blomgren, M. (2013). Behavioral treatments for children and adults who stutter: A review. *Psychology Research and Behavior Management, 6,* 9–19.

Blomgren, M., & Goberman, A.M. (2007). Revisiting speech rate and utterance length manipulations in stuttering speakers. *Journal of Communication Disorders, 41,* 159–178.

Blomgren, M., Nagarajan, S.S., Lee, J.N., Li, T., & Alvord, L. (2003). Preliminary results of a functional MRI study of brain activation patterns in stuttering and nonstuttering speakers during a lexical access task. *Journal of Fluency Disorders, 28,* 337–357.

Blood, G.W. (1985). Laterality differences in child stutterers: Heterogeneity, severity levels, and statistical treatments. *Journal of Speech and Hearing Disorders, 50*(1), 66–72.

Blood, G.W., & Blood, I.M. (1984). Central auditory function in young stutterers. *Perceptual Motor Skills, 59,* 699–705.

Blood, G.W., Blood, I.M., & Tellis, G. (2000). Auditory processing and cluttering in young children. *Perceptual Motor Skills, 90*(2), 631–639.

Blood, I.M. (1996). Disruptions in auditory and temporal processing in adults who stutter. *Perceptual and Motor Skills, 82,* 242–244.

Bloodstein, O. (1958). Stuttering as anticipatory struggle reaction. In J. Eisenson (Ed.), *Stuttering: A symposium* (pp. 1–69). Harper & Row.

Bloodstein, O. (1960). The development of stuttering: I. Changes in nine basic features. *Journal of Speech and Hearing Disorders, 25,* 219–237.

Bloodstein, O. (1961). Stuttering in families of adopted stutterers. *The Journal of Speech and Hearing Disorders, 26,* 395–396.

Bloodstein, O. (1969). *A handbook on stuttering.* National Easter Seal Society for Crippled Children and Adults.

Bloodstein, O. (1970). Stuttering and normal nonfluency a continuity hypothesis. *British Journal of Disorders of Communication, 5*(1), 30–39.

Bloodstein, O. (1987). *A handbook on stuttering* (4th ed.). National Easter Seal Society.

Bloodstein, O. (1995). *A handbook on stuttering* (5th ed.). Singular Publishing

Bloodstein, O. (2006). Some empirical observations about early stuttering: A possible link to language development. *Journal of Communication Disorders, 39*(3), 185–191.

Bloodstein, O., & Bernstein Ratner, N. (2008). *A handbook on stuttering* (6th ed.). Delmar Learning.

Bloodstein, O., Bernstein Ratner, N., & Brundage, S.B. (2021). *A handbook on stuttering* (7th ed.). Plural Publishing Inc.

Bluemel, C. (1931). Primary and secondary stuttering. *Quarterly Journal of Speech, 18,* 178–200.

Boberg, E. (1981). *Maintenance of fluency.* Elsevier.

Boberg, E., & Kully, D. (1985). *Comprehensive stuttering program.* College-Hill Press.

Boberg, E., & Kully, D. (1994a). Long-term results of an intensive treatment program for adults and adolescents who stutter. *Journal of Speech and Hearing Research, 37,* 1050–1059.

Boberg, E., & Kully, D. (1994b). The comprehensive stuttering program. *Journal of Fluency Disorders, 19*(3), 155.

Boehmler, R. M. (1958). Listener responses to nonfluencies. *Journal of Speech & Hearing Research, 1*, 132–141.

Boey, R.A., Van de Heyning, P.H., Wuyts, F.L., Heylen, L., Stoop, R., & De Bodt, M.S. (2009). Awareness and reactions of young stuttering children aged 2–7 years old towards their speech disfluency. *Journal of Communication Disorders, 42*(5), 334–346.

Boey, R.A., Wuyts, F.L., Van de Heyning, P.H., De Bodt, M.S., & Heylen, L. (2007). Characteristics of stuttering-like disfluencies in Dutch-speaking children. *Journal of Fluency Disorders, 32*(4), 310–329.

Bohland, J.W., Bullock, D., & Guenther, F.H. (2010). Neural representations and mechanisms for the performance of simple speech sequences. *Journal of Cognitive Neuroscience, 22*(7), 1504–1529.

Bohr, J.W.F. (1963). The effects of electronic and external control methods on stuttering: A review of some research. *Journal of South African Logopedic Society, 10*, 4–13.

Bolinger, D.L. (1958). A theory of pitch accent in English. *Word, 14*, 109–149.

Bona, J. (2019). Clustering of disfluencies in typical, fast and cluttered speech. *Clinical Linguistics and Phonetics, 33*(5), 393–405.

Bonin, B., Ramig, P., & Prescott, T. (1985). Performance differences between stuttering and nonstuttering subjects on a sound fusion task. *Journal of Fluency Disorders, 10*, 291–300.

Boome, E.J., & Richardson, M.H. (1931). *The nature and treatment of stammering*. Methuen.

Boomer, D S. (1970). Psycholinguistics; experiments in spontaneous speech: Frieda Goldman Eisler Academic Press, London & New York 1968. viii, 169 pp. 50 s. *Lingua, 25*(C), 152–164. https://doi.org/10.1016/0024-3841(70)90028-8

Bortfeld, H., Leon, S. D., Bloom, J.E., Schober, M.F., & Brennan, S.E. (2001). Disfluency rates in conversation: Effects of age, relationship, topic, role, and gender. *Language and Speech, 44*(2), 123–147.

Boscolo, B., Bernstein Ratner, N., & Rescorla, L. (2002). Fluency of school-aged children with a history of specific expressive language impairment: An exploratory study. *American Journal of Speech – Language Pathology, 11*, 41–49.

Bothe, A.K. (Ed.). (2004). *Evidence-based treatment of stuttering: Empirical bases and clinical applications*. Psychology Press.

Bowers, A., Saltuklaroglu, T., & Kalinowski, J. (2012). Autonomic arousal in adults who stutter prior to various reading tasks intended to elicit changes in stuttering frequency. *International Journal of Psychophysiology, 83*, 45–55.

Boyle, M.P. (2018). Enacted stigma and felt stigma experienced by adults who stutter. *Journal of Communication Disorders, 73*, 50–61.

Brady, J.P. (1998). Drug-induced stuttering: A review of the literature. *Journal of Clinical Psychopharmacology. 18*(1), 50–54.

Brady, J.P., & Berson, J. (1975). Stuttering, dichotic listening, and cerebral dominance. *Archives of General Psychiatry, 32*, 1449–1452.

Breitenfeldt, D. H., & Lorenz, D. R. (1989). *Successful stuttering management program (SSMP) for adolescent and adult stutterers*. Cheney: Eastern Washington University School of Health Sciences.

Bridgman, K., Onslow, M., O'Brian, S., Jones, M., & Block, S. (2016). Lidcombe program webcam treatment for early stuttering: A randomized controlled trial. *Journal of Speech, Language, and Hearing Research, 59*(5), 932–939.

Brignell, A., Krahe, M., Downes, M., Kefalianos, E., Reilly, S., & Morgan, A.T. (2020). A systematic review of interventions for adults who stutter. *Journal of Fluency Disorders, 64*, 1057–66.

Briley, P.M. (2017). An exploration of anticipation of stuttering in adults. *Journal of Speech Pathology and Therapy, 2*, 123. https://doi.org/10.4172/2472-5005.1000123

Brin, M.F., Stewart, C., Blitzer, A., & Diamond, B. (1994). Laryngeal botulinum toxin injections for disabling stuttering in adults. *Neurology, 44*(12), 2262–2262.

Broadbent, B.E., & Gregory, M. (1964). Accuracy of recognition for speech presented to the right and left ears. *Quarterly Journal of Experimental Psychology, 16*, 359–360.

Brocklehurst, P.H., & Corley, M. (2011). Investigating the inner speech of people who stutter: Evidence for (and against) the Covert Repair Hypothesis. *Journal of Communication Disorders, 44*, 246–260.

Brown, S.F. (1937). The influence of grammatical function on the incidence of stuttering. *Journal of Speech Disorders, 2*, 207–215.

Brown, S.F. (1938). Stuttering with relation to word accent and word position. *The Journal of Abnormal and Social Psychology, 33*(1), 112–120.

Brown, S.F. (1945). The loci of stutterings in the speech sequence. *Journal of Speech Disorders, 10*(3), 181–192.

Brundage, S.B., Corcoran, T., Wu, C., & Sturgill, C. (2016). Developing and using big data archives to quantify disfluency and stuttering in bilingual children. *Seminars in Speech and Language, 37*(2), 117–127.

Brutten, G.J., & Dunham, S. (1989). The communication attitude test: A normative study of grade school children. *Journal of Fluency Disorders, 14*, 371–377.

Brutten, G.J., & Miller, R. (1988). The disfluencies of normally fluent black first graders. *Journal of Fluency Disorders, 13*(4), 291–299.

Brutten, G.J., & Vanryckeghem, M. (2003). *Behavior assessment battery: A multi-dimensional and evidence-based approach to diagnostic and therapeutic decision making for children who stutter.* Stichting Integratie Gehandicapten & Acco Publishers.

Brutten, G.J., & Vanryckeghem, M. (2006). *Behavioral assessment battery for school-age children who stutter.* Plural Publishing.

Brutten, G.J., & Vanryckeghem, M. (2007). *Behavior assessment battery for school-age children who stutter.* Plural Publishing.

Byrd, C. (2018). Assessing bilingual children: Are their disfluencies indicative of stuttering or a byproduct of navigating two languages? *Seminars in Speech and Language, 39*(4), 324–332.

Byrd, C.T., Bedore, L.M., & Ramos, D. (2015). The disfluent speech of bilingual Spanish – English children: Considerations for differential diagnosis of stuttering. *Language, Speech, and Hearing Services in Schools, 46*(1), 30–43.

Byrd, C.T., McGill, M., & Usler, E. (2015). Nonword repetition and phoneme elision in adults who do and do not stutter: Vocal versus nonvocal performance differences. *Journal of Fluency Disorders, 44*, 17–31.

Byrd, C.T., Watson, J., Bedore, L., & Mullis, A. (2015). Identification of stuttering in bilingual Spanish-English speaking children. *Contemporary Issues in Communication Sciences and Disorders, 42*, 72–87.

Campbell, J.H., & Hill, D. (1987). *Systematic disfluency analysis.* Northwestern University.

Canter, G.J. (1971). Observations on neurogenic stuttering: A contribution to differential diagnosis. *International Journal of Language & Communication Disorders, 6*(2), 139–143.

Chang, S.E., Angstadt, M., Chow, H.M., Etchell, A.C., Garnett, E.O., Choo, A.L., Kessler, D., Welsh, R.C., & Sripada, C. (2018). Anomalous network architecture of the resting brain in children who stutter. *Journal of Fluency Disorders, 55*, 46–67.

Chang, S.E., Erickson, K.I., Ambrose, N.G., Hasegawa-Johnson, M.A., & Ludlow, C.L. (2008). Brain anatomy differences in childhood stuttering. *Neuroimage, 39*, 1333–1244.

Chang, S.E., Zhu, D.C., Choo, A.L., & Angstadt, M. (2015). White matter neuroanatomical differences in young children who stutter. *Brain, 138*(3), 694–711.

Chaudhary, C., Maruthy, S., Guddattu, V., & Krishnan, G. (2021). A systematic review on the role of language-related factors in the manifestation of stuttering in bilinguals. *Journal of Fluency Disorders, 68*. https://doi.org/10.1016/j.jfludis.2021.105829

Chengappa, S.K., & Kumar, R. (2008). Normative & clinical data on the Kannada version of Western Aphasia Battery (WAB-K). *Language in India, 8*(6).

Cherry, E.C., & Sayers, B.M. (1956). Experiments on the total inhibition of stuttering by external control, and some clinical results. *Journal of Psychosomatic Research, 1*, 233–246.

Cherry, E.C., Sayers, B.M., & Marland, P. (1955). Experiments on the complete suppression of stammering. *Nature, 176*, 874–875.

Choi, J., Conture, E.G., Walden, T.A., Lambert, W.E., & Tumanova, V. (2013). Behavioral inhibition and childhood stuttering. *Journal of Fluency Disorders, 38*, 171–183.

Ciabarra, A.M., Elkind, M.S., Roberts, J.K., Marshall, R.S., & York-Presbyterian, N. (2000). Subcortical infarction resulting in acquired stuttering. *Journal of Neurology, Neurosurgery & Psychiatry, 69*(4), 546–549. https://doi.org/10.1136/JNNP.69.4.546

Cimorell-Strong, J.M., Gilbert, H.R., & Frick, J.V. (1983). Dichotic speech perception: A comparison between stuttering and nonstuttering children. *Journal of Fluency Disorders, 8*(1), 77–91.

Civier, O., Bullock, O., Max, L., & Guenther, F.H. (2013). Computational modeling of stuttering caused by impairments in basal ganglia thalamo-cortical circuit involved in syllable selection and initiation. *Brain and Language, 126*, 263–278.

Clarke, H. (1971). The importance of linguistics for the study of speech hesitation. The perception of language. In D. Horton & J. Jenkins (Eds.), *The proceedings of the symposium*. Charles. E. Merrill.

Cocomazzo, N., Block, S., Carey, B., O'Brian, S., Onslow, M., Packman, A., & Iverach, L. (2012). Camperdown Program for adults who stutter: A student training clinic phase I trial. *International Journal of Language & Communication Disorders, 47*(4), 365–372.

Connally, E.L., Ward, D., Howell, P., & Watkins, K.E. (2014). Disrupted white matter in language and motor tracts in developmental stuttering. *Brain and Language, 131*, 25–35.

Conture, E.G. (1982). Stuttering in young children. *Journal of Developmental and Behavioral Pediatrics, 3*, 163–169.

Conture, E.G. (1990a). Childhood stuttering: What is it and who does it? *ASHA Reports Series (American Speech-Language-Hearing Association), 18*, 2–14.

Conture, E.G. (1990b). *Stuttering*. Prentice Hall.

Conture, E.G. (2001). *Stuttering: Its nature, diagnosis, and treatment*. Pearson College Division.

Conture, E.G., & Guitar, B.E. (1993). Evaluating efficacy of treatment of stuttering: School-age children. *Journal of Fluency Disorders, 18*(2–3), 253–287.

Conture, E.G., Walden, T.A., Arnold, H.S., Graham, C.G., Hartfield, K.N., & Karrass, J. (2006). Communication emotional model of stuttering. In N. Bernstein Ratner & J. Tetnowski (Eds.), *Current issues in stuttering research and practice* (pp. 17–46). Erlbaum.

Cook, K., & Millard, S.K. (2018). The most important therapy outcomes for school-aged children who stutter: An exploratory study. *American Journal of Speech-Language Pathology, 27*(3S), 1152–1163.

Cook, M. (1971). The incidence of filled pauses in relation to part of speech. *Language and Speech, 14*(2), 135–139.

Cook, M., Smith, J., & Lalljee, M.G. (1974). Filled Pauses and Syntactic Complexity: *Language and Speech, 17*(1), 11–16.

Cooper, E.B. (1972). Recovery from stuttering in a junior and senior high school population. *Journal of Speech and Hearing Research, 15*(3), 632–638.

Cooper, E.B., & Cooper, C.S. (1991). A fluency disorders prevention program for preschoolers and children in the primary grades. *American Journal of Speech-Language Pathology, 1*(1), 28–31.

Costa, L. M. O., Martins-Reis, V. O., & Celeste, L. C. (2016). Methods of analysis of speech rate: A pilot study. *CoDAS, 28*(1), 41–45.

Craig, A.R. (1998). Relapse following treatment for stuttering: A critical review and correlative data. *Journal of Fluency Disorders, 23*(1), 1–30.

Craig, A.R., & Andrews, G. (1985). The prediction and prevention of relapse in stuttering: The value of self-control techniques and locus of control measures. *Behavior Modification, 9*(4), 427–442.

Craig, A.R., Franklin, J.A., & Andrews, G. (1984). A scale to measure locus of control of behaviour. *British Journal of Medical Psychology, 57*(2), 173–180.

Craig, A.R., & Hancock, K. (1995). Self-reported factors related to relapse following treatment for stuttering. *Australian Journal of Human Communication Disorders, 23*(1), 48–60.

Craig, A.R., Hancock, K., Tran, Y., Craig, M., & Peters, K. (2002). Epidemiology of stuttering in the community across the entire life span. *Journal of Speech, Language, and Hearing Research, 45*, 1097–1105.

Craig, A.R., & Tran, Y. (2005). The epidemiology of stuttering: The need for reliable estimates of prevalence and anxiety levels over the lifespan. *Advances in Speech Language Pathology, 7*(1), 41–46.

Craig-McQuaide, A., Akram, H., Zrinzo, L., & Tripoliti, E. (2014, November). A review of brain circuitries involved in stuttering. *Frontiers in Human Neuroscience, 8*, 1–20. https://doi.org/10.3389/fnhum.2014.00884

Cream, A., Onslow, M., Packman, A., & Llewellyn, G. (2003). Protection from harm: The experience of adults after therapy with prolonged-speech. *International Journal of Language & Communication Disorders, 38*(4), 379–395.

Cuadrado, E.M., & Weber-Fox, C.M. (2003). Atypical syntactic processing in individuals who stutter: Evidence from event-related brain potentials and behavioral measures. *Journal of Speech and Hearing Research, 46*, 960–976.

Culatta, R., & Leeper, L. (1989). The differential diagnosis of disfluency. *NSSLHA Journal, 17*, 59–64.

Curlee, R.F. (1990). *Stuttering and related disorders of fluency*. Thieme Medical Publishers.

Curry, F., & Gregory, H. (1969). The performance of stutterers on dichotic listening tasks thought to reflect cerebral dominance. *Journal of Speech and Hearing Research, 12*, 73–81.

Cykowski, M.D., Fox, P.T., Ingham, R.J., Ingham, J.C., & Robin, D.A. (2010). A study of the reproducibility and etiology of diffusion anisotropy differences in developmental stuttering: A potential role for impaired myelination. *Neuroimage, 52*, 1495–1504.

Daliri, A., & Max, L. (2018). Stuttering adults' lack of pre-speech auditory modulation normalizes when speaking with delayed auditory feedback. *Cortex, 99*, 55–68.

Dalton, P. (2018). Some developments in individual personal construct therapy with adults who stutter. In C. Levy (Ed.), *Stuttering therapies – practical approaches* (pp. 47–60). Routledge.

Dalton, P., & Hardcastle, W. J. (1989). *Disorders of fluency*. Wiley-Blackwell.

Daly, D.A. (1993). Cluttering: Another fluency syndrome. In R. F. Curlee (Ed.), *Stuttering and related disorders of fluency*. Thieme Medical Publishers.

Daly, D.A. (2006). *Predictive cluttering inventory*. Retrieved June 12, 2022, from https://drive.google.com/file/d/188NTu5Qz5iZ7wjgwxkR5g-y8s0MDxPfs/view

Daly, D.A., & Burnett, M. (1999). Cluttering: Traditional views and new perspectives. In R.F. Curlee (Ed.), *Stuttering and related disorders of fluency* (2nd ed.). Thieme Medical Publishers.

Darley, F.L. (1955). The relationship of parental attitudes and adjustments to the development of stuttering. In W. Johnson (Ed.), *Stuttering in children and adults* (pp. 74–152). University of Minnesota Press.

Darmody, T., O'Brien, S., Rogers, K., Onslow, M., Jacobs, C., McEwen, A., Lowe, R., Packman, A., & Menzies, R. (2022). Stuttering, family history and counselling: A contemporary database. *Journal of Fluency Disorders, 73*. https://doi.org/10.1016/j.jfludis.2022.105925

Dayalu, V.N., Kalinowski, J., Stuart, A., Holbert, D., & Rastatter, M. P. (2002). Stuttering frequency on content and function words in adults who stutter: A concept revised. *Journal of Speech, Language and Hearing Research, 45*(5), 871–878.

De Nil, L.F. (1999). Stuttering: A neurophysiologic perspective. In N. Bernstein Ratner & E.C. Healey (Eds.), *Stuttering research and practice: Bridging the gap* (pp. 85–102). Lawrence Erlbaum.

De Nil, L.F. (2004). Recent developments in brain imaging research in stuttering. In H.P. Maassen & R. Kent (Eds.), *Speech motor control in normal and disordered speech* (pp. 113–137). Oxford University Press.

De Nil, L.F., Jokel, R., & Rochon, E. (2007). Etiology, symptomatology, and treatment of neurogenic stuttering. In E. Conture & R. Curlee (Eds.), *Stuttering and related disorders of fluency* (3rd ed., pp. 326–343). Thieme Medical Publishers.

de Sonneville-Koedoot, C., Stolk, E., Rietveld, T., & Franken, M.C. (2015). Direct versus indirect treatment for preschool children who stutter: The RESTART randomized trial. *PLOS ONE*. https://doi.org/10.1371/journal.pone.0133758.

Dechamma, D., & Maruthy, S. (2018). Envelope modulation spectral (EMS) analyses of solo reading and choral reading conditions suggest changes in speech rhythm in adults who stutter. *Journal of Fluency Disorders, 58*, 47–60.

Decker, T.N., Healey, E.C., & Howe, S.W. (1982). Brainstem auditory electrical response characteristics of stutterers and nonstutterers: A preliminary report. *Journal of Fluency Disorders, 7*, 385–401.

DeJoy, D.A., & Gregory, H.H. (1985). The relationship between age and frequency of disfluency in preschool children. *Journal of Fluency Disorders, 10*(2), 107–122.

Dietrich, S. (1997). Central auditory processing in people who stutter. *Journal of Fluency Disorders, 2*(22), 148.

Dietrich, S., Barry, S.J., & Parker, D.E. (1995). Middle latency auditory evoked responses in males who stutter. *Journal of Speech, Language, and Hearing Research, 38*, 5–17.

Donnan, G.A. (1979). Stuttering as a manifestation of stroke. *Medical Journal of Australia, 1*(2), 44–45. https://doi.org/10.5694/J.1326-5377.1979.TB111968.X

Dorman, M.F., & Porter, R.J. (1975). Hemispheric lateralization for speech perception in stutterers. *Cortex, 11*, 81–85.

Downie, A.W., Low, J.M., & Lindsay, D.D. (1981). Speech disorder in Parkinsonism -usefulness of delayed auditory feedback in selected cases. *British Journal of Disorders of Communication, 16*(2), 135–139.

Druce, T., Debney, S., & Byrt, T. (1997). Evaluation of an intensive treatment program for stuttering in young children. *Journal of Fluency Disorders, 22*, 169–186.

Druker, K., Hennessey, N., Mazzucchelli, T., & Beilby, J. (2019). Elevated attention deficit hyperactivity disorder symptoms in children who stutter. *Journal of Fluency Disorders, 59*, 80–90.

Dryden, W., & Branch, R. (2008). *Fundamentals of rational emotive behaviour therapy: A training handbook.* John Wiley & Sons.

Duffy, J. (2005). *Motor speech disorders* (2nd ed.). Elsevier, Mosby.

Duffy, J.R. (1995). *Motor speech disorders. Substrates, differential diagnosis, and management.* Mosby, St Louis.

Dworkin, J.P., Culatta, R.A., Abkarian, G.G., & Meleca, R.J. (2002). Laryngeal anesthetization for the treatment of acquired disfluency: A case study. *Journal of Fluency Disorders*, *27*(3), 215–226.

Dworzynski, K., Howell, P., & Natke, U. (2003). Predicting stuttering from linguistic factors for German speakers in two age groups. *Journal of Fluency Disorders*, *28*(2), 95–113.

Dworzynski, K., Remington, A., Rijsdijk, F., Howell, P., & Plomin, R. (2007). Genetic etiology in cases of recovered and persistent stuttering in an unselected, longitudinal sample of young twins. *American Journal of Speech-Language Pathology*, *16*, 169–178.

Eggers, K., De Nil, L.F., & Van der Bergh, B.R. (2010). Temperament dimensions in stuttering and typically developing children. *Journal of Fluency Disorders*, *35*, 355–372.

Eggers, K., De Nil, L.F., & Van den Bergh, B.R. (2013). Inhibitory control in childhood stuttering. *Journal of Fluency Disorders*, *38*, 1–13.

Eggers, K., Millard, S.K., & Kelman, E. (2022). Temperament, anxiety, and depression in school-age children who stutter. *Journal of Communication Disorders*, *97*, 106218. https://doi.org/10.1016/j.jcomdis.2022.106218.

Eggers, K., Van Eerdenburg, S., & Byrd, C.T. (2020). Speech disfluencies in bilingual Yiddish-Dutch speaking children. *Clinical Linguistics and Phonetics*, *34*(6), 576–592.

Eichorn, N., & Fabus, R. (2018). Assessment of fluency disorders in children and adults. In C. Stein & R. Fabus (Eds.), *A guide to clinical assessment and professional report writing in speech-language pathology* (2nd ed.). SLACK, Inc.

Eisenson, J. (1958). A perseverative theory of stuttering. In J. Eisenson (Ed.), *Stuttering: A symposium* (pp. 223–272). Harper & Row.

Eisenson, J. (1975). Stuttering as perseverative behavior. In J. Eisenson (Ed.), *Stuttering: A second symposium* (pp. 401–452). Harper & Row.

Elliott, R.L., & Thomas, B.J. (1985). A case report of alprazolam-induced stuttering. *Journal of Clinical Psychopharmacology*, *5*(3), 159–160.

Ellis, A. (1974). *Humanistic psychotherapy. The rational-emotive approach*. McGraw-Hill.

Ellis, C., & Rittman, M. (2009, Fall). Disfluency: An exploratory study of the effects of subcortical stroke. *Contemporary Issues in Communication Science and Disorders*, *36*, 149–156. https://doi.org/10.1044/CICSD_36_F_149

Embrechts, M., Ebben, H., Franke, P., & van de Poel, C. (2000). Temperament: A comparison between children who stutter and children who do not stutter. In *Proceedings of the third world congress on fluency disorders: Theory, research, treatment, and self-help*, Nyborg, Denmark.

Enderby, P.M., & Palmer, R. (2008). *Frenchay dysarthria assessment*. Pro-ed.

Erickson, R. L. (1969). Assessing communication attitudes among stutterers. *Journal of Speech & Hearing Research*, *12*(4), 711–724.

Evesham, M., & Fransella, F. (1985). Stuttering relapse: The effect of a combined speech and psychological reconstruction programme. *International Journal of Language & Communication Disorders*, *20*(3), 237–248.

Fagan, L.B. (1931). Graphic stuttering. *Psychology Monographs*, *43*, 67–71.

Fagnani, C., Fibiger, S., Skytthe, A., & Hjelmborg, J. V. B. (2009). Heritability and genetic relationship of adult self-reported stuttering, cluttering and childhood speech-language disorders. *Logopedia*, *38*, 71–100.

Fagnani, C., Fibiger, S., Skytthe, A., & Hjelmborg, J.V.B. (2011). Heritability and environmental effects for self-reported periods with stuttering: A twin study from Denmark. *Logopedics Phoniatrics Vocology*, *36*(3), 114–120.

Fairbanks, G. (1954). Systematic research in experimental phonetics – I. A theory of the speech mechanism as a servomechanism. *Journal of Speech and Hearing Disorders*, *19*, 133–139.

Falkowski, G.L., Guilford, A.M., & Sandler, J. (1982). Effectiveness of a modified version of airflow therapy: Case studies. *Journal of Speech and Hearing Disorders*, 47(2), 160–164.

Fanning, J. (2018, October 12–13). Cluttering across the lifespan: Overview of assessment and treatment. In *Paper presented at the OSHA annual conference*. www.oregonspeechand hearing.org/event-3038478.

Fant, C.G.M. (1958). *Acoustic theory of speech production*. Royal institute of Technology, Div. of Telegraphy telephony, Rep. No. 10. Presented in mimeographed form.

Feldman, H. M., & Messick, C. (2009). Language and speech disorders. In W. B. Carey, A. C. Crocker, W. L. Coleman, E. R. Elias, & H. M. Feldman (Eds.), *Developmental-behavioral pediatrics* (4th ed., pp. 717–729). Saunders.

Felsenfeld, S., Kirk, M., Zhu, G., Statham, D., Neale, M., & Martin, N. (2000). A study of the genetic and environmental etiology of stuttering in a selected twin sample. *Behavioral Genetics*, 30(5), 359–366.

Felsenfeld, S., & Plomin, R. (1997). Epidemiological and offspring analyses of developmental speech disorders using data from the Colorado Adoption Project. *Journal of Speech, Language, and Hearing Research*, 40(4), 778–791.

Ferrand, C.T., Gilbert, H.R., & Blood, G.W. (1991). Selected aspects of central processing and vocal motor function in stutterers and nonstutterers. *Journal of Fluency Disorders*, 16, 101–115.

Fiez, J., & Raichle, M. (1997). Linguistic processing. In J. Schmahmann (Ed.), *The cerebellum and cognition* (pp. 233–254). Academic Press.

Finitzo, T., Pool, K.D., Freeman, F.J., Devous, M.D., & Watson, B.C. (1991). Cortical dysfunction in developmental stutterers. In H. F. M. Peters et al. (Eds.), *Speech motor control and stuttering* (pp. 251–261). Elsevier.

Finn, P. (1996). Establishing the validity of recovery from stuttering without formal treatment. *Journal of Speech, Language, and Hearing Research*, 39(6), 1171–1181.

Finn, P. (1997). Adults recovered from stuttering without formal treatment: Perceptual assessment of speech normalcy. *Journal of Speech, Language, and Hearing Research*, 40(4), 821–831.

Finn, P. (2004). Establishing the validity of stuttering treatment effectiveness: The fallibility of clinical experience. *Perspectives on Fluency and Fluency Disorders*, 14(2), 9–12.

Fiorin, M., Marconato, E., Palharini, T.A., Picoloto, L.A., Frizzo, A.C.F., Cardoso, A.C.V., & de Oliveira, C.M.C. (2021). Impact of auditory feedback alterations in individuals with stuttering. *Brazilian Journal of Otorhinolaryngology*, 87(3), 247–254.

Fisher, S.E., Vargha-Khadem, F., Watkins, K.E., Monaco, A.P., & Pembrey, M.E. (1998). Localisation of a gene implicated in a severe speech and language disorder. *Nature Genetics*, 18(2), 168–170.

Foundas, A.L., Bollich, A.M., Corey, D.M., Hurley, M., & Heilman, K.M. (2001). Anomalous anatomy of speech language areas in adults with persistent developmental stuttering. *Neurology*, 57, 207–215.

Foundas, A.L., Bolich, A.M., Feldman, J., Corey, D.M., Hurley, M., Lemen, L.C., & Heilman, K.M. (2004). Aberrant auditory processing and atypical planum temporal in developmental stuttering. *Neurology*, 63, 1640–1646.

Foundas, A.L., Corey, D.M., Angeles, V., Bollich, A.M., Crabtree-Hartman, E., & Heilman, K.M. (2003). Atypical cerebral laterality in adults with persistent developmental stuttering. *Neurology*, 61, 1378–1385.

Fox, P.T., Ingham, R.J., Ingham, J.C., Hirsch, T.B., Downs, J.H., Martin, C., Jerabek, P., Glass, T., & Lancaster, J.L. (1996). A PET study of the neural systems of stuttering. *Nature*, 382, 158–162.

Franken, M.C., Bovers, L., Peters, H.F.M., & Webster, R.L. (1995). Perceptual rating instrument for speech evaluation of stutterers. *Journal of Speech and Hearing Research, 38*(2), 280–288.

Franken, M.C., & Laroes, E. (2021). *RESTART-DCM method* (Revised ed.). https://www.restartdcm.nl

Franken, M.C.J., Kielstra-Van der Schalk, C.J., & Boelens, H. (2005). Experimental treatment of early stuttering: A preliminary study. *Journal of Fluency Disorders, 30*(3), 189–199.

Fransella, F. (1972). *Personal change and reconstruction.* Academic Press.

Freund, H. (1966). *Psychopathology and the problems of stuttering.* Charles C Thomas.

Frigerio-Domingues, C., & Drayna, D. (2017). Genetic contributions to stuttering: The current evidence. *Molecular Genetics and Genomic Medicine, 5*(2), 95–102.

Fry, D.B. (1955). Duration and intensity as physical correlates of linguistic stress. *The Journal of the Acoustical Society of America, 27*, 765–768.

Furlanis, G., Busan, P., Formaggio, E., Menichelli, A., Lunardelli, A., Ajcevic, M., Pesavento, V., & Manganotti, P. (2023). Stuttering-like dysfluencies as a consequence of long COVID-19. *Journal of Speech, Language, and Hearing Research.* https://doi.org/10.1044/2022_JSLHR-22-00381

Gahl, S. (2020). Bilingualism as a purported risk factor for stuttering: A close look at a seminal study (Travis et al., 1937). *Journal of Speech, Language, and Hearing Research, 63*, 3680–3684.

Geetha, Y. V. (2007). Introduction to management of fluency disorders. In V. Basavaraj (Ed.), *Assessment and management of fluency disorders* (pp. 47–57). All India Institute of Speech and Hearing.

George, V.M., & Bajaj, G. (2020). Fluency disorders. In G. Shirly, S.K. Kunnath, V.M. George, & A. Varghese (Eds.). *Communication disorders: Illustrated in ICF framework* (1st ed., pp. 177–207). National Institute of Speech and Hearing & Department of Social Justice, Government of Kerala.

Gerwin, K.L., Walsh, B., & Tichenor, S.E. (2022). Nonword repetition performance differentiates children who stutter with and without concomitant speech sound and developmental language disorders. *Journal of Speech, Language, and Hearing Research, 65*(1), 96–108.

Gifford, M.F. (1940). *How to overcome stammering.* Prentice Hall.

Gillam, R.B., Logan, K.J., & Pearson, N.A. (2009). *Test of childhood stuttering (TOCS).* Pro-Ed.

Glauber, I.P. (1982). *Stuttering: A psychoanalytic understanding.* Human Sciences Press.

Godai, U., Tatarelli, R., & Bonanni, G. (1976). Stuttering and tics in twins. *Acta Geneticae Medicae et Gemellologiae, 25*, 369–375.

Goldiamond, I. (1965). Stuttering and fluency as manipulatable operant response classes. In L. Krasner & P.L. Ullmann (Eds.), *Research in behaviour modification* (pp. 106–156). Holt, Rinehart & Winston.

Goldman-Eisler, F. (1958). The predictability of words in context and the length of pauses in speech. *Language and Speech, 1*(3), 226–231.

Goral-Polrola, J., Zielinska, J., Jastrezebowska, G., & Tarkowski, Z. (2016). Cluttering: Specific communication disorder. *Acta Neuropsychologica, 14*(1), 1–15.

Gough, P.M., Connally, E.L., Howell, P., Ward, D., Chesters, J., & Watkins, K.E. (2018). Planum temporale asymmetry in people who stutter. *Journal of Fluency Disorders, 55*, 94–105.

Grabe, E.L., & Low, E.L. (2002). Durational variability in speech and the Rhythm Class Hypothesis. *Laboratory Phonology, 7*, 515–546. https://doi.org/10.1515/9783110197105.2.515/HTML

Gregory, H.H. (1964). Stuttering and auditory central nervous system disorder. *Journal of Speech and Hearing Research, 7*, 335–341.

Gruber, L., & Powell, R.L. (1974). Responses of stuttering and non-stuttering children to a dichotic listening task. *Perceptual and Motor Skills, 38*(1), 263–264.

Guenther, F.H., Ghosh, S.S., & Tourville, J.A. (2006). Neural modeling and imaging of the cortical interactions underlying syllable production. *Brain and Language, 96*(3), 280–301.

Guillaume, J.G., Mazars, G., & Mazars, Y. (1957). Epileptic medication in certain types of stuttering. *Revue Neurologique, 99*, 59–62.

Guitar, B. (2006). *Stuttering: An integrated approach to its nature and treatment* (3rd ed.). Williams & Wilkins.

Guitar, B. (2013). *Stuttering: An integrated approach to its nature and treatment* (4th ed.). Philadelphia: Lippincott Williams and Wilkins.

Guitar, B. (2019). *Stuttering: An integrated approach to its nature and treatment* (5th ed.). Lippincott Williams and Wilkins.

Guitar, B., & Bass, C. (1978). Stuttering therapy: The relation between attitude change and long-term outcome. *Journal of Speech and Hearing Disorders, 43*(3), 392–400.

Guitar, B., & Grims, S. (1977, November). Developing a scale to assess communication attitudes in children who stutter. In *Paper presented at the annual meeting of the American speech-language-hearing association*, Atlanta, GA.

Guo, L.Y., Tomblin, J.B., & Samelson, V. (2008). Speech disruptions in the narratives of English-speaking children with specific language impairment. *Journal of Speech, Language and Hearing Research, 51*(3), 722–738.

Guttormsen, L.S., Yaruss, J.S., & Naess, K-A.B. (2020). Caregivers' perceptions of stuttering impact in young children: Agreement in mothers', fathers' and teachers' ratings. *Journal of Communication Disorders, 86*(2). 106001. https://doi.org/10.1016/j.jcomdis.2020.106001

Hall, J.W., & Jerger, J. (1978). Central auditory function in stutterers. *Journal of Speech and Hearing Research, 21*(2), 324–337.

Hall, P.K. (1977). The occurrence of disfluencies in language-disordered school-age children. *Journal of Speech and Hearing Disorders, 42*(3), 364–369.

Ham, R. (1999). *Clinical management of stuttering in older children and adults*. Apsen.

Hampton, A., & Weber-Fox, C. (2008). Non-linguistic auditory processing in stuttering: Evidence from behavior and event-related potentials. *Journal of Fluency Disorders, 33*, 253–273.

Harms, M., & Malone, J. (1939). The relationship of hearing acuity to stammering. *Journal of Speech Disorders, 4*, 363–370.

Harrison, E., Onslow, M., Andrews, G., Packman, A., & Webber, M. (1998). *Control of stuttering with prolonged speech: Preliminary outcome of a one-day instatement program*. Singular Publishing Group.

Harrison, J. (2004). Two very different cases of adult onset stuttering. In A. Packman, A. Meltzer, & H.F.M. Peters (Eds.), *Theory, research and therapy in fluency disorders. Proceedings of the 4th world congress on fluency disorders* (pp. 499–504). Nijmegen University Press.

Hausman, E. (2019). *Effects of stuttering frequency, speaking rate and treatment on speech naturalness in adults who stutter* [Honors theses, Western Michigan University].

Hayhow, R. (2018). Personal construct therapy with children who stutter and their families. In C. Levy (Ed.), *Stuttering therapies – practical approaches* (pp. 1–18). Routledge.

Haynes, W.O., & Hood, S.B. (1977). Language and disfluency variables in normal speaking children from discrete chronological age groups. *Journal of Fluency Disorders, 2*(1), 57–74.

Healey, E.C. (2007). A multidimensional approach to the assessment of children who stutter. *Perspectives on Fluency and Fluency Disorders, 17*(3), 6–9.

Healey, E.C., & Howe, S.W. (1987). Speech shadowing characteristics of stutterers under diotic and dichotic conditions. *Journal of Communication Disorders, 20*, 493–506.

Healey, E.C., Trautman, L.S., & Susca, M. (2004, Spring). Clinical applications of a multidimensional approach for the assessment and treatment of stuttering. *Contemporary Issues in Communication Science and Disorders, 31*, 40–48.

Hegde, M.N. (2007). *Treatment protocols for stuttering*. Plural Publishing Inc.

Hegde, M.N., & Hartman, D.E. (1979a). Factors affecting judgements of fluency: I. Interjections. *Journal of Fluency Disorders, 4*, 1–11.

Hegde, M.N., & Hartman, D.E. (1979b). Factors affecting judgements of fluency: II. Word repetitions. *Journal of Fluency Disorders, 4*, 13–22.

Helgadóttir, F.D., Menzies, R.G., Onslow, M., Packman, A., & O'Brian, S. (2014). A standalone Internet cognitive behaviour therapy treatment for social anxiety in adults who stutter: CBTpsych. *Journal of Fluency Disorders, 41*, 47–54.

Helm, N.A. (1979). Management of palilalia with a pacing board. *Journal of Speech and Hearing Disorders, 44*(3), 350–353.

Helm-Estabrooks, N. (1999). Stuttering associated with acquired neurological disorders. In *Stuttering and related disorders of fluency* (Vol. 3, pp. 255–268). Thieme Medical Publishers.

Helm-Estabrooks, N., & Kaplan, E. (1989). *Boston stimulus board: Clinician's guide*. Riverside Publishing Company (Houghton Mifflin Company).

Hewat, S., Unicomb, R., Dean, I., & Cui, G. (2018). Treatment of childhood stuttering using the Lidcombe program in mainland China: Case studies. *Speech, Language and Hearing, 23*(2), 1–11.

Hirnstein, M., Stuebs, J., Moe, A., & Hausman, M. (2022). Sex/gender differences in verbal fluency and verbal episodic memory: A meta-analysis. *Perspectives on Psychological Science*, 17456916221082116. https://doi.org/10.1177/17456916221082116

Howell, P. (2004). The assessment of some contemporary theories of stuttering that apply to spontaneous speech. *Contemporary Issues in Communicative Sciences and Disorders, 31*, 122–139.

Howell, P., & Au-Yeung, J. (2002). The EXPLAN theory of fluency control applied to the diagnosis of stuttering. *Amsterdam Studies in the Theory and History of Linguistic Science Series, 4*, 75–94.

Howell, P., & Au-Yeung, J. (2007). Phonetic complexity and stuttering in Spanish. *Clinical Linguistics and Phonetics, 21*(2), 111–127.

Howell, P., Au-Yeung, J., & Sackin, S. (1999). Exchange of stuttering from function words to content words with age. *Journal of Speech, Language and Hearing Research, 42*(2), 345–354.

Howell, P., Au-Yeung, J., & Sackin, S. (2000). Internal structure of content words leading to lifespan differences in phonological difficulty in stuttering. *Journal of Fluency Disorders, 25*(1), 1–20.

Howell, P., & Davis, S. (2011). The epidemiology of cluttering with stuttering. In D. Ward & K. Scaler Scott (Eds.), *Cluttering: A handbook of research, intervention and education* (pp. 3–28). Psychology Press.

Howell, P., Davis, S., & Williams, R. (2009). The effects of bilingualism on stuttering during late childhood. *Archives of Diseases in Childhood, 94*, 42–46.

Howell, P., Davis, S., & Williams, S.M. (2006). Auditory abilities of speakers who persisted, or recovered, from stuttering. *Journal of Fluency Disorders, 31*, 257–270.

Howell, P., Rosen, S., Hanigan, G., & Rustin, L. (2000). Auditory backward-masking performance by children who stutter and its relation to disfluency rate. *Perceptual and Motor Skills, 90*, 355–363.

Howell, P., & Williams, M. (2004). Development of auditory sensitivity in children who stutter and fluent children. *Ear and Hearing, 25*, 265–274.

Howie, P. (1981). Concordance for stuttering in monozygotic and dizygotic twin pairs. *Journal of Speech and Hearing Research, 24*, 317–321.

Hubbard, C.P., & Yairi, E. (1988). Clustering of disfluencies in the and nonstuttering preschool children. *Journal of Speech, Language, and Hearing Research, 31*(2), 228–233.

Hubble, M.A., Duncan, B.L., & Miller, S.D. (1999). *The heart and soul of change: What works in therapy*. American Psychological Association. https://doi.org/10.1037/11132-000

Ilkhani, Z., Shafiee, B., Jafari, N., & Dehkordi, S.H. (2019). Effectiveness of the Westmead therapeutic method on preschool children with stuttering. *Koomesh Journal, 22*(1), 138–144.

Indu, V. (1990). *Some aspects of fluency in children (4–5 yrs)* [Master's dissertation, All India Institute of Speech and Hearing, Mysuru].

Ingham, J.C. (2003). Evidence-based treatment of stuttering: I. Definition and application. *Journal of Fluency Disorders, 28*(3), 197–207.

Ingham, R.J. (1984). *Stuttering and behaviour therapy: Current status and experimental foundations*. College Hill Press.

Ingham, R.J. (1987). *Residential prolonged speech stuttering therapy manual*. Department of Speech and Hearing Sciences, University of California Santa Barbara.

Ingham, R.J., & Andrews, G. (1973). Behaviour therapy and stuttering: A review. *Journal of Speech and Hearing Disorder, 38*(4), 405–441.

Ingham, R.J., & Bothe, A.K. (2001). Recovery from early stuttering: Additional issues within the Onslow & Packman-Yairi & Ambrose (1999) exchange. *Journal of Speech, Language and Hearing Research, 44*(4), 862–867.

Ingham, R.J., & Cordes, A.K. (1997). Self-measurement and evaluating stuttering treatment efficacy. In R.F. Curlee & G.M. Siegel (Eds.), *Nature and treatment of stuttering: New directions* (2nd ed., pp. 413–437). Allyn & Bacon.

Ingham, R.J., & Cordes, A.K. (1998). Treatment decisions for young children who stutter: Further concerns and complexities. *American Journal of Speech-Language Pathology, 7*(3), 10–19.

Ingham, R.J., Finn, P., & Bothe, A.K. (2005). "Roadblocks" revisited: Neural change, stuttering treatment, and recovery from stuttering. *Journal of Fluency Disorders, 30*(2), 91–107.

Ingham, R.J., Fox, P.T., & Ingham, J.C. (1994). Brain image investigation of the speech of stutterers and nonstutterers. *American Speech-Language and Hearing Association, 36*, 188.

Ingham, R.J., Fox, P.T., Ingham, J.C., Zamarripa, F., Martin, C., Jerabek, P., & Cotton, J. (1996). Functional-lesion investigation of developmental stuttering with Positron Emission Tomography. *Journal of Speech and Hearing Research, 39*, 1208–1227.

Ingham, R.J., Gow, M., & Costello, J.M. (1985). Stuttering and speech naturalness: Some additional data. *Journal of Speech and Hearing Disorders, 50*(2), 217–219.

Ingham, R.J., Grafton, S.T., Bothe, A.K., & Ingham, J.C. (2012). Brain activity in adults who stutter: Similarities across speaking tasks and correlations with stuttering frequency and speaking rate. *Brain and Language, 122*, 11–24.

Ingham, R.J., Ingham, J.C., Bothe, A.K., Wang, Y., & Kilgo, M. (2015). Efficacy of the modifying phonation intervals (MPI) stuttering treatment program with adults who stutter. *American Journal of Speech-Language Pathology, 24*(2), 256–271.

Ingham, R.J., Ingham, J.C., Onslow, M., & Finn, P. (1989). Stutterers' self ratings of speech naturalness: Assessing effects and reliability. *Journal of Speech and Hearing Research, 32*(2), 419–431.

Ingham, R.J., & Onslow, M. (1985). Measurement and modification of speech naturalness during stuttering therapy. *Journal of Speech and Hearing Disorders, 50*(3), 261–281.

Ingham, R.J., & Packman, A.C. (1978). Perceptual assessment of normalcy of speech following stuttering therapy. *Journal of Speech and Hearing Research, 21*(1), 63–73.

Ingham, R.J., & Packman, A.C. (1979). A further evaluation of the speech of stutterers during chorus and non-chorus reading conditions. *Journal of Speech and Hearing Research, 22*, 784–793.

Ingham, R.J., Sato, W., Finn, P., & Belknap, H. (2001). The modification of speech naturalness during rhythmic stimulation treatment of stuttering. *Journal of Speech, Language and Hearing Research, 44*(4), 841–52

Iverach, L., Jones, M., O'Brian, S., Block, S., Lincoln, M., Harrison, E., Hewat, S., Cream, A., Menzies, R., Packman, A., & Onslow, M. (2009). The relationship between mental health disorders and treatment outcomes among adults who stutter. *Journal of Fluency Disorders*, *34*(1), 29–43.

Iverach, L., O'Brian, S., Jones, M., Block, S., Lincoln, M., Harrison, E., Hewat, S., Menzies, R.G., Packman, A., & Onslow, M. (2009). Prevalence of anxiety disorders among adults seeking speech therapy for stuttering. *Journal of Anxiety Disorders*, *23*(7), 928–934.

Iverach, L., O'Brian, S., Jones, M., Block, S., Lincoln, M., Harrison, E., Hewat, S., Menzies, R.G., Packman, A., & Onslow, M. (2010). The five factor model of personality applied to adults who stutter. *Journal of Communication Disorders*, *43*(2), 120–132.

Jancke, L., Hanggi, J., & Steinmetz, H. (2004). Morphological brain differences between adult stutterers and non-stutterers. *BMC Neurology*, *4*, 23.

Jasper, H.H. (1932). A laboratory study of diagnostic indices of bilateral neuromuscular organization in stutterers and normal speakers. *Psychology Monographs*, *43*, 172–174.

Jassem, W.J., Morton, J., & Steffen-Batog, M. (1968). The perception of stress in synthetic speech like stimuli by Polish listeners, *Speech Analysis and Synthesis*, *1*, 289–308.

Jayaram, M. (1981). Grammatical factors in stuttering. *Journal of the Indian Institute of Science*, *63*(B), 141–147.

Jayaram, M. (1984). Distribution of stuttering in sentences: Relationship to sentence length and clause position. *Journal of Speech and Hearing Research*, *27*, 338–341.

Jayaram, M., & Savithri, S.R. (1993). *Fluency disorders: Assessment and management*. ISHA Monograph. ISHA.

Johnson, C.A., Liu, Y., Waller, N., & Chang, S.E. (2022). Tract profiles of the cerebellar peduncles in children who stutter. *Brain Structure and Function*, *227*(5), 1773–1787.

Johnson, W. (1942). A study of the onset and development of stuttering. *Journal of Speech & Hearing Disorders*, *7*, 251–257.

Johnson, W., & Associates (1959). *The onset of stuttering: Research findings and implications*. University of Minnesota Press.

Johnson, W., & Colley, W.H. (1945). The relationship between frequency and duration of stuttering. *Journal of Speech and Hearing Disorders*, *10*, 35–38.

Johnson, W., & Knott, J.R. (1937). Studies in the psychology of stuttering: I. The distribution of moments of stuttering in successive readings of the same material. *Journal of Speech Disorders*, *2*(1), 17–19.

Jokel, R., Nil, L. de, & Sharpe, K. (2007). Speech disfluencies in adults with neurogenic stuttering associated with stroke and traumatic brain injury. *Journal of Medical Speech-Language Pathology*, *15*(3), 243–262.

Jones, M., Onslow, M., Packman, A., O'Brian, S., Hearne, A., Williams, S., Ormond, T., & Schwarz, I. (2008). Extended follow-up of a randomized controlled trial of the Lidcombe Program of early stuttering intervention. *International Journal of Language and Communication Disorders*, *43*(6), 649–661.

Jossinger, S., Sares, A., Zislis, A., Sury, D., Gracco, V., & Ben-Shachar, M. (2022). White matter correlates of sensorimotor synchronization in persistent developmental stuttering. *Journal of Communication Disorders*, *95*, 106169.

Kalinowski, J., Armson, J., Roland-Mieszkowski, M., Stuart, A., & Gracco, V.L. (1993). Effects of alterations in auditory feedback and speech rate on stuttering frequency. *Language and Speech*, *36*(1), 1–16.

Kalinowski, J., Nobel, S., Armson, J., & Stuart, A. (1994). Pre-treatment and post-treatment speech naturalness ratings of adults with mild and severe stuttering. *American Journal of Speech and Language Pathology*, *3*(2), 61–66.

Kanchan, S. (1997). *Multidimensional speech naturalness scale for stutterers* [Master's Dissertation, All India Institute of Speech and Hearing, Mysuru].

Kang, C., Riazuddin, S., Mundorff, J., Krasnewich, D., Friedman, P., Mullikin, J.C., & Drayna, D. (2010). Mutations in the lysosomal enzyme-targeting pathway and persistent stuttering. *The New England Journal of Medicine, 362*(8), 677–685.

Karuppalli, S., & Bhat, J. (2016). *Manipal manual of adolescent language assessment.* Manipal University Press.

Kaul, V., Lale, M., Ashley, S., & Kelkar, P. (2022). Perceived naturalness of typical and cluttered speech: A comparative study. *Disabilities and Impairments, 36*(1), 31–42.

Kekade, N., & Valame, D. (2014). Auditory temporal processing in children with Stuttering. *Journal of the Indian Speech Language and Hearing Association, 28*(2), 41–46.

Kelkar, P. (2022, May 27–30). *Two finger feedback (TFF): A new rate control strategy for persons who clutter.* In *Paper presented at the joint world congress for stuttering and cluttering*, Montreal, Canada.

Kelkar, P., Jyotsna, K., & Maruthy, S. (2020). Construction and validation of a short version of the Impact Scale for Assessment of Cluttering and Stuttering (ISACS-s). In *Poster presented at the Annual conference of the Indian speech and hearing association*, Chandigarh.

Kelkar, P., & Mukundan, G. (2015). Development of an impact scale for assessment of fluency disorders. *Disabilities and Impairments, 29*(2), 109–115.

Kelkar, P., & Mukundan, G. (2016). Impact of fluency disorders: A comparison of perceptions of typical speakers and persons with fluency disorders. *Speech, Language and Hearing, 19*(1), 10–16.

Kelkar, P., Sanghi, M., & Chaudhari, S. (2018, July). Development and validation of an Impact Scale for Assessment of Cluttering and Stuttering (ISACS): Preliminary data. In *Paper presented at the Joint world congress on fluency disorders*, Hiroshima, Japan.

Kelkar, P.Y. (2017). An adapted Indian version of the stutterers' Self-ratings of reactions to speech situations: A mixed methods study. *Journal of Indian Speech Language & Hearing Association, 31*(2), 37.

Kelly, E.M., & Conture, E.G. (1992). Speaking rates, response time latencies, and interrupting behaviors of young stutterers, nonstutterers, and their mothers. *Journal of Speech and Hearing Research, 35*, 1256–1267.

Kelly, G.A. (1955). *The psychology of personal constructs.* Norton.

Kelman, E., & Nicholas, A. (2020). *Palin parent – child interaction therapy for early childhood stammering* (2nd ed.). Routledge.

Kertesz, A. (1982). *Western aphasia battery.* Grune & Stratton.

Keyhoe, T.D. (1998). Computers and electronic devices for stuttering therapy. In E.C. Healey & H.F.M. Peters (Eds.), *Proceedings of the 2nd world congress on fluency disorders* (pp. 262–266). Nijmegen University Press.

Khedr, E., El-Nasser, W.A., Abdel Haleem, E.K., Bakr, M.S., & Trakhan, M.N. (2000). Evoked potentials and electroencephalography in stuttering. *Folia Phoniatrica et Logopaedica, 52*, 178–186.

Kidd, K. (1977). A genetic perspective on stuttering. *Journal of Fluency Disorders, 2*, 259–269.

Kidd, K., Kidd, J.R., & Records, M.A. (1978). The possible causes of the sex ratio in stuttering and its implications. *Journal of Fluency Disorders, 3*(1), 13–23.

Kiefte, M., & Armson, J. (2008). Dissecting choral speech: Properties of the accompanist critical to stuttering reduction. *Journal of Communication Disorders, 41*, 33–48.

Kimura, D. (1961). Cerebral dominance and the perception of verbal stimuli. *Canadian Journal of Psychology, 15*, 166–171.

Kloth, S.A., Kraaimaat, F.W., Janssen, P.E.G.G.Y., & Brutten, G.J. (1999). Persistence and remission of incipient stuttering among high-risk children. *Journal of Fluency Disorders, 24*(4), 253–265.

Koenraads, S.P.C., van der Schroeff, M.P., van Ingen, G., Lamballais, S., Tiemeier, H., de Jong, R.B., White, T., Franken, M.C., & Muetzel, R.L. (2020). Structural brain differences in pre-adolescents who persist in and recover from stuttering. *NeuroImage: Clinical, 27*, 102334. https://doi.org/10.1016/j.nicl.2020.102334.

Kolk, H., & Postma, A. (1997). Stuttering as a covert repair hypothesis. In R.F. Curlee & G.M. Siegel (Eds.), *Nature and treatment of stuttering: New directions* (pp. 182–203). Allyn & Bacon.

Kools, J.A., & Berryman, J.D. (1971). Differences in disfluency behavior between male and female nonstuttering children. *Journal of Speech and Hearing Research, 14*(1), 125–130.

Koushik, S., Shenker, R., & Onslow, M. (2009). Follow-up of 6–10-year-old stuttering children after Lidcombe program treatment: A phase I trial. *Journal of Fluency Disorders, 34*(4), 279–290.

Kowal, S., O'Connell, D.C., & Sabin, E.J. (1975). Development of temporal patterning and vocal hesitations in spontaneous narratives. *Journal of Psycholinguistic Research, 4*(3), 195–207.

Kramer, M.B., Green, D., & Guitar, B. (1987). A comparison of stutterers and nonstutterers on a masking level differences and synthetic sentence identification task. *Journal of Communication Disorders, 20*, 379–390.

Krishnan, G., & Tiwari, S. (2011). Revisiting the acquired neurogenic stuttering in the light of developmental stuttering. *Journal of Neurolinguistics, 24*(3), 383–396.

Kroll, R.M., De Nil, L.F., Kapur, S., & Houle, S. (1997). A positron emission tomography investigation of post-treatment brain activation in stutterers. In *Proceedings of the third speech motor production and fluency disorders*, Amsterdam.

Kuhr, A., & Rustin, L. (1985). The maintenance of fluency after intensive in-patient therapy: Long-term follow-up. *Journal of Fluency Disorders, 10*(3), 229–236.

Kully, D., & Boberg, E. (1991). Therapy for school-age children. *Seminars in Speech and Language, 12*(4), 291–300.

Kully, D., Langevin, M., & Lomheim, H. (2007). Intensive treatment of stuttering in adolescents and adults. In E.G. Conture & R.F. Curlee (Eds.), *Stuttering and related disorders of fluency* (3rd ed., pp. 213–232). Thieme.

Kvenseth, H.B. (2007, May). Cluttering: Helene's personal experiences. In K. Bakker, L.J. Raphael, & F.L. Myers (Eds.), *Proceedings of the first world congress on cluttering* (pp. 50–53). International Cluttering Association, Katarino, Bulgaria. Retrieved January 29, 2015, from http://associations.missouristate.edu/ica/.

La Salle, L. (2010). When is it cluttering and when is it cluttering-plus? In *Plenary session at the international cluttering online conference, April 14–May 5*. Retrieved April 28, 2021, from www.mnsu.edu/comdis/ica1/papers/lasalle1c.html.

Lakkanna, S., Venkatesh, K., Bhat., J., & Karuppalli, S. (2021). *Assessment of language development*. Manipal University Press.

Lan, J., Song, M., Pan, C., Zhuang, G., Wang, Y., Ma, W., Chu, Q., Lai, Q., Xu, F., Li, Y., Liu, L., & Wang, W. (2009). Association between dopaminergic genes (SLC6A3 and DRD2) and stuttering among Han Chinese. *Journal of Human Genetics, 54*(8), 457–460.

Langevin, M., & Boberg, E. (1996). Results of intensive stuttering therapy with adults who clutter and stutter. *Journal of Fluency Disorders, 21*(3–4), 315–327.

Langevin, M., & Kully, D. (2012). The comprehensive stuttering program and its evidence base. In S. Jelčić Jakšić & M. Onslow (Eds.), *The science and practice of stuttering treatment: A symposium* (pp. 115–129). Wiley-Blackwell. https://doi.org/10.1002/9781118702796.ch9

Langevin, M., Kully, D., Teshima, S., Hagler, P., & Prasad, N.N. (2010). Five-year longitudinal treatment outcomes of the ISTAR Comprehensive Stuttering Program. *Journal of Fluency Disorders, 35*(2), 123–140.

Langova, J., & Moravek, M. (1964). Some results of experimental examinations among stutterers and clutterers. *Folia Phoniatrica, 162,* 290–296.

LaSalle, L.R., & Conture, E.G. (1995). Clustering of between- and within-word disfluencies in the speech of children who do and do not stutter. *Journal of Speech and Hearing Research, 38,* 965–999.

Lattermann, C., Euler, H.A., & Neumann, K. (2008). A randomized controlled trial to investigate the impact of the Lidcombe Program on early stuttering in German-speaking preschoolers. *Journal of Fluency Disorders, 33*(1), 52–65.

Leadholm, B.J., & Miller, J.F. (1994). *Language sample analysis: The Wisconsin guide.* Wisconsin Department of Public Instruction. https://files.eric.ed.gov/fulltext/ED371528.pdf

Lebrun, Y., & Leleux, C. (1985). Acquired stuttering following right brain damage in dextrals. *Journal of Fluency Disorders, 10*(2), 137–141.

Lebrun, Y., Leleux, C., & Retif, J. (1987). Neurogenic stuttering. *Acta Neurochirurgica, 85*(3), 103–109.

Leder, S.B. (1996). Adult onset of stuttering as a presenting sign in a parkinsonian-like syndrome: A case report. *Journal of Communication Disorders, 29*(6), 471–478.

Lehiste, I. (1968). Vowel quality in word and utterances in Estonian. In *Congressus secundus internationalis finno-ugristarum, Helsinki, 1965* (pp. 293–303). Societas Finno-Ugrica.

Levelt, W. (1989). *Speaking: From intention to articulation.* MIT Press.

Levy, C. (1983). Group therapy with adults. In P. Dalton (Ed.), *Approaches to the treatment of stuttering* (pp. 136–163). Croom Helm.

Lewis, C., Packman, A., Onslow, M., Simpson, J.M., & Jones, M. (2008). A phase II trial of telehealth delivery of the Lidcombe Program of early stuttering intervention. *American Journal of Speech-Language Pathology, 17*(2), 139–149.

Lickley, R. (2017). *Disfluency in typical and stuttered speech.* https://core.ac.uk/download/pdf/155779398.pdf

Lieberman, P. (1960). Some acoustic correlates of word stress in American English. *Journal of the Acoustical Society of America, 32,* 451–454.

Liebetrau, R.M., & Daly, D.A. (1981). Auditory processing and perceptual abilities of "organic" and "functional" stutterers. *Journal of Fluency Disorders, 6*(3), 219–231.

Lincoln, M.A., & Onslow, M. (1997). Long-term outcome of early intervention for stuttering. *American Journal of Speech-Language Pathology, 6*(1), 51–58.

Lincoln, M.A., Onslow, M., Lewis, C., & Wilson, L. (1996). A clinical trial of an operant treatment for school-age children who stutter. *American Journal of Speech-Language Pathology, 5*(2), 73–85.

Logan, K. (2020). *Fluency disorders: Stuttering, cluttering and related fluency problems* (2nd ed.). Plural publishing, Inc.

Logan, K. (2005). Improving communicative functioning with school-aged children who stutter. In R. Lees & C. Stark (Eds.), *The treatment of stuttering in the young school-aged child* (pp. 108–139). Whurr Publishers.

Logan, K., & LaSalle, L. (1999). Grammatical characteristics of children's conversational utterances that contain disfluency clusters. *Journal of Speech, Language, and Hearing Research, 42,* 80–91.

Lotzmann, G. (1961). On the use of varied delay times in stammerers. *Folia Phoniatrica, 13,* 276–310.

Louko, L., Edwards, M.L., & Conture, E.G. (1990). Treating children who exhibit co-occurring stuttering and disordered phonology. In R. Curlee (Ed.), *Stuttering and related disorders of fluency* (pp. 124–138). Thieme Medical Publishers.

Low, E.L. (2006). A review of recent research on speech rhythm: Some insights for language acquisition, language disorders and language teaching. In R. Hughes (Ed.), *Spoken*

English, TESOL and applied linguistics. Palgrave Macmillan. https://doi.org/10.1057/9780230584587_5

Ludlow, C.L., Rosenberg, J., Salazar, A., Grafman, J., & Smutok, M. (1987). Site of penetrating brain lesions causing chronic acquired stuttering. *Annals of Neurology, 22*(1), 60–66.

Lundie, M., Erasmus, Z., Zsilavecz, U., & van der Linde, J. (2014). Compilation of a preliminary checklist for the differential diagnosis of neurogenic stuttering. *The South African Journal of Communication Disorders, 61*(1). https://doi.org/10.4102/SAJCD.V61I1.64

Luterman, D. (1991). *Counseling the communicatively disordered and their families.* Pro-Ed.

MacDermot, K.D., Bonora, E., Sykes, N., Coupe, A.M., Lai, C.S., Vernes, S.C., Vargha-Khadem, F., McKenzie, F., Smith, R., Monaco, A., & Fisher, S.E. (2005). Identification of FOXP2 truncation as a novel cause of developmental speech and language deficits. *American Journal of Human Genetics, 76*(6), 1074–1080.

MacFarlane, W.B., Hanson, M., Walton, W., & Mellon, C.D. (1991). Stuttering in five generations of a single family: A preliminary report including evidence supporting a sex-modified mode of transmission. *Journal of Fluency Disorders, 16,* 117–123.

Macleod, J., Kalinowski, J., Stuart, A., & Armson, J. (1955). Effect of single and combined altered auditory feedback on stuttering frequency at two speech rates. *Journal of Communication Disorders, 28,* 217–228.

Maguire, G.A., Nguyen, D.L., Simonson, K.C., & Kurz, T.L. (2020). The pharmacologic treatment of stuttering and its neuropharmacologic basis. *Frontiers in Neuroscience, 14,* 158. https://doi.org/10.3389/fnins.2020.00158

Maguire, G.A., Riley, G.D., Franklin, D.L., Wu, J., Ortiz, T., Johnson, T., & Gottschalk, L.A. (2000). The dopamine hypothesis of stuttering and its treatment implications. *International Journal of Neuropsychopharmacology, 3*(1), 18. https://doi.org/10.1017/S1461145700009998

Mahesh, S., & Raju, R. (2020). The effect of syllable complexity on speech disfluencies of Kannada speaking adults who stutter. *Journal of the All India Institute of Speech and Hearing, 39,* 23–30.

Mahr, G., & Leith, W. (1992). Psychogenic stuttering of adult onset. *Journal of Speech and Hearing Research, 35,* 283–286.

Maner, K.J., Smith, A., & Grayson, L. (2000). Influences of utterance length and complexity on speech motor performance in children and adults. *Journal of Speech, Language, and Hearing Research, 43*(2), 560–573.

Manning, W.H. (2001). *Clinical decision making in fluency disorders* (2nd ed.). Singular Publishing Group.

Manning, W.H. (2009). *Clinical decision making in fluency disorders* (3rd ed.). Cengage Learning.

Manning, W.H., & DiLollo, A. (2018). *Clinical decision making in fluency disorders* (4th ed.). Plural Publishing.

Mansson, H. (2000). Childhood stuttering: Incidence and development. *Journal of Fluency Disorders, 25*(1), 47–57.

Market, K.E., Montague, J.C., Buffalo, M.D., & Drummond, S.S. (1990). Acquired stuttering: Descriptive data and treatment outcome. *Journal of Fluency Disorders, 15*(1), 21–33.

Marshall, R.C., & Starch, S.A. (1984). Behavioral treatment of acquired stuttering. *Australian Journal of Human Communication Disorders, 12*(1), 87–92.

Martin, R.R., & Haroldson, S.K. (1979). Effects of five experimental treatments on stuttering. *Journal of Speech and Hearing Research, 22*(1), 132–146.

Martin, R.R., & Haroldson, S.K. (1981). Stuttering identification: Standard definition and moment of stuttering. *Journal of Speech, Language, and Hearing Research, 24*(1), 59–63.

Martin, R.R., & Haroldson, S.K. (1992). Stuttering and speech naturalness: Audio and audiovisual judgments. *Journal of Speech, Language, and Hearing Research, 35*(3), 521–528.

Martin, R.R., Haroldson, S.K., & Triden, K.A. (1984). Stuttering and speech naturalness. *Journal of Speech and Hearing Disorders, 49*(1), 53–58.

Martin, R.R., Kuhl, P., & Haroldson, S. (1972). An experimental treatment with two preschool stuttering children. *Journal of Speech and Hearing Research, 15*, 743–752.

Martin, R.R., Johnson, L., Siegel, G., & Haroldson, S. (1985). Auditory stimulation, rhythm, and stuttering. *Journal of Speech and Hearing Research, 28*, 487–495.

Martyn, M.M., & Sheehan, J. (1968). Onset of stuttering and recovery. *Behaviour Research and Therapy, 6*(3), 295–307.

Maruthy, S., Raj, N., Geetha, M.P., & Sindhu Priya, C. (2015). Disfluency characteristics of Kannada-English bilingual adults who stutter. *Journal of Communication Disorders, 56*, 19–28.

Masumi, E., Kashani, Z.A., Hassanpour, N., & Kamali, M. (2015). The effect of syllable structure on the frequency of disfluencies in adults with stuttering. *Middle East Journal of Rehabilitation Health, 2*(2), e26436. https://doi.org/10.17795/mejrh-26436

Max, L., Caruso, A.J., & Vandevenne, A. (1997). Decreased stuttering frequency during repeated readings: A motor learning perspective. *Journal of Fluency Disorders, 22*, 1–17.

Max, L., Kadri, M., Mitsuya, T., & Balasubramanian, V. (2019). Similar within-utterance loci of dysfluency in acquired neurogenic and persistent developmental stuttering. *Brain and Language, 189*, 1–9.

Mazzucchi, A., Moretti, G., Carpeggiani, P., Parma, M., & Paini, P. (1981). Clinical observations on acquired stuttering. *British Journal of Disorders of Communication, 16*(1), 19–30.

McClellan, J., & King, M.C. (2010). Genetic heterogeneity in human disease. *Cell, 141*(2), 210–217.

McDonough, A.N., & Quesal, R.W. (1988). Locus of control orientation of stutterers and nonstutterers. *Journal of Fluency Disorders, 13*(2), 97–106.

McFarland, D.H., & Moore, W.H., Jr. (1982). Alpha asymmetries during an electromyographic biofeedback procedure for stuttering. In *Annual convention of the American speech-language-hearing association*, Toronto, Canada.

McGill, M., Sussman, H., & Byrd, C.T. (2016). From grapheme to phonological output: Performance of adults who stutter on a word jumble task. *PLOS ONE, 11*(3), e0151107. https://doi.org/10.1371/journal.pone.0151107

Menzies, R.G., O'Brian, S., Onslow, M., Packman, A., St Clare, T., & Block, S. (2008). An experimental clinical trial of a cognitive-behavior therapy package for chronic stuttering. *Journal of Speech, Language and Hearing Research, 51*(6), 1451–1464.

Menzies, R.G., O'Brian, S., Packman, A., Jones, M., Helgadóttir, F.D., & Onslow, M. (2019). Supplementing stuttering treatment with online cognitive behavior therapy: An experimental trial. *Journal of Communication Disorders, 80*, 81–91.

Menzies, R.G., Onslow, M., Packman, A., & O'Brian, S. (2009). Cognitive behaviour therapy for adults who stutter: A tutorial for speech-language pathologists. *Journal of Fluency Disorders, 34*(3), 187–200.

Menzies, R.G., Packman, A., Onslow, M., O'Brian, S., Jones, M., & Helgadóttir, F.D. (2019). In-clinic and standalone Internet cognitive behaviour therapy treatment for social anxiety in stuttering: A randomized trial of iGlebe. *Journal of Speech, Language, and Hearing Research, 62*(6), 1614–1624.

Merriam-Webster. (n.d.). Disorder. In *Merriam-Webster.com dictionary*. Retrieved February 11, 2022, from www.merriam-webster.com/dictionary/disorder

Messenger, M., Onslow, M., Packman, A., & Menzies, R. (2004). Social anxiety in stuttering: Measuring negative social expectancies. *Journal of Fluency Disorders, 29*(3), 201–212.

Messenger, M., Packman, A., Onslow, M., Menzies, R., & O'Brian, S. (2015). Children and adolescents who stutter: Further investigation of anxiety. *Journal of Fluency Disorders, 46*, 15–23.

Metz, D.E., Schiavetti, N., & Sacco, P.R. (1990). Acoustic and psychophysical dimensions of the perceived speech naturalness of non-stutterers and post-treatment stutterers. *Journal of Speech and Hearing Disorders, 55*(3), 516–525.

Meyers, S.C. (1986). Qualitative and quantitative differences and patterns of variability in disfluencies emitted by preschool stutterers and nonstutterers during dyadic conversations. *Journal of Fluency Disorders, 11*(4), 293–306.

Meyers, S.C., Ghatak, L.R., & Woodford, L. (1990). Case descriptions of non-fluency and loci: Initial and follow-up conversations with three preschool children. *Journal of Fluency Disorders, 14*, 383–398.

Meyers, S.C., Hughes, L.F., & Schoeny, Z.G. (1989). Temporal-phonemic processing skills in adult stutterers and nonstutterers. *Journal of Speech, Language, and Hearing Research, 32*(2), 274–280.

Millard, S.K., Edwards, S., & Cook, F.M. (2009). Parent-child interaction therapy: Adding to the evidence. *International Journal of Speech-Language Pathology, 11*(1), 61–76.

Millard, S.K., Nicholas, A., & Cook, F.M. (2008). Is parent – child interaction therapy effective in reducing stuttering? *Journal of Speech, Language, and Hearing Research, 51*, 636–650.

Millard, S.K., Zebrowski, P., & Kelman, E. (2018). Palin parent– child interaction therapy: The bigger picture. *American Journal of Speech-Language Pathology, 27*(3S), 1211–1223.

Misaghi, E., Zhang, Z., Gracco, V.L., De Nil, L.F., & Beal, D.S. (2018). White matter tractography of the neural network for speech-motor control in children who stutter. *Neuroscience Letters, 668*, 37–42.

Molt, L. (1996). An examination of various aspects of auditory processing in clutterers. *Journal of Fluency Disorders, 21*, 215–226.

Molt, L.F., & Guilford, A.M. (1979). Auditory processing and anxiety in stutterers. *Journal of Fluency Disorders, 4*, 255–267.

Moncur, J.P. (1952). Parental domination in stuttering. *Journal of Speech and Hearing Disorders, 17*(2), 155–165.

Monroe, S., & Simmons, A. (1991). Diathesis-stress theories in the context of life stress research: Implications for the depressive disorders. *Psychological Bulletin, 110*, 406–425.

Montgomery, B.M., & Fitch, J.L. (1988). The prevalence of stuttering in the hearing-impaired school age population. *Journal of Speech and Hearing Disorders, 53*, 131–135.

Moore, W. (1984). Hemispheric alpha asymmetries during an electromyographic biofeedback procedure for stuttering: A single-subject experimental design. *Journal of Fluency Disorders, 9*, 143–162.

Morgan, M. D., Cranford, J. L., & Burk, K. (1997). P300 event-related potentials in stutterers and nonstutterers. *Journal of Speech, Language and Hearing Research, 40*(6), 1334–1340.

Morton, J., & Jassem, W. (1965). Acoustic correlates of stress. *Language & Speech, 8*, 159–187.

Mouradian, M.S., Paslawski, T., & Shuaib, A. (2000). Return of stuttering after stroke. *Brain and Language, 73*(1), 120–123.

Murza, K.A., & Nye, C. (2009). The Lidcombe program demonstrates positive results for German preschoolers who stutter. *Evidence-Based Communication Assessment and Intervention, 3*(1), 15–18.

Myers, F. (1996). Annotations on research and clinical perspectives on cluttering since 1964. *Journal of Fluency Disorders, 21*, 187–199.

Myers, F.L. (2011). Treatment of cluttering: A cognitive-behavioral approach centered on rate control. In D. Ward & K. Scaler Scott (Eds.), *Cluttering: A handbook of research, intervention and education* (pp. 152–174). Psychology Press.

Myers, F.L., & Wall, M.J. (1981). Issues to consider in the differential diagnosis of normal childhood nonfluencies and stuttering. *Journal of Fluency Disorders, 6*(3), 189–195. https://doi.org/10.1016/0094-730X(81)90001-2

Nagapoornima, M. (1990). *Disfluencies in children (3–4 years)* [Master's dissertation, All India Institute of Speech and Hearing, Mysuru].

Natke, U. (2000). Stottern Reduktion unter verzögerter und frequenz verschobener auditiver Rückmeldung (Reduction of stuttering frequency using frequency shifted and delayed auditory feedback). *Folia Phoniatrica et Logopaedica, 52,* 151–159.

Natke, U., Grosser, J., Sandreiser, P., & Kaveram, K.T. (2002). The duration component of the stress effect in stuttering. *Journal of Fluency Disorders, 27,* 305–318.

Natke, U., Sandrieser, P., Pietrowsky, R., & Kalveram, K.T. (2006). Disfluency data of German preschool children who stutter and comparison children. *Journal of Fluency Disorders, 31*(3), 165–176.

Natke, U., Sandrieser, P., van Ark, M., Pietrowsky, R., & Kalveram, K.T. (2004). Linguistic stress, within-word position, and grammatical class in relation to early childhood stuttering. *Journal of Fluency Disorders, 29*(2), 109–222.

Neaves, A.I. (1970). To establish a basis for prognosis in stammering: (An abridged version of a thesis presented for the Fellowship of the College of Speech Therapists). *British Journal of Disorders of Communication, 5*(1), 46–58.

Neef, N.E., Anwander, A., Bütfering, C., Schmidt-Samoa, C., Friederici, A.D., Paulus, W., & Sommer, M. (2018). Structural connectivity of right frontal hyperactive areas scales with stuttering severity. *Brain, 14*(1), 191–204.

Neiders, G.K. (2011). *Theoretical development of a proposed Rational Emotive Behaviour Therapy based model to treat persons with Chronic Perseverative Stuttering Syndrome* (Publication No.3537793) [Doctoral dissertation, Argosy University/Seattle]. ProQuest Dissertations and Theses Global.

Neiders, G.K., & Ross, W. (2013). *From stuttering to fluency: Manage your emotions and live more fully.* Createspace Independent Pub.

Newman, P.W., Bunderson, K., & Brey, R.H. (1985). Brainstem electrical responses of stutterers and normals by sex, ears, and recovery. *Journal of Fluency Disorders, 10,* 59–67.

Newman, R.S., & Bernstein Ratner, N. (2007). The role of selected lexical factors on confrontation naming accuracy, speed, and fluency in adults who do and do not stutter. *Journal of Speech, Language, and Hearing Research, 50*(1), 196–213.

Neumann, K., Euler, H.A., Zens, R., Piskernik, B., Packman, A., Louis, K.O.S., Kell, C.A., Amir, O., Blomgren, M., Aumont Boucand, V., Eggers, K., Fibiger, S., Fourches, A., Franken, J.P.M-C., & Finn, P. (2019). "Spontaneous" late recovery from stuttering: Dimensions of reported techniques and causal attributions. *Journal of Communication Disorders, 81,* 105915. https://doi.org/10.1016/j.jcomdis.2019.105915

Neumann, K., Preibisch, C., Euler, H.A., von Gudenberg, A.W., Lanfermann, H., Gall, V., & Giraud, A.L. (2005). Cortical plasticity associated with stuttering therapy. *Journal of Fluency Disorders, 30,* 23–39.

Newton, K.R., Blood, G.W., & Blood, I.M. (1986). Simultaneous and staggered dichotic word and digit tests with stutterers and nonstutterers. *Journal of Fluency Disorders, 11*(3), 201–216.

Nip, I.S., Green, J.R., & Marx, D.B. (2009). Early speech motor development: Cognitive and linguistic considerations. *Journal of Communication Disorders, 42*(4), 286–298.

Nippold, M.A. (2018). Stuttering in preschool children: Direct versus indirect treatment. *Language, Speech, and Hearing Services in Schools, 49*(1), 4–12.

Nippold, M.A., Schwarz, I.E., & Jescheniak, J.D. (1991). Narrative ability in school-age stuttering boys: A preliminary investigation. *Journal of Fluency Disorders, 16*(5–6), 289–308.

Novelli, A. (2018). *Speech naturalness before and following treatment in adults who stutter* [Honors theses. 3015]. https://scholarworks.wmich.edu/honors_theses/3015

Ntourou, K., Conture, E.G., & Lipsey, M.W. (2011). Language abilities of children who stutter: A meta-analytical review. *American Journal of Speech Language Pathology*, *20*(3), 163–179.

Ntourou, K., Conture, E.G., & Walden, T.A. (2013). Emotional reactivity and regulation in preschool-age children who stutter. *Journal of Fluency Disorders*, *38*(3), 1–25.

O'Brian, S., Onslow, M., Cream, A., & Packman, A. (2003). The Camperdown program: Outcomes of a new prolonged-speech treatment model. *Journal of Speech and Hearing Research*, *46*(4), 933–946.

O'Brian, S., Smith, K., & Onslow, M. (2014). Webcam delivery of the Lidcombe program for early stuttering: A phase I clinical trial. *Journal of Speech, Language, and Hearing Research*, *57*(3), 825–830.

Onslow, M. (1996). *Behavioral management of stuttering*. Singular Publishing Group.

Onslow, M. (2021). *Stuttering and its treatment – Eleven lectures*. Australian Stuttering Research Centre.

Onslow, M., Andrews, C., & Lincoln, M. (1994). A control/experimental trial of an operant treatment for early stuttering. *Journal of Speech and Hearing Research*, *37*(6), 1244–1259.

Onslow, M., Costa, L., Andrews, C., Harrison, E., & Packman, A. (1996). Speech outcomes of a prolonged-speech treatment for stuttering. *Journal of Speech, Language, and Hearing Research*, *39*(4), 734–749.

Onslow, M., Costa, L., & Rue, S. (1990). Direct early intervention with stuttering: Some preliminary data. *Journal of Speech and Hearing Disorders*, *55*(3), 405–416.

Onslow, M., Hayes, B., Hutchins, L., & Newman, D. (1992). Speech naturalness and prolonged-speech treatments for stuttering: Further variables and data. *Journal of Speech, Language, and Hearing Research*, *35*(2), 274–282.

Onslow, M., & Ingham, R. J. (1987). Speech quality measurement and the management of stuttering. *The Journal of Speech and Hearing Disorders*, *52*(1), 2–17.

Onslow, M., Stocker, S., Packman, A., & McLeod, S. (2009). Speech timing in children after the Lidcombe program of early stuttering intervention. *Clinical Linguistics and Phonetics*, *16*(1), 21–33.

Onslow, M., Webber, M., Harrison, E., Arnott, S., Bridgman, K., Carey, B., Sheedy, S., O'Brian, S., MacMillan, V., & Lloyd, W. (2021). *The Lidcombe Program treatment guide*. www.uts.edu.au/asrc/resources

Ooki, S. (2005). Genetic and environmental influences on stuttering and tics in Japanese twin children. *Twin Research and Human Genetics*, *8*(1), 69–75.

Op't Hof, J., & Uys, R. (1974). A Clinical Delineation of Tachyphemia (Cluttering): A case of dominant inheritance. *South African Medical Journal*, *38*(48), 1624–1628.

Ornstein, A.F., & Manning, W. H. (1985). Self-efficacy scaling by adult stutterers. *Journal of Communication Disorders*, *18*(4), 313–320.

Orton, S.T. (1927). Studies in stuttering. *Archives of Neurology and Psychiatry*, *18*, 671–672.

Orton, S.T., & Travis, L.E. (1929). Studies in stammering. IV. Studies of action currents in stutterers. *Archives of Neurology and Psychiatry*, *21*, 61–68.

Oxford. (n.d.). Theory. In *Oxford learner's dictionaries*. Retrieved February 11, 2022, from www.oxfordlearnersdictionaries.com/definition/american_english/theory

Packman, A., & Attanasio, J.S. (2010). A model of the mechanisms underpinning early interventions for stuttering. In *Annual convention of the American speech-language and hearing association*, Philadelphia, USA.

Packman, A., & Attanasio, J.S. (2017). *Theoretical issues in stuttering*. Routledge.

Packman, A., & Kuhn, L. (2009). Looking at stuttering through the lens of complexity. *International Journal of Speech-Language Pathology*, *11*(1), 77–82.

Packman, A., Onslow, M., & Menzies, R. (2000). Novel speech patterns and the treatment of stuttering. *Disability and Rehabilitation*, *22*(1–2), 65–79.

Packman, A., Onslow, M., & Van Doorn, J. (1997). Linguistic stress and the rhythm effect in stuttering. In W. Hulstijn et al. (Eds.), *Speech production: Motor control, brain research and fluency disorders* (pp. 473–478). Elsevier Science.

Packman, A., Onslow, M., Reilly, S., Attanasio, J., & Shenker, R. (2009). Stuttering and bilingualism. *Archives of Disease in Childhood, 94*(3), 248.

Packman, A., Onslow, M., Richard, F., & Van Doorn, J. (1996). Syllabic stress and variability: A model of stuttering. *Clinical Linguistics and Phonetics, 10*(3), 235–263.

Park, J., & Logan, K.J. (2015). The role of temporal speech cues in facilitating the fluency of adults who stutter. *Journal of Fluency Disorders, 46*, 41–55.

Pelczarski, K.M., Tendera, A., Dye, M., & Loucks, T.M. (2018). Delayed phonological encoding in stuttering: Evidence from eye tracking. *Language and Speech, 6*, 475–493.

Pelczarski, K.M., & Yaruss, J.S. (2014). Phonological encoding of young children who stutter. *Journal of Fluency Disorders, 39*, 12–24.

Pellowski, M.W., & Conture, E.G. (2002). Characteristics of speech disfluency and stuttering behaviors in 3-and 4-year-old children. *Journal of Speech, Language, and Hearing Research, 45*(1), 20–34.

Pellowski, M.W., & Conture, E.G. (2005). Lexical priming in picture naming of young children who do and do not stutter. *Journal of Speech, Language and Hearing Research, 48*(2), 278–294.

Penttilä, N., & Korpijaakko-Huuhka, A.M. (2015). New guidelines for assessing neurogenic stuttering. *Procedia – Social and Behavioral Sciences, 193*, 310–313.

Perkins, W.H. (1973). Replacement of stuttering with normal speech: I. Rationale. *Journal of Speech and Hearing Disorders, 38*(3), 283–294.

Perkins, W.H., Bell, J., Johnson, L., & Stocks, J. (1979). Phone rate and the effective planning time hypothesis of stuttering. *Journal of Speech, Language, and Hearing Research, 22*(4), 747–755.

Perkins, W.H., Rudas, J., Johnson, L., & Bell, J. (1976). Stuttering: Discoordination of phonation with articulation and respiration. *Journal of Speech and Hearing Research, 19*, 509–522.

Peters, T., & Guitar, B. (1991). *Stuttering: An integrated approach to its nature and treatment.* Lippincott Williams and Wilkins.

Pierce, C.M., & Lipcon, H.H. (1959). Clinical and encephalographic findings. *Military Medicine, 12*, 511–519.

Pike, K. (1945). *The intonation of American English.* University of Michigan Press.

Pindzola, R.H., & White, D.T. (1986). A protocol for differentiating the incipient stutterer. *Language, Speech, and Hearing Services in Schools, 17*(1), 2–15.

Pinsky, S.D., & McAdam, D.W. (1980). Electroencephalographic and dichotic indices of cerebral laterality in stutterers. *Brain and Language, 11*(2), 374–397.

Plexico, L., Manning, W.H., & DiLollo, A. (2005). A phenomenological understanding of successful stuttering management. *Journal of Fluency Disorders, 30*(1), 1–22.

Pool, K.D., Devous, M.D., Sr., Freeman, F.J., Watson, B.C., & Finitzo, T. (1991). Regional cerebral blood flow in developmental stutterers. *Archives of Neurology, 48*, 509–512.

Postma, A., & Kolk, H. (1993). The covert repair hypothesis: Prearticulatory repair processes in normal and stuttered disfluencies. *Journal of Speech, Language and Hearing Research, 36*(3), 472–487.

Preibisch, C., Neumann, K., Raab, P., Euler, H.A., von Gudenberg, A.W., & Gall, V. (2003). Evidence for compensation for stuttering by the right frontal operculum. *Neuroimage, 20*, 1356–1364.

Preus, A. (1981). *Identifying subgroups of stutterers.* Scandinavian University Press.

Preus, A. (1996). Cluttering and stuttering: Related, different or antagonistic disorders? In F. L. Myers & K.O. St Louis (Eds.), *Cluttering: A clinical perspective* (pp. 55–70). Singular Publishing Group.

Priyanka, K., & Maruthy, S. (2019). Cross-linguistic generalization of fluency to untreated language in bilingual adults who stutter. *Journal of Indian Speech Language & Hearing Association, 33*(1), 23.

Quader, S.E. (1977). Dysarthria: An unusual side effect of tricyclic antidepressants. *British Medical Journal, 2*(6079), 97. https://doi.org/10.1136/BMJ.2.6079.97

Quinn, P.T. (1972). Stuttering – cerebral dominance and dichotic word test. *Medical Journal of Australia, 2*, 639–642.

Rajendraswamy. (1991). *Some aspects of fluency in children (6–7 years)* [Master's dissertation, All India Institute of Speech and Hearing, Mysuru].

Rajupratap, S. (1991). Production of word stress in children – 3–4 years. In M. Jayaram & S. R. Savithri (Eds.), *Research at AIISH, dissertation abstracts, Vol. III, 11*. All India Institute of Speech and Hearing.

Rakesh, C.V. (2021). *Efficacy of prolonged speech and pause and talk techniques in school-aged children with stuttering: A comparison* [Unpublished doctoral thesis, University of Mysore].

Ram, A.B., & Savithri, S.R. (2007). Disfluencies in 5.1 to 6 year old Kannada speaking children. *Journal of All India Institute of Speech and Hearing, 26*(1), 3–8.

Rastatter, M.P., Stuart, A., & Kalinowski, J. (1998). Quantitative electroencephalogram of posterior cortical areas of fluent and stuttering participants during reading with normal and altered auditory feedback. *Perceptual and Motor Skills, 87*(2), 623–633.

Rathika, R., Kanaka, G., Sunila, J., & Rajashekhar, B. (2012). Disfluencies in typically developing Tamil; speaking children 4–8 years. *Languages in India, 12*, 479–497.

Ratusnik, D.L., Kiriluk, E., Melnick, C., & Ratusnik, R. (1979). Relationship among race, social status, and sex of preschoolers' normal dysfluencies: A cross-cultural investigation. *Language, Speech, and Hearing Services in Schools, 10*(3), 171–177.

Rautakoski, P., Hannus, T., Simberg, S., Sandnabba, N.K., & Santtila, P. (2012). Genetic and environmental effects on stuttering: A twin study from Finland. *Journal of Fluency Disorders, 37*(3), 202–210.

Raza, M.H., Gertz, E.M., Mundorff, J., Lukong, J., Kuster, J., Schäffer, A.A., & Drayna, D. (2013). Linkage analysis of a large African family segregating stuttering suggests polygenic inheritance. *Human Genetics, 132*(4), 385–396.

Raza, M.H., Riazuddin, S., & Drayna, D. (2010). Identification of an autosomal recessive stuttering locus on chromosome 3q13.2–3q13.33. *Human Genetics, 128*(4), 461–463.

Records, M.A., Heimbuch, R.C., & Kidd, J.R. (1977). Handedness and stuttering: A dead horse? *Journal of Fluency Disorders, 2*, 271–282.

Rehder, P. (1968). *Beitrage zur Erforschung der serbokroatischen prosodie*, Slavistische Beitrage 31. Veriag otto sagner.

Reichel, I. (2010). Treating the person who clutters and stutters. In K. Bakker, L. Raphael, & F. Myers (Eds.), *Proceedings of the first world conference on cluttering* (pp. 99–107). International Cluttering Association, Katarino, Bulgaria.

Reichel, I.K., Ademola-Sokoya, G., Bakhtiar, M., Barrett, H., Bona, J., Busto-Marolt, L., Caesar, N.N., Diaz, C., Haj-Tas, M., Lilian, D., Makauskienė, V., Miyamoto, S., Shah, E., Bian de Touzet, B., & Yasin, S.A. (2014). Frontiers of cluttering across continents: Research, clinical practices, self-help, and professional preparation. *Perspectives on Global Issues in Communication Sciences and Related Disorders, 4*(2), 42–50.

Reichel, I.K., Ademola-Sakoya, G., Boucand, V. A., Bona, J., Carmona, J., Cosyns, M., Filatova, Y., Haj-Tas, M., Kelkar, P., Remman, R., Miyamoto, S., Ozdemir, S., Sanghi, S., Schnell, A., Biain de Touzet, B., & Yang, S.L. (2019). A decade of collaboration among international representatives of the International Cluttering Association. *SIG 17 Global Issues in Communication Sciences and Related Disorders, 4*(6), 1573–1580.

Reilly, S., Onslow, M., Packman, A., Cini, E., Conway, L., Ukoumunne, O.C., Bavin, E.L., Prior, M., Eadie, P., Block, S., & Wake, M. (2013). Natural history of stuttering to 4 years of age: A prospective community-based study. *Pediatrics, 132*(3), 460–467.

Reilly, S., Onslow, M., Packman, A., Wake, M., Bavin, E.L., Prior, M., Eadie, P., Cini, E., Bolzonello, C., & Ukoumunne, O.C. (2009). Predicting stuttering onset by the age of 3 years: A prospective, community cohort study. *Pediatrics, 123,* 270–277.

Rentschler, G.J., Driver, L.E., & Callaway, E.A. (1984). The onset of stuttering following drug overdose. *Journal of Fluency Disorders, 9*(4), 265–284.

Riaz, N., Steinberg, S., Ahmad, J., Pluzhnikov, A., Riazuddin, S., Cox, N.J., & Drayna, D. (2005). Genomewide significant linkage to stuttering on chromosome 12. *American Journal of Human Genetics, 76*(4), 647–651.

Richels, C., Buhr, A., Conture, E., & Ntourou, K. (2010). Utterance complexity and stuttering on function words in preschool age children who stutter. *Journal of Fluency Disorders, 35*(3), 314–331.

Richels, C., & Conture, E.G. (2010). Indirect treatment of childhood stuttering: Diagnostic predictors of treatment outcome. In B. Guitar & R.J. McCauley (Eds.), *Treatment of stuttering: Established and emerging interventions* (pp. 18–55). Lippincott Williams & Wilkins.

Rigault, A. (1962). Role de la frequence, de l'intensite et de la duree vocaliques dans la perception de l'accent en francais. In *Proceedings of the 4th international congress of phonetic sciences, Helsinki, 1961* (pp. 735–748). Mouton & Co.

Riley, G.D. (1981). *The stuttering prediction instrument for young children.* Pro-Ed.

Riley, G.D. (1994). *Stuttering severity instrument for children and adults.* Pro-Ed Austin.

Riley, G.D. (2009). *SSI-4: Stuttering severity instrument* (4th ed.). Pro-Ed.

Riley, G.D., & Riley, J. (1986). Oral motor dis-coordination among children who stutter. *Journal of Fluency Disorders, 11*(4), 335–344.

Ringo, C.C., & Dietrich, S. (1995). Neurogenic stuttering: An analysis and critique. *Journal of Medical Speech-Language Pathology, 3*(2), 111–122.

Ritto, A.P., Juste, F.S., Stuart, A., Kalinowski, J., & Andrade, C.R.F. (2016). Randomized clinical trial: The use of SpeechEasy® in stuttering treatment. *International Journal of Language and Communication Disorders, 51,* 769–774.

Roberts, P.M., Meltzer, A., & Wilding, J. (2009). Disfluencies in non-stuttering adults across sample lengths and topics. *Journal of Communication Disorders, 42*(6), 414–427.

Rocha, M.S., Yaruss, J.S., & Rato, J.R. (2019). Temperament, executive functioning, and anxiety in school-age children who stutter. *Frontiers in Psychology, 10,* 2244. https://doi.org/10.3389/fpsyg.2019.02244

Rodgers, N.H., & Jackson, E.S. (2021). Temperament is linked to avoidant responses to stuttering anticipation. *Journal of Communication Disorders, 93,* 106139.

Rommel, D. (2001). The influence of psycholinguistic variables on stuttering in childhood. In *Fluency disorders: Theory, research, treatment, and self-help.* Third World Congress of Fluency Disorders, Nyborg, Denmark.

Rosal, A.G.C., Cordeiro, A.A.D.A., & Queiroga, B.A.M.D. (2013). Phonological awareness and phonological development in children of public and private schools. *Revista Cefac, 15*(4), 837–846.

Rosenbek, J.C. (1984). Stuttering secondary to nervous system damage. In R.F. Curlee & W.H. Perkins (Eds.), *Nature and treatment of stuttering: New directions.* (pp. 31–48). College Hill

Rosenbek, J.C., Messert, B., Collins, M., & Wertz, R.T. (1978). Stuttering following brain damage. *Brain and Language, 6*(1), 82–96.

Roth, C., Aronson, A., & Davis, L. (1989). Clinical studies in psychogenic stuttering of adult onset. *Journal of Speech and Hearing Disorders, 54,* 634–646.

Rousey, C.L., Goetzinger, C.P., & Dirks, D. (1959). Sound localization ability of normal, stuttering, neurotic, and hemiplegic subjects. *AMA Archives of General Psychiatry, 1,* 640–645.

Rousseau, I., Onslow, M., Packman, A., & Jones, M. (2008). Comparisons of audio and audiovisual measures of stuttering frequency and severity in preschoolage children. *American Journal of Speech- Language Pathology, 17,* 173–178.

Rousseau, I., Packman, A., Onslow, M., Harrison, E., & Jones, M. (2007). An investigation of language and phonological development and the responsiveness of preschool-age children to the Lidcombe program. *Journal of Communication Disorders, 40*(5), 382–397.

Rubow, R.T., Rosenbek, J.C., & Schumacher, J.G. (1986). Stress management in the treatment of neurogenic stuttering. In *Biofeedback and self-regulation* (Vol. 11, Issue 1, pp. 77–78). Plenum Publishing Corporation.

Runyan, C.M., & Runyan, S.E. (1986). A fluency rules therapy program for young children in the public schools. *Language, Speech, and Hearing Services in Schools, 17*(4), 276–284.

Runyan, C.M., & Runyan, S.E. (1999). Therapy for school-aged stutterers: An update on the fluency rules program. In R. Curlee (Ed.), *Stuttering and related disorders of fluency* (2nd ed., pp. 101–123). Thieme.

Runyan, C.M., & Runyan, S.E. (2007). Therapy for school-aged stutterers: An update on the fluency rules program. In E.G. Conture & R. Curlee (Eds.), *Stuttering and related disorders of fluency* (3rd ed., pp. 100–114). Thieme Medical Publishers.

Ryan, B.P., & Van Kirk, B. (1974). The establishment, transfer, and maintenance of fluent speech in 50 stutterers using delayed auditory feedback and operant procedures. *Journal of Speech and Hearing Disorders, 39*(1), 3–10.

Sackett, D.L., Rosenberg, W.M.C., Gray, J.A.M., Haynes, R.B., & Richardson, W.S. (1996). Evidence-based medicine: What it is and what it isn't. *British Medical Journal, 312,* 71–72.

Sakhai, F., Darouie, A., Anderson, J.D., Dastjerdi-Kazemi, M., Golmohammadi, G., & Bakhshi, E. (2021). A comparison of the performance of Persian speaking children who do and do not stutter on three nonwords repetition tasks. *Journal of Fluency Disorders, 67*(105825).

Sanghi, M., Pandey, S., & Shah, H. (2009). Gene- environment interaction in speech and language development- a case study of monozygotic twins. *Journal of All India Institute of Speech and Hearing, 28*(1), 19–24.

Sanghi, M., Tambay, M., Wadia, D., Nandurkar, A., & Mohite, J. (2021). *MISHA test of communication development in Marathi.* Indian Speech and Hearing Association -Maharashtra Branch.

Sasisekaran, J., Brady, A., & Stein, J. (2013). A preliminary investigation of phonological encoding skills in children who stutter. *Journal of Fluency Disorders, 38,* 45–58.

Sasisekaran, J., & Byrd, C.T. (2013). Nonword repetition and phoneme elision skills in school-age children who do and do not stutter. *International Journal of Language and Communication Disorders, 48*(6), 625–639.

Sasisekaran, J., & Weathers, E. (2019). Disfluencies and phonological revisions in a nonword repetition task in school-age children who stutter. *Journal of Communication Disorders, 81,* 105917.

Sasisekaran, J., & Weisberg, S. (2014). Practice and retention of nonwords in adults who stutter. *Journal of Fluency Disorders, 41,* 55–71.

Savithri, S.R. (1987). Some acoustic and perceptual correlates of stress in Kannada. In *Proceedings of the national symposium on acoustics, special edition* (p. 209).

Savithri, S.R. (1999). Perceptual cues of word stress in Kannada. *Journal of the Acoustical Society of India, 25,* 1–4.

Savithri, S.R. (2019). Development of fluency in children. *Journal of the All India Institute of Speech & Hearing, 38*(1), 1–15.

Savithri, S.R., Goswamy, S., & Kedarnath, D. (2007). Speech rhythm in Indo – Aryan and Dravidian language. In *Proceedings of the international symposium on frontiers of research on speech and music* (pp. 170–174).

Savithri, S.R., Sreedevi, N., Jayakumar, T., & Kavya, V. (2010). Development of speech rhythm in Kannada speaking children. *Journal of All India Institute of Speech and Hearing, 29*(2), 175–180.

Sawyer, J., & Yairi, E. (2006). The effect of sample size on the assessment of stuttering severity. *American Journal of Speech Language Pathology, 15*(1), 36–44.

Scaler Scott, K. (2011). Cluttering and autism spectrum disorders. In D. Ward & K. Scaler Scott (Eds.), *Cluttering: A handbook of research, intervention and education* (pp. 115–134). Psychology Press.

Schlosser, R. W., & Raghavendra, P. (2004). Evidence-based practice in augmentative and alternative communication. *Augmentative and Alternative Communication, 20*(1), 1–21.

Schwartz, M. (1976). *Stuttering solved*. Lippincott.

Sebastian, S., Mathew, J., Sundaresan, R., Gowri, M., & Micheal, R. (2000). Speech intelligibility and communication related quality of life in tracheoesophageal speakers. *International Journal of Phonosurgery and Laryngology, 10*(2), 33–39.

Seth, D. (2020). *Efficacy of response cost treatment in preschool children who stutter* [Unpublished doctoral thesis, University of Mysore].

Seth, D., & Maruthy, S. (2019). Effect of phonological and morphological factors on speech disfluencies of Kannada speaking preschool children who stutter. *Journal of Fluency Disorders, 61*, 105707. https://doi.org/10.1016/j.jfludis.2019.105707.

Shames, G.H., & Florence, C.L. (1980). *Stutter-free speech: A goal for therapy*. Charles E. Merrill.

Shapiro, D.A. (1999). *Stuttering intervention: A collaborative journey to fluency freedom*. Pro-Ed.

Shearer, W. M., & Williams, J. D. (1965). Self-recovery from stuttering. *Journal of Speech and Hearing Disorders, 30*(3), 288–290.

Sheehan, J.G. (1953). Theory and treatment of stuttering as an approach-avoidance conflict. *Journal of Psychology, 36*, 27–49.

Sheehan, J.G. (1958). Conflict theory of stuttering. In J. Eisenson (Ed.), *Stuttering: A symposium*. Harper & Row.

Sheehan, J.G. (1970). *Stuttering: Research and therapy*. Harper & Row.

Sheehan, J.G. (1975). Conflict theory and avoidance reduction therapy. In J. Eisenson (Ed.), *Stuttering: A second symposium* (pp. 97–198). Harper & Row.

Sheehan, J.G., & Martyn, M.M. (1966). Spontaneous recovery from stuttering. *Journal of Speech and Hearing Research, 9*(1), 121–135.

Shenker, R.C., & Santayana, G. (2018, September). What are the options for the treatment of stuttering in preschool children? *Seminars in Speech and Language, 39*(4), 313–323.

Shugart, Y.Y., Mundorff, J., Kilshaw, J., Doheny, K., Doan, B., Wanyee, J., & Drayna, D. (2004). Results of a genome-wide linkage scan for stuttering. *American Journal of Medical Genetics, Part A, 124A*(2), 133–135.

Shumak, I.C. (1955). A speech rating sheet for stutterers. In W. Johnson & R.R. Leutenegger (Eds.), *Stuttering in children and adults: Thirty years of research at the University of Iowa* (pp. 341–347). University of Minnesota Press.

Siegel, G.M. (2000). Demands and capacities or demands and performance? *Journal of Fluency Disorders, 25*(4), 321–327.

Silverman, F.H. (1981). Relapse following stuttering therapy. In N. J. Lass (Ed.), *Speech and language: Advances in basic research and practice* (Vol. 5, pp. 51–78). Academic Press.

Silverman, F.H. (1992). *Stuttering and other fluency disorders*. Prentice Hall.

Simpson, F. (2006). *Mount Wilga high level language test* (Revised). Retrieved September 4, 2022, from https://silo.tips/download/mount-wilga-high-level-language-test-page-version-by-fiona-simpson

Slorach, N., & Noehr, B. (1973). Dichotic listening in stuttering and dyslalic children. *Cortex*, *9*(3), 295–300.

Smith, A. (1999). Stuttering: A unified approach to a multifactorial, dynanlic disorder. In N. Bernstein Ratner & E. C. Healey (Eds.), *Stuttering research and practice: Bridging the gap* (pp. 27–44). Lawrence Erlbaum Associates.

Smith, A., & Goffman, L. (2004). Interaction of motor and language factors in the development of speech production. In B. Maasen et al. (Eds.), *Speech motor control in normal and disordered speech* (pp. 227–252). Oxford University Press.

Smith, A., & Kelly, E. (1997). *Stuttering: A dynamic, multifactorial model* (2nd ed.). Allyn & Bacon.

Smith, A., McCauley, R.J., & Guitar, B. (2000). Development of the Teacher Assessment of Student Communicative Competence (TASCC) in grades 1 through 5. *Communication Disorders Quarterly*, *22*, 3–11.

Smith, A., & Weber, C. (2017). How stuttering develops: The multifactorial dynamic pathways theory. *Journal of Speech, Language and Hearing Research*, *60*, 2483–2505.

Smith, M., & Howell, P. (2013). Stuttering patterns in Japanese and English preschool-aged and school-aged children: As a progress report (analyses and conditions of speech disorders-focusing on stuttering and articulation disorders). *Journal of the Phonetic Society of Japan*, *17*(2), 83–89.

Smits-Bandstra, S.M., & Yovetich, W.S. (2003). Treatment effectiveness for school age children who stutter. *Revue d'orthophonie et d'audiologie*, *27*(2), 125–133.

Soderberg, G.A. (1969). Delayed auditory feedback and the speech of stutterers: A review of studies. *Journal of Speech and Hearing Disorders*, *34*, 20–29.

Sommer, M., Koch, M.A., Paulus, W., Weiller, C., & Buchel, C. (2002). Disconnection of speech-relevant brain areas in persistent developmental stuttering. *Lancet*, *360*, 380–383.

Sommer, M., Waltersbacher, A., Schlotmann, A., Schroder, H., & Strzelczyk, A. (2021). *Frontiers in Human Neuroscience*, *15*. https://doi.org/10.3389/fnhum.2021.645292.

Sommers, R.K., Brady, W.A., & Moore, W.R. (1975). Dichotic ear preference of stuttering children and adults. *Perceptual and Motor Skills*, *41*, 931–938.

Soroker, N., Bar-Israel, Y., Schechier, I., & Solzi, P. (1990). Stuttering as a manifestation of right-hemispheric subcortical stroke. *European Neurology*, *30*(5), 268–270.

St Claire, T., Menzies, R.G., Onslow, M., Packman, A., Thompson, R., & Block, S. (2009). Unhelpful thoughts and beliefs linked to social anxiety in stuttering: Development of a measure. *International Journal of Language & Communication Disorders*, *44*(3), 338–351.

St Louis, K.O. (1992). On defining cluttering. In F.L. Myers & K.O. St Louis (Eds.), *Cluttering: A clinical perspective*. Far Communications.

St Louis, K.O. (2001). *Living with stuttering: Stories, basics, resources and hope*. Populore.

St Louis, K.O. (2005). *St. Louis inventory of life perspectives and speech/language difficulty (SL ILP-S/L)*. Populore.

St Louis, K.O. (2006). Measurement issues in fluency disorders. In N. Bernstein Ratner & J. Tetnowski (Eds.), *Current issues in stuttering research and practice* (pp. 61–86). Lawrence Erlbaum, Inc.

St Louis, K.O., Coskun, M., Ozdemir, S., Topbas, S., Goranova, E., & Filatova, Y. (2007, May). Public attitudes towards cluttering and stuttering: USA, Turkey, Bulgaria and Russia. In K. Bakker, L.J. Raphael, & F.L. Myers (Eds.), *Proceedings of the first world congress on cluttering* (pp. 190–198). International Cluttering Association, Katarino, Bulgaria. Retrieved January 29, 2015, from http://associations.missouristate.edu/ica/.

St Louis, K.O., Filatova, Y., Coskun, M., Topbas, S., Ozdemir, S., Georgieva, D., McCaffrey, E., & George, R.D. (2010). Identification of cluttering and stuttering by the public in four countries. *International Journal of Speech-Language Pathology*, *12*(6), 508–519.

St Louis, K.O., Filatova, Y., Coskun, M., Topbas, S., Ozdemir, S., Georgieva, D., McCaffrey, E., & George, R.D. (2011). Public attitudes towards cluttering and stuttering in four countries. In E.L. Simon (Ed.), *Psychology of Stereotypes* (pp. 81–113). Nova Science Publishers, Inc.

St Louis, K.O., & McCaffrey, E. (2005, November). Public awareness of cluttering and stuttering: Preliminary results. In *Poster presented at the 2005 ASHA convention*, San Diego, CA.

St Louis, K.O., & Myers, F.L. (1998). A synopsis of cluttering and its treatment. In *Paper presented at the international stuttering awareness day online conference*. Retrieved April 2, 2021, from www.mnsu.edu/comdis/isad/papers/stlouis.html.

St Louis, K.O., Myers, F.L., Bakker, K., & Raphael, L.J. (2007). Understanding and treating cluttering. In E. Conture & R. Curlee (Eds.), *Stuttering and related disorders of fluency* (pp. 297–325). Thieme Medical Publishers.

St Louis, K.O., Myers, F.L., Cassidy, L.J., Michael, A.J., Penrod, S.M., Litton, B.A. et al. (1996). Efficacy of delayed auditory feedback for treating cluttering: Two case studies. *Journal of Fluency Disorders*, *21*, 305–314.

St Louis, K.O., Raphael, L.J., Myers, F., & Bakker, K. (2003). Cluttering updated. *The ASHA Leader*, *8*(21), 4–5 & 20–23.

St Louis, K.O., Reichel, I.K., Yaruss, J.S., & Lubker, B.B. (2009). Construct and concurrent validity of a prototype questionnaire to survey public attitudes towards stuttering. *Journal of Fluency Disorders*, *34*(1), 11–28.

St Louis, K.O., & Schulte, K. (2011). Defining cluttering: The lowest common denominator. In D. Ward & K. Scaler Scott (Eds.), *Cluttering: A handbook of research, intervention and education* (pp. 233–253). Psychology Press.

Stager, S.V. (1990). Heterogeneity in stuttering: Results from auditory brainstem response testing. *Journal of Fluency Disorders*, *15*, 9–19.

Stager, S.V., Jeffries, J.J., & Braun, A.R. (2003). Common features of fluency evoking conditions studied in stuttering subject sand controls: An H(2)12O PET study. *Journal of Fluency Disorders*, *28*, 319–335.

Starkweather, C.W. (1987). *Fluency and stuttering*. Prentice Hall.

Starkweather, C.W., & Gottwald, S.R. (1990). The demands and capacities model II: Clinical applications. *Journal of Fluency Disorders*, *15*(3), 143–157.

Starkweather, C.W., & Gottwald, S.R. (2000). The demands and capacities model. *Journal of Fluency Disorders*, *25*, 369–375.

Stoppler, M. (2021). *Medical definition of prevalence*. Retrieved January 28, 2022, from www.medicinenet.com/prevalence/definition.htm.

Striefler, M., & Gumpertz, F. (1955). Cerebral potentials in stuttering and cluttering. *Confinia Neurologica*, *15*, 771–780.

Strub, R.L., Black, F.W., & Naeser, M.A. (1987). Anomalous dominance in sibling stutterers: Evidence from CT scan asymmetries, dichotic listening, neuropsychological testing, and handedness. *Brain and Language*, *30*(2), 338–350.

Stuart, A., Frazier, C.L., Kalinowski, J., & Vos, P.W. (2008). The effect of frequency altered feedback on stuttering duration and type. *Journal of Speech, Language, and Hearing Research*, *51*, 889–897.

Stuart, A., & Kalinowski, J. (2004). The perception of speech naturalness of post-therapeutic and altered auditory feedback speech of adults with mild and sever stuttering. *Folia Phoniatrica et Logopaedica*, *56*(6), 347–357.

Stuart, A., Kalinowski, J., Armson, J., Stenstrom, R., & Jones, K. (1996). Fluency effect of frequency alterations of plus/minus one-half and one-quarter octave shifts in auditory feedback of people who stutter. *Journal of Speech and Hearing Research, 39*, 396–401.

Stuart, A., Kalinowski, J., & Rastatter, M.P. (1997). Effect of monoaural and binaural altered auditory feedback on stuttering frequency. *Journal of Acoustical Society of America, 101*(6), 3806–3809.

Subramanian, A. (1997). Naturalness ratings of stutterers' speech. In M. Jayaram & S.R. Savithri (Eds.), *Research at AIISH: Dissertation abstracts: Vol. II.1.2003.*

Sudhi, N., John, M., & Geetha, Y.V. (2010). Age and gender differences in persons with stuttering. *Journal of the All India Institute of Speech and Hearing, 29*(2), 131–138. http://203.129.241.91/jaiish/index.php/aiish

Sugathan, N., & Maruthy, S. (2020). Nonword repetition and identification skills in Kannada speaking school-aged children who do and do not stutter. *Journal of Fluency Disorders, 63*, 105745.

Sugathan, N., & Maruthy, S. (2021). Predictive factors for persistence and recovery of stuttering in children: A systematic review. *International Journal of Speech Language Pathology, 23*(4), 359–371.

Supprian, T., Retz, W., & Deckert, J. (1999). Clozapine-Induced Stuttering: Epileptic Brain Activity? *American Journal of Psychiatry, 156*(10), 1663–1664.

Suresh, R., Ambrose, N., Roe, C., Pluzhnikov, A., Wittke-Thompson, J., & C-Y Ng., M. (2006). New complexities in the genetics of stuttering: Significant sex-specific linkage signals. *American Journal of Human Genetics, 78*(4), 554–563.

Sussman, H.M., & MacNeilage, P.F. (1975). Hemispheric specialization for speech production and perception in stutterers. *Neuropsychologia, 13*(1), 19–26.

Suvi, N., & Leipakka, T. (2012). *Neurogeeninen änkytys suljetun aivovamman jälkeen. Monitapaustutkimus.* https://trepo.tuni.fi/handle/10024/83975

Tani, T., & Sakai, Y. (2011). Analysis of five cases with neurogenic stuttering following brain injury in the basal ganglia. *Journal of Fluency Disorders, 36*(1), 1–16.

Teesson, K., Packman, A., & Onslow, M. (2003). The Lidcombe behavioral data language of stuttering. *Journal of Speech, Language, and Hearing Research, 46*(4), 1009–2003.

Teshima, S., Langevin, M., Hagler, P., & Kully, D. (2010). Post-treatment speech naturalness of comprehensive stuttering program clients and differences in ratings among listener groups. *Journal of Fluency Disorders, 35*(1), 44–58.

Theys, C., van Wieringen, A., Sunaert, S., Thijs, V., & de Nil, L.F. (2011). A one year prospective study of neurogenic stuttering following stroke: Incidence and co-occurring disorders. *Journal of Communication Disorders, 44*(6), 678–687.

Tichenor, S., & Yaruss, J.S. (2020). Repetitive negative thinking, temperament, and adverse impact in adults who stutter. *American Journal of Speech-Language Pathology, 29*(1), 201–215.

Toscher, M.M., & Rupp, R.R. (1978). A study of the central auditory processes in stutterers using the Synthetic Sentence Identification (SSI) Test battery. *Journal of Speech and Hearing Research, 21*(4), 779–792.

Tourville, J.A., & Guenther, F.H. (2011). The DIVA model: A neural theory of speech acquisition and production. *Language and Cognitive Processes, 26*(7), 952–981.

Trager, G.L., & Smith, H.L. (1951). *Outline of English structure.* Battenburg Press.

Trajkovski, N., Andrews, C., O'Brian, S., Onslow, M., & Packman, A. (2006). Treating stuttering in a preschool child with syllable-timed speech: A case report. *Behaviour Change, 23*(4), 270–277.

Trajkovski, N., Andrews, C., Onslow, M., O'Brian, S., Packman, A., & Menzies, R. (2011). A phase II trial of the Westmead program: Syllable-timed speech treatment for preschool children who stutter. *International Journal of Speech-Language Pathology, 13*(6), 500–509.

Trajkovski, N., Andrews, C., Onslow, M., Packman, A., O'Brian, S., & Menzies, R. (2009). Using syllable-timed speech to treat preschool children who stutter: A multiple baseline treatment. *Journal of Fluency Disorders, 34*(1), 1–10.

Trajkovski, N., O'Brian, S., Onslow, M., Packman, A., Lowe, R., Menzies, R., Jones, M., & Reilly, S. (2019). A three-arm randomized controlled trial of Lidcombe Program and Westmead Program early stuttering interventions. *Journal of Fluency Disorders, 61*, 1–8.

Travis, L.E. (1928). A comparative study of the performances of stutterers and normal speakers in mirror tracing. *Psychological Monographs, 39*, 45–51.

Travis, L.E. (1931). *Speech pathology*. Appleton-Century.

Travis, L.E., & Herren, R.Y. (1929). Studies in stuttering. V: A study of simultaneous antitropic movements of the hands of stutterers. *Archives of Neurology and Psychiatry, 22*, 487–494.

Travis, L.E., Johnson, W., & Shover, J. (1937). The relation of bilingualism to stuttering: A survey of the East Chicago, Indiana, schools. *Journal of Speech Disorders, 2*(3), 185–189.

Travis, L.E., Malamud, W., & Thayer, L.R. (1934). The relationship between physical habitus and stuttering. *The Journal of Abnormal and Social Psychology, 29*(2), 132–140.

Tumanova, V., Conture, E.G., Lambert, E.W., & Walden, T.A. (2014). Speech disfluencies of preschool-age children who do and do not stutter. *Journal of Communication Disorders, 49*, 25–41.

Turgut, N., Utku, U., & Balci, K. (2002). A case of acquired stuttering resulting from left parietal infarction. *Acta Neurologica Scandinavica, 105*(5), 408–410.

Usler, E., & Weber-Fox, C. (2015). Neurodevelopment for syntactic processing distinguishes childhood stuttering recovery vs. persistence. *Journal of Neurodevelopmental Disorders, 7*(1), 3–4.

Uysal, H.T., & Kose, A. (2021). The investigation of the validity and reliability of the Turkish version of the Wright and Ayre Stuttering Self-Rating Profile (WASSP). *International Journal of Language and Communication Disorders, 56*(3), 653–661.

Valente, A.R.S., & Jesus, L.M. (2011). Characteristics of stuttering-like disfluencies in Portuguese school age children. In *9th Congress for people who stutter (ISA) and 2nd Latin American congress on stuttering (AAT)*.

Van Beijsterveldt, C.E., Felsenfeld, S., & Boomsma, D.I. (2010). Bivariate genetic analyses of stuttering and nonfluency in a large sample of 5-year-old twins. *Journal of Speech, Language, and Hearing Research, 53*(3), 609–619.

Van Borsel, J. (2011). Cluttering and down syndrome. In D. Ward & K. Scaler Scott (Eds.), *Cluttering: A handbook of research, intervention and education* (pp. 90–99). Psychology Press.

Van Borsel, J., Drummond, D., & de Britto Pereira, M.M. (2010). Delayed auditory feedback and acquired neurogenic stuttering. *Journal of Neurolinguistics, 23*(5), 479–487.

Van Borsel, J., Meirlaen, A., Achten, R., Vingerhoets, G., & Santens, P. (2009). Acquired stuttering with differential manifestation in different languages: A case study. *Journal of Neurolinguistics, 22*(2), 187–195. https://doi.org/10.1016/J.JNEUROLING.2008.10.003

Van Borsel, J., Moeyart, J., Mostaert, C., Rosseel, R., Van Loo, E., & Van Renterghem, T. (2006). Prevalence of stuttering in regular and special school populations in Belgium based on teacherperceptions. *Folia Phoniatrica et Logopaedica, 58*, 289–302.

Van Borsel, J., Reunes, G., & Van-Den-Bergh, N. (2003). Delayed auditory feedback in stuttering. Clients as consumers. *International Journal of Language & Communication Disorders, 38*(2), 119–129.

Van Borsel, J., & Taillieu, C. (2001). Neurogenic stuttering versus developmental stuttering: An observer judgement study. *Journal of Communication Disorders, 34*(5), 385–395.

Van Borsel, J., van der Made, S., & Santens, P. (2003). Thalamic stuttering: A distinct clinical entity? *Brain and Language, 85*(2), 185–189.

Van Borsel, J., & Vandermeulen, A. (2008). Cluttering in down syndrome. *Folia Phoniatrica et Logopedica, 60*(6), 312–317.

van der Merwe, B., Robb, M.P., Lewis, J.G., & Ormond, T. (2011). Anxiety measures and salivary cortisol responses in preschool children who stutter. *Contemporary Issues in Communication Science and Disorders, 38,* 1–10.

Van Eerdenbrugh, S., Packman, A., Onslow, M., O'Brian, S., & Menzies, R. (2016). Development of an internet version of the Lidcombe Program of early stuttering intervention: A trial of Part I. *International Journal of Speech-Language Pathology, 20*(2), 216–225.

Van Riper, C. (1935). The quantitative measurement of laterality. *Journal of Experimental Psychology, 17,* 327–332.

Van Riper, C. (1937). The preparatory set in stuttering. *Journal of Speech Disorders, 2,* 149–154.

Van Riper, C. (1971). *The nature of stuttering.* Prentice Hall.

Van Riper, C. (1982). *The nature of stuttering* (2nd ed.). Prentice Hall.

Van Riper, C. (1984). *Speech correction: An introduction to speech language pathology and audiology.* Allyn & Bacon.

Van Riper, C. (1990). *Treatment of stuttering.* Prentice Hall.

Van Riper, C., & Erickson, R. L. (1996). *Speech correction: An introduction to speech pathology and audiology* (9th ed.). Allyn and Bacon.

van Zaalen, Y. (2009). *Cluttering identified. differential diagnostics between cluttering, stuttering and learning disability.* Ph.D. thesis, Utrecht, Zuidam. https://dspace.library.uu.nl.

van Zaalen, Y., Myers, F., Ward, D., & Bennett, E. (2008). *The cluttering assessment protocol.* Retrieved May 12, 2018, from https://associations.missouristate.edu/ica/Resources/cluttering_assessment.htm#:~:text=Cluttering%20assessment%20should%20include%20different,nature%20of%20the%20speaking%20task.

van Zaalen, Y., & Reichel, I. (2014). Cluttering treatment: Theoretical considerations and treatment planning. *Perspectives on Global Issues in Communication Sciences and Related Disorders, 4*(2), 57–62.

van Zaalen, Y., & Reichel, I. (2015). *Cluttering: Current views on its nature, assessment and treatment.* iUniverse Publishing.

van Zaalen, Y., & Reichel, I. (2017). Prevalence of cluttering in two European countries: A pilot study. *Perspectives of ASHA Special Interest Groups SIG 17, 2*(1), 1–8.

van Zaalen, Y., Ward, D., Nederveen, A.J., Grolman, W., Wijnen, F., De Jonckere, P. (2009). Cluttering and stuttering: Different disorders. A neuroimaging study. *Unpublished manuscript.* Retrieved March 27, 2021, from www.researchgate.net/publication/236658098_Cluttering_Stuttering_different_disorders_A_neuro-imaging_study.

van Zaalen, Y., Wijnen, F., & Dejonckere, P. (2009a). Language planning disturbances in children who clutter or have learning disabilities. *International Journal of Speech Language Pathology, 11,* 496–508.

van Zaalen, Y., Wijnen, F., & Dejonckere, P. (2009b). A test of speech motor control on word level productions: The SPA test (Dutch: Screening Pittige Articulatie). *International Journal of Speech-Language Pathology, 11*(1), 26–33.

van Zaalen, Y., Wijnen, F., & Djonckere, P. (2011). The assessment of cluttering: Rationale, tasks and interpretation. In D. Ward & K. Scaler Scott (Eds.), *Cluttering: A handbook of research, intervention and education* (pp. 137–151). Psychology Press.

Vanryckeghem, M., & Brutten, G.J. (2007). *Communication attitude test for preschool and kindergarten children who stutter (KiddyCAT).* Plural Publishing.

Vanryckeghem, M., & Brutten, G.J. (2011). The Big CAT: A normative and comparative investigation of the communication attitude of nonstuttering and stuttering adults. *Journal of Communication Disorders, 44*(2), 200–206.

Vanryckeghem, M., & Brutten, G.J. (2018). *The behavior assessment battery for adults who stutter.* Plural Publishing.

Vanryckeghem, M., & Brutten, G.J. (2020). *The behavior assessment battery for school-age children who stutter* (Testna Baterija Za Oceno osnovnošolskih otrok, ki jecljajo). Center za Komunikacijo, Portoroz, Slovenia. ISBN 978-961-94141-8-7.

Vanryckeghem, M., Brutten, G.J., & Hernandez, L.M. (2005). A comparative investigation of the speech-associated attitude of preschool and kindergarten children who do and do not stutter. *Journal of Fluency Disorders, 30*(4), 307–318.

Vanryckeghem, M., Hylebos, C., Brutten, G.J., & Peleman, M. (2001). The relationship between communication attitude and emotion of children who stutter. *Journal of Fluency Disorders, 26*(1), 1–15.

Vanryckeghem, M., Matthews, M., & Xu, P. (2017). Speech situation checklist – revised: Investigation with adults who do not stutter and treatment-seeking adults who stutter. *American Journal of Speech-Language Pathology, 26*(4), 1129–1140.

Vargha-Khadem, F., Watkins, K., Alcock, K., Fletcher, P., & Passingham, R. (1995). Praxic and nonverbal cognitive deficits in a large family with a genetically transmitted speech and language disorder. *Proceedings of the National Academy of Sciences of the United States of America, 92*(3), 930–933.

Veerabhadrappa, R.C., Krishnakumar, J., Vanryckeghem, M., & Maruthy, S. (2021). Communication attitude of Kannada-speaking adults who do and do not stutter. *Journal of Fluency Disorders, 70*(1), 105866. https://doi.org/10.1016/j.jfludis.2021.105866

Veerabhadrappa, R.C., Vanryckeghem, M., & Maruthy, S. (2021a). Communication attitude of Kannada-speaking school-age children who do and do not stutter. *Folia Phoniatrica et Logopaedica, 73*(2), 126–133.

Veerabhadrappa, R.C., Vanryckeghem, M., & Maruthy, S. (2021b). The speech situation checklist – Emotional reaction: Normative and comparative study of Kannada-speaking children who do and do not stutter. *International Journal of Speech-Language Pathology, 23*(5), 559–568.

Vincent, I., Grela, B.G., & Gilbert, H.R. (2012). Phonological priming in adults who stutter. *Journal of Fluency Disorders, 37*(2), 91–105.

Viswanath, N., Lee, H.S., & Chakraborty, R. (2004). Evidence for a major gene influence on persistent developmental stuttering. *Human Biology, 76*(3), 401–412.

Vong, E., Wilson, L., & Lincoln, M. (2016). The Lidcombe Program of early stuttering intervention for Malaysian families: Four case studies. *Journal of Fluency Disorders, 49*, 29–39.

Wada, J., & Rasmussen, T. (1960). Intracarotid injection of sodium amytal for the lateralizarion of cerebral speech dominance: Experimental and clinical observations. *Journal of Neurology and Neurosurgery, 17*, 266–282.

Wagaman, J.R., Miltenberger, R.G., & Arndorfer, R.E. (1993). Analysis of a simplified treatment for stuttering in children. *Journal of Applied Behavior Analysis, 26*, 53–61.

Wakaba, Y.Y. (1997, August 18–22). Research on temperament of stuttering children with early onset. In *2nd World congress on fluency disorders*, San Francisco, USA.

Walden, T.A., Frankel, C.B., Buhr, A.P., Johnson, K.N., Conture, E.G., & Karrass, J.M. (2012). Dual diathesis-stressor model of emotional and linguistic contributions to developmental stuttering. *Journal of Abnormal Child Psychology, 40*(4), 633–644.

Walker, C., & Black, J. (1950). *The intrinsic intensity of oral phrases* (Joint Project Report No. 2). Pensacola, Fla.: Naval Air Station, U.S. Naval School of Aviation Medicine.

Ward, D. (2006). *Stuttering and cluttering: Frameworks for understanding and treatment*. Psychology Press.

Ward, D. (2010a). Cluttering: The bad, the good, and the misunderstood. *In Proceedings of the world congress on cluttering* (pp. 31–37). International Cluttering Association, Katarino, Bulgaria.

Ward, D. (2010b). Stuttering and normal nonfluency: Cluttering spectrum behavior as a functional descriptor of abnormal fluency. In K. Bakker, L. Raphael, & F. Myers (Eds.), *Proceedings of the first world conference on cluttering* (pp. 261–267). Katarino, Bulgaria. http://associations.missouristate.edu/ICA.

Ward, D. (2011a). Motor speech control and cluttering. In D. Ward & K. Scaler Scott (Eds.), *Cluttering: A handbook of research, intervention and education* (pp. 34–44). Psychology Press.

Ward, D. (2011b). Scope and constraint in the diagnosis of cluttering: Combining two perspectives. In D. Ward & K. Scaler Scott (Eds.), *Cluttering: A handbook of research, intervention and education* (pp. 254–262). Psychology Press.

Ward, D. (2018). *Stuttering and cluttering* (2nd ed.). Psychology Press.

Ward, D., Connally, E.L., Pliatsikas, C., Bretherton-Furness, J., & Watkins, K.E. (2015). The neurological underpinnings of cluttering: Some initial findings. *Journal of Fluency Disorders, 43,* 1–16.

Watkins, K.E., Dronkers, N.F., & Vargha-Khadem, F. (2002). Behavioural analysis of an inherited speech and language disorder: Comparison with acquired aphasia. *Brain, 125*(3), 452–464.

Watkins, K.E., Smith, S., Davis, S., & Howell, P. (2008). Structural and functional abnormalities of the motor system in developmental stuttering. *Brain, 131*(1), 50–59.

Watson, B.C., & Freeman, F.J. (1997). Brain imaging contributions. In R.F. Curlee & G.M. Siegel (Eds.), *Nature and treatment of stuttering: New directions* (pp. 143–166). Allyn and Bacon.

Watson, B.C., Pool, K.D., Devous, M.D., Freeman, F.J., & Finitzo, T. (1992). Brain blood flow related to acoustic laryngeal reaction time in adult developmental stutterers. *Journal of Speech and Hearing Research, 35,* 555–561.

Weber-Fox, C. (2001). Neural systems for sentence processing in stuttering. *Journal of Speech, Language and Hearing Research, 44,* 814–825.

Weber-Fox, C., Spencer, R.M.C., Spruill III, J.E., & Smith, A. (2004). Phonologic processing in adults who stutter: Electrophysiological and physiological evidence. *Journal of Speech, Language and Hearing Research, 47*(6), 1244–1258.

Webster, R.L. (1980). Evolution of a target-based behavioural therapy for stuttering. *Journal of Fluency Disorders, 5*(3), 303–320.

Webster, W. (1987). What hurried hands reveal about "tangled tongues": A neuropsychological approach to understanding stuttering. *Human Communication Canada, 11,* 11–18.

Webster, W.G. (1993). Hurried hands and tangled tongues: Implications of current research for the management of stuttering. In E. Boberg (Ed.), *Neuropsychology of stuttering* (pp. 73–127). The University of Alberta Press.

Webster, W.G. (1998). Brain models and the clinical management of stuttering. *Journal of Speech-Language Pathology and Audiology, 22*(4), 220–230

Weiss, D. (1964). *Cluttering*. Prentice Hall.

West, R. (1958). An agnostic's speculations about stuttering. In J. Eisenson (Ed.), *Stuttering: A symposium*. Harper & Row.

Westin, K., Buddenhagen, R.G., & Obrecht, D.H. (1966). An experimental analysis of relative importance of pitch quantity and intensity as cues to phonemic distinctions in southern Swedish. *Language and Speech, 9,* 114–126.

Wexler, K.B. (1982). Developmental disfluency in 2-, 4-, and 6-year-old boys in neutral and stress situations. *Journal of Speech and Hearing Research, 25*(2), 229–234.

Williams, D., & Kent, L. (1958). Listeners' evaluations of speech interruptions. *Journal of Speech and Hearing Research, 1,* 124–136.

Williams, M.J. (2006). *Children who stutter: Easy, difficult, or slow to warm up?* Annual Convention of American Speech-Language and Hearing Association.

Wilson, L., Onslow, M., & Lincoln, M. (2004). Telehealth adaptation of the Lidcombe program of early intervention: Five case studies. *American Journal of Speech-Language Pathology, 13*(1), 81–93.

Wingate, M.E. (1964a). Recovery from stuttering. *Journal of Speech and Hearing Disorders, 29*(3), 312–321.

Wingate, M.E. (1964b). A standard definition of stuttering. *Journal of Speech and Hearing Disorders, 29*, 484–489.

Wingate, M.E. (1984). Fluency, disfluency, dysfluency, and stuttering. *Journal of Fluency Disorders, 9*(2), 163–168.

Wingate, M.E. (1988). *The structure of stuttering: A psycholinguistic study.* Springer-Verlag.

Winslow, M., & Guitar, B. (1994). The effects of structured turn-taking on disfluencies: A case study. *Language, Speech, and Hearing Services in Schools, 25*, 251–257.

Wittke-Thompson, J.K., Ambrose, N., Yairi, E., Roe, C., Cook, E.H., Ober, C., & Cox, N.J. (2007). Genetic studies of stuttering in a founder population. *Journal of Fluency Disorders, 32*(1), 33–50.

Wood, F., Stump, D., McKeehan, A., Sheldon, S., & Proctor, J. (1980). Patterns of regional cerebral blood flow during attempted reading aloud by stutterers both on and off Haloperidol medication: Evidence for inadequate left frontal activation during stuttering. *Brain and Language, 9*, 141–144.

Woolf, G. (1967). Assessment of stuttering as struggle, avoidance and expectancy. *British Journal of Disorders of Communication, 2*, 158–177.

World Health Organization (WHO). (2001). *International classification of functioning, disability and health.* World Health Organisation.

World Health Organization (WHO). (2016). *The international statistical classification of diseases and health related states- tenth revision* (5th ed.). World Health Organisation.

Wright, L., & Ayre, A. (2000). *WASSP: The Wright and Ayre stuttering self-rating profile.* Speechmark Publishing Limited.

Wright, L., Ayre, A., & Grogan, S. (1998). Outcome measurement in adult stuttering therapy: A self-rating profile. *International Journal of Language and Communication Disorders, 33*, 378–383.

Wu, J.C., Maguire, G., Riley, G., Fallon, J., LaCasse, L., Chin, S., Klein, Tang, C., & Cadwell, S., & Lottenberg, S. (1995). A positron emission tomography deoxyglucose study of developmental stuttering. *Neuroreport, 6*, 501–505.

Wu, J.C., Maguire, G., Riley, G., Lee, A., Keator, D., Tang, C., Fallon, J., & Najafi, A. (1997). Increased dopamine activity associated with stuttering. *Neuroreport, 8*(3), 767–770.

Wyatt, G.L. (1969). *Language learning and communication disorders in children.* Free Press.

Yairi, E. (1981). Disfluencies of normally speaking two-year-old children. *Journal of Speech and Hearing Research, 24*(4), 490–495.

Yairi, E. (1982). Longitudinal studies of disfluencies in two-year-old children. *Journal of Speech and Hearing Research, 25*(1), 155–160.

Yairi, E. (1997). Disfluency characteristics of childhood stuttering. In R.F. Curlee & G.M. Siegel (Eds.), *Nature and treatment of stuttering: New directions* (pp. 49–78). Allyn &Bacon.

Yairi, E. (2007). Subtyping stuttering I: A review. *Journal of Fluency Disorders, 32(3)*, 165–196.

Yairi, E., & Ambrose, N. (1992). A longitudinal study of stuttering in children: A preliminary report. *Journal of Speech, Language, and Hearing Research, 35*(4), 755–760.

Yairi, E., & Ambrose, N. (1999). Early childhood stuttering: I. Persistency and recovery rates. *Journal of Speech, Language, and Hearing Research, 42*(5), 1097–1112.

Yairi, E., & Ambrose, N. (2005). *Early childhood stuttering: For clinicians by clinicians*. Pro-Ed.

Yairi, E., & Ambrose, N. (2013). Epidemiology of stuttering: 21st century advances. *Journal of Fluency Disorders, 38*(2), 66–87.

Yairi, E., Ambrose, N., & Cox, N. (1996). Genetics of stuttering: A critical review. *Journal of Speech and Hearing Research, 39*, 771–784.

Yairi, E., Ambrose, N., Paden, E.P., & Throneburg, R.N. (1996). Predictive factors of persistence and recovery: Pathways of childhood stuttering. *Journal of Communication Disorders, 29*(1), 51–77.

Yairi, E., & Lewis, B. (1984). Disfluencies at the onset of stuttering. *Journal of Speech, Language, and Hearing Research, 27*(1), 154–159.

Yairi, E., & Seery, C. (2014). *Stuttering: Foundations and clinical applications* (2nd ed.). Pearson Education.

Yairi, E., & Seery, C. (2023). *Stuttering: Foundations and clinical applications* (3rd ed.). Plural Publishing.

Yamini, B.K. (1990). *Disfluencies in children (5–6 years)* [Master's dissertation, All India Institute of Speech and Hearing, Mysuru].

Yang, Y., Jia, F., Fox, P.T., Siok, W.T., & Tan, L.H. (2018). Abnormal neural response to phonological working memory demands in persistent developmental stuttering. *Human Brain Mapping, 40*, 214–225.

Yaruss, J.S. (1997a, Spring). Clinical measurement of stuttering behaviors. *Contemporary Issues in Communication Science and Disorders, 24*, 27–38.

Yaruss, J.S. (1997b). Utterance timing and childhood stuttering. *Journal of Fluency Disorders, 22*, 263–286.

Yaruss, J.S. (1998). Describing the consequences of disorders: Stuttering and the international classification of impairments, disabilities, and handicaps. *Journal of Speech, Language, and Hearing Research, 41*(2), 249–257.

Yaruss, J.S. (2007). Application of the ICF in fluency disorders. *Seminars in Speech and Language, 28*(4), 312–322.

Yaruss, J.S., Coleman, C., & Quesal, R.W. (2010). *OASES- S: Overall assessment of the speaker's experience of stuttering – school- age* (Ages 7–12). Pearson Assessments.

Yaruss, J.S., & Conture, E.G. (1996). Stuttering and phonological disorders in children: Examination of the Covert Repair Hypothesis. *Journal of Speech and Hearing Research, 39*, 349–364.

Yaruss, J.S., Logan, K.J., & Conture, E.G. (1995). Speaking rate and diadochokinetic abilities of children who stutter. In *Stuttering: Proceedings of the first world congress of fluency disorders*, Nijmegen, The Netherlands.

Yaruss, J.S., & Quesal, R.W. (2004). Stuttering and the International Classification of Functioning, Disability, and Health (ICF): An update. *Journal of Communication Disorders, 37*(1), 35–52.

Yaruss, J.S., & Quesal, R.W. (2006). Overall assessment of the speaker's experience of stuttering (oases): Documenting multiple outcomes in stuttering treatment. *Journal of Fluency Disorders, 31*(2), 90–115.

Yaruss, J.S., Quesal, R.W., & Coleman, C. (2010). *OASES- T: Overall assessment of the speaker's experience of stuttering – teenagers* (Ages 13–17). Pearson Assessments.

Zebrowski, P.M. (1991). Duration of the speech disfluencies of beginning stutterers. *Journal of Speech, Language, and Hearing Research, 34*(3), 483–491.

Zebrowski, P.M. (1994). Duration of sound prolongation and sound/syllable repetition in children who stutter: Preliminary observations. *Journal of Speech, Language, and Hearing Research, 37*(2), 254–263.

Zebrowski, P.M., & Kelly, E.M. (2002). *Manual of stuttering intervention*. Singular Publishing Group.

Zengin-Bolatkale, H., Conture, E.G., & Walden, T.A. (2015). Sympathetic arousal of young children who stutter during a stressful picture naming task. *Journal of Fluency Disorders, 46*, 24–40.

Zhao, L., & Lian, M. (2021). Lexical planning in people who stutter: A defect in lexical encoding or the planning scope? *Frontiers in Psychology, 12*, 581304.

Zimmerman, S., Kalinowski, J., Stuart, A., & Rastatter, M. (1997). Effect of altered auditory feedback on people who stutter during scripted telephone conversations. *Journal of Speech, Language, and Hearing Research, 40*(5), 1130–113.

Zimmermann, G. (1980). Stuttering: A disorder of movement. *Journal of Speech and Hearing Research, 23*, 122–136.

Zimmermann, G.N., Smith, A., & Hanley, J.M. (1981). Stuttering: In need of a unifying conceptual framework. *Journal of Speech and Hearing Research, 24*, 25–31.

Appendix A

Detailed information gathering

Santosh Maruthy

Date:		Interviewer:	

Participant's info			
Participant's name		□ Male □ Female	
Relation to the participant (if the informant is not the participant)	□ Mother □ Father □ Relative (specify): □ Other (specify):	Age at time of initial visit (years, months)	
		Stuttering age of onset (years, months)	
Place of birth:		Child lives with:	□ Own parents □ Foster parents □ Other relative
Complete address:		Telephone number: Best time to call:	
		Referred by:	
Native language and other languages			
What is the primary language that you speak at home?			
What other languages are you (is your child) exposed to?			
Do you (does your child) experience more stuttering in one of the languages you know?			
If yes (for the previous question), which one?			

(Continued)

(Continued)

General Speech – Language, Hearing, Orofacial
As far as you know do you (does your child) have any other speech, language, feeding or hearing problems? ☐ Speech (e.g. unable to speak clearly) ☐ Language (e.g. unable to form complete sentences) ☐ Feeding and/or swallowing ☐ Hearing (e.g. does not respond consistently to sounds)
Do you (does your child) have problems related to reading and writing?

Accompanying conditions
Developmental
Have you (has your child) been diagnosed with any known developmental condition? (e.g. Attention Deficit, Autism Spectrum Disorder, etc.)
Emotional
Do you (does your child) have any diagnosed emotional/psychological problems?
Medical
Are you (is your child) on any medications? If so, what are the names, and what are they for?
List illnesses, allergies, injuries, surgeries (if any) in the past/present.
List physical disabilities, if any.
Vision normal? ☐ Y ☐ N
Are you (is your child) right-handed ☐ left-handed ☐ both ☐
Do other members of the family have speech, language or reading problems or learning disabilities? If so, please describe.
Did you (your child) attend therapy for stuttering previously? If yes, how long?

For a child participant	
Grade level:	
School:	
Fathers name and age:	
Father's occupation:	
Mother's name and age:	
Mother's occupation	

(Continued)

(Continued)

Siblings		
Name	Age	Speech – Language – Hearing problems

History and development of stuttering
Do other individuals in the family stutter, or did any stutter but recover? Who and when?
Give the exact age at which stuttering was first noticed.
What is the time gap between previous therapy and present interview?
Describe any situations or conditions that you associate with the onset of stuttering.
What were the first signs of stuttering (if an adolescent or adult does not remember, they can ask parents or siblings)? Approximately how long did each block seem to last?
Has the type of stuttering and the severity of the stuttering changed over time?
Was the stuttering easy, or was there struggle at the time when the stuttering was first noticed? Has that changed over time?
Were the words that were stuttered at the beginning of sentences, or were they scattered throughout the sentence? Has that changed over time?
When stuttering first began, was there any avoidance of sounds/words/situations? Has that changed over time?

(Continued)

History and development of stuttering
When stuttering was first noticed, what was your (your child's) reaction? (Select the reactions below that apply) ☐ Awareness that speech was different? ≤ Indifference to it? ☐ Surprise? ☐ Anger or frustration? ☐ Fear of stuttering again? ☐ Shame? ☐ Other?
Which of these reactions have changed over time? ☐ Awareness that speech was different? ☐ Indifference to it? ☐ Surprise? ☐ Anger or frustration? ☐ Fear of stuttering again? ☐ Shame? ☐ Other? In what way?
What attempts (if any) have been made to treat the stuttering problem? Be as detailed as possible.
Do you feel that stuttering interferes with any of the following? (Select the ones below that apply) ☐ Social relationships ☐ School life ☐ Job opportunities ☐ Success on the job ☐ Daily life

List the type of dysfluencies: (frequency and duration)

Secondary behaviours:

Breathing pattern:

Normal respiration during rest, speech: Present/absent

(Observe for any shallow breathing, audible inhalations/exhalations, gasping, arhythmical breathing during speaking)

Rate of speech:

Administration of standardized tests: (SSI-4, OASES-A, etc., based on the individual requirement)

Test results:

Provisional diagnosis:
Diagnostic formulation:

Recommendations:

Appendix B

Impact Scale for Assessment of Cluttering and Stuttering (ISACS)

Pallavi Kelkar

Administration:

Although the written instructions given to the respondent in the form are self-explanatory, it is recommended that the clinician orally instruct the respondent as well to ensure complete understanding. Along the same lines, presence of the clinician while the respondent fills the form helps to clarify any queries that might arise while filling the form and ensures that no items are missed.

Scoring: <u>Items 1, 3 and 7 are to be reverse scored.</u> For example, a rating of 1 is converted to 5, a rating of 4 to 2, and a rating of 3 would remain the same. After reverse scoring these items, the clinician just needs to add all the Likert ratings to give a total (raw) score.

The raw score is then converted to a **total (percent) score** using the formula:

$$\frac{Total\ score\ obtained \times 100}{\left(Number\ of\ items\ attempted \times 5\right)}$$

A rating of 5 being the maximum possible rating on each Likert scale, multiplying it by number of items attempted would give the total possible score. **Subscale (percent) scores** can be calculated in a similar manner.

These total and subscale scores can provide the clinician with a profile of the respondent in terms of the bio psychosocial model of the International Classification of Functioning, Disability and Health. This profile as well as individual item scores can serve as pointers to plan goals for intervention or counselling. The scores can also serve as a baseline for outcomes assessment to check whether the therapy approach used is successfully reducing the impact of the fluency disorder and improving quality of life.

The ISACS (B) is scored exactly like ISACS (A), but gives the profile of the person with the fluency disorder through the eyes of their significant other. Discrepancies in profiles on the two forms can be addressed with appropriate counselling. The ISACS (B) also helps the clinician identify barriers and facilitators for improvement.

Impact Scale for Assessment of Cluttering and Stuttering (ISACS)–[A]

Instructions for the respondent

This is a scale which will help us examine different aspects of speech and the effect it has on the way one goes about one's daily life. Please read each statement carefully and circle the appropriate number. If a statement does not apply to you (e.g. "Advancing in your career" when you are not working yet), you may leave it and move on to the next statement. But try not to leave out any statement as far as possible.

Identifying information:

Name: **Age:**   **Gender:**

Education:

Occupation:

Section I (Body functions)

Do you think you speak . . . ?

		Extremely	Very	Somewhat	A little	Not at all
1.	fast	1	2	3	4	5
2.	with pauses, emphasis wherever necessary	1	2	3	4	5
3.	in a flat/monotonous voice	1	2	3	4	5
4.	with a smooth, uninterrupted flow of words	1	2	3	4	5
5.	with clear enunciation of words	1	2	3	4	5
6.	with a proper idea of what you want to say	1	2	3	4	5

How often do you think you . . . ?

		Never	Rarely	Sometimes	Often	Always
7.	sound natural (like everybody else)	1	2	3	4	5
8.	have general body tension while speaking	1	2	3	4	5
9.	have trouble finding words	1	2	3	4	5
10.	have trouble following a long narrative	1	2	3	4	5
11.	attend therapy for improving speech	1	2	3	4	5
12.	use techniques/strategies for improving speech	1	2	3	4	5

Section II (Personal contextual factors)

BEHAVIORAL

How often do you do the following?

		Never	Rarely	Sometimes	Often	Always
1.	Using unnecessary facial grimaces, eye blinks, etc., while speaking	1	2	3	4	5
2.	Using gestures as a substitute for speaking (smiling, nodding)	1	2	3	4	5
3.	Adding an extra or unnecessary sound, word or phrase to help yourself get started (e.g. "I mean", "you know")	1	2	3	4	5
4.	Speaking with great struggle and effort	1	2	3	4	5
5.	Avoiding meeting new people	1	2	3	4	5
6.	Avoiding activities wherever speaking would be a challenging task	1	2	3	4	5
7.	Avoiding certain sounds/words while speaking	1	2	3	4	5
8.	Mumbling while speaking	1	2	3	4	5
9.	Speaking out of turn	1	2	3	4	5
10.	Speaking in a socially inappropriate manner	1	2	3	4	5

COGNITIVE

How often do you experience the following thoughts?

		Never	Rarely	Sometimes	Often	Always
11.	Thinking that you have a speech problem	1	2	3	4	5
12.	Thinking that your speech will never be good enough	1	2	3	4	5
13.	Thinking that you would not be able to speak well (before a speaking situation)	1	2	3	4	5
14.	Thinking that people unnecessarily criticize your speech	1	2	3	4	5
15.	Thinking that you care a lot about the way you speak	1	2	3	4	5
16.	Thinking that people do not listen well when you speak	1	2	3	4	5
17.	Thinking that speaking is very difficult	1	2	3	4	5

AFFECTIVE

How much do you experience each of the following emotions when you think about your speech?

		Not at all	*A little*	*Somewhat*	*Very*	*Extremely*
18.	Self-consciousness	1	2	3	4	5
19.	Anger	1	2	3	4	5
20.	Sadness	1	2	3	4	5
21.	Shame	1	2	3	4	5
22.	Nervousness	1	2	3	4	5
23.	Frustration	1	2	3	4	5
24.	Defensiveness	1	2	3	4	5
25.	Embarrassment	1	2	3	4	5
26.	Guilt	1	2	3	4	5
27.	Loneliness	1	2	3	4	5
28.	Helplessness	1	2	3	4	5

Section III (Activities and environmental factors)

How difficult do you think the following situations would be for you?

	Not at all difficult	*Not very difficult*	*Somewhat difficult*	*Very difficult*	*Extremely difficult*
1. Starting a conversation with one person	1	2	3	4	5
2. Narrating for 2–3 minutes	1	2	3	4	5
3. Introducing oneself to a group of people	1	2	3	4	5
4. Continuing a one-to-one conversation for 10–15 minutes	1	2	3	4	5
5. Continuing a conversation with a group of people for 10–15 minutes	1	2	3	4	5
6. Debating with one person	1	2	3	4	5
7. Participating in a group discussion or debate	1	2	3	4	5
8. Speaking over the telephone	1	2	3	4	5
9. Asking a stranger for directions	1	2	3	4	5
10. Speaking to a person in authority	1	2	3	4	5
11. Chatting with friends	1	2	3	4	5
12. Having a relaxed conversation with a neighbour	1	2	3	4	5
13. Speaking to a colleague/classmate	1	2	3	4	5
14. Speaking to family members	1	2	3	4	5
15. Speaking to someone you know who you have met after a long time	1	2	3	4	5
16. Speaking with members of the extended family	1	2	3	4	5
17. Forming a good impression on someone of the same age group but of the opposite sex	1	2	3	4	5
18. Ordering food in a restaurant	1	2	3	4	5

(Continued)

(Continued)

	Not at all difficult	Not very difficult	Somewhat difficult	Very difficult	Extremely difficult
19. Asking a bus conductor for a ticket	1	2	3	4	5
20. Making an inquiry over a counter	1	2	3	4	5
21. Telling a joke to a group of people	1	2	3	4	5
22. Talking to a child	1	2	3	4	5
23. Speaking to a large crowd over a microphone	1	2	3	4	5
24. Talking to the family doctor	1	2	3	4	5

How do you think the attitudes of the following people would be towards you?

		Extremely positive	Very positive	Somewhat positive	Not very positive	Not at all positive
25.	Family members	1	2	3	4	5
26.	Relatives	1	2	3	4	5
27.	Friends	1	2	3	4	5
28.	Neighbours	1	2	3	4	5
29.	Colleagues/classmates	1	2	3	4	5
30.	Acquaintances	1	2	3	4	5
31.	Superiors	1	2	3	4	5
32.	Subordinates	1	2	3	4	5
33.	Strangers	1	2	3	4	5

How much would the attitudes of the following people matter to you?

		Not at all	A little	Somewhat	A lot	Extremely
34.	Family members	1	2	3	4	5
35.	Relatives	1	2	3	4	5
36.	Friends	1	2	3	4	5
37.	Neighbours	1	2	3	4	5
38.	Colleagues/classmates	1	2	3	4	5
39.	Acquaintances	1	2	3	4	5
40.	Superiors	1	2	3	4	5
41.	Subordinates	1	2	3	4	5
42.	Strangers	1	2	3	4	5

Section IV (Participation/QoL)

How much (if at all) according to you is your speech negatively affecting the following:

		Not at all	A little	Somewhat	A lot	Extremely
1.	Relationships with family members	1	2	3	4	5
2.	Relationships with extended family	1	2	3	4	5
3.	Relationships with friends	1	2	3	4	5
4.	Relationships with colleagues	1	2	3	4	5
5.	Relationships with superiors	1	2	3	4	5
6.	Relationships with neighbours	1	2	3	4	5
7.	Intimate relationships	1	2	3	4	5
8.	Forming new relationships	1	2	3	4	5
9.	School life	1	2	3	4	5
10.	College life	1	2	3	4	5
11.	Getting a suitable job	1	2	3	4	5
12.	Maintaining a job	1	2	3	4	5
13.	Professional relationships	1	2	3	4	5
14.	Advancing in a career	1	2	3	4	5
15.	Social life	1	2	3	4	5
16.	Feeling content with life	1	2	3	4	5
17.	Feeling confident about oneself	1	2	3	4	5
18.	Feeling in control of one's own life	1	2	3	4	5

Number of statements attempted:
Total score:

Impact Scale for Assessment of Cluttering and Stuttering (ISACS) –[B]

Instructions for the respondent

This is a scale which will help us examine different aspects of speech and the effect it has on the way one goes about one's daily life. Please read each statement carefully and circle the appropriate number. If a statement does not apply to this person (e.g. "Advancing in their career" when they are not working yet), you may leave it and move on to the next statement. But try not to leave out any statement as far as possible.

Identifying information:

Name: **Age:**   **Gender:**

Education:

Occupation:

Informing about (name):

Section I (Body functions)

Do you think this person speaks . . . ?

		Extremely	Very	Somewhat	A little	Not at all
1.	fast	1	2	3	4	5
2.	with pauses, emphasis wherever necessary	1	2	3	4	5
3.	in a flat/monotonous voice	1	2	3	4	5
4.	with a smooth, uninterrupted flow of words	1	2	3	4	5
5.	with clear enunciation of words	1	2	3	4	5
6.	with a proper idea of what they want to say	1	2	3	4	5

How often do you think this person . . . ?

		Never	Rarely	Sometimes	Often	Always
7.	sounds natural (like everybody else)	1	2	3	4	5
8.	has general body tension while speaking	1	2	3	4	5
9.	has trouble finding words	1	2	3	4	5
10.	has trouble following a long narrative	1	2	3	4	5
11.	attends therapy for improving speech	1	2	3	4	5
12.	uses techniques/strategies for improving speech	1	2	3	4	5

Section II (Personal contextual factors)

BEHAVIOURAL

How often do you think this person does the following?

		Never	Rarely	Sometimes	Often	Always
1.	Using unnecessary facial grimaces, eye blinks, etc., while speaking	1	2	3	4	5
2.	Using gestures as a substitute for speaking (smiling, nodding)	1	2	3	4	5
3.	Adding an extra or unnecessary sound, word or phrase to help yourself get started (e.g. "I mean", "you know")	1	2	3	4	5
4.	Speaking with great struggle and effort	1	2	3	4	5
5.	Avoiding meeting new people	1	2	3	4	5
6.	Avoiding activities wherever speaking would be a challenging task	1	2	3	4	5
7.	Avoiding certain sounds/words while speaking	1	2	3	4	5
8.	Mumbling while speaking	1	2	3	4	5
9.	Speaking out of turn	1	2	3	4	5
10.	Speaking in a socially inappropriate manner	1	2	3	4	5

COGNITIVE

How often do you think this person experiences the following thoughts?

		Never	Rarely	Sometimes	Often	Always
11.	Thinking that they have a speech problem	1	2	3	4	5
12.	Thinking that their speech will never be good enough	1	2	3	4	5
13.	Thinking that they would not be able to speak well (before a speaking situation)	1	2	3	4	5
14.	Thinking that people unnecessarily criticize their speech	1	2	3	4	5
15.	Thinking that they care a lot about the way they speak	1	2	3	4	5
16.	Thinking that people do not listen well when they speak	1	2	3	4	5
17.	Thinking that speaking is very difficult	1	2	3	4	5

AFFECTIVE

How much do you think this person experiences each of the following emotions when they think about their speech?

		Not at all	A little	Somewhat	Very	Extremely
18.	Self-consciousness	1	2	3	4	5
19.	Anger	1	2	3	4	5
20.	Sadness	1	2	3	4	5
21.	Shame	1	2	3	4	5
22.	Nervousness	1	2	3	4	5
23.	Frustration	1	2	3	4	5
24.	Defensiveness	1	2	3	4	5
25.	Embarrassment	1	2	3	4	5
26.	Guilt	1	2	3	4	5
27.	Loneliness	1	2	3	4	5
28.	Helplessness	1	2	3	4	5

Section III (Activities and environmental factors)

How difficult do you think the following situations would be for this person?

	Not at all difficult	Not very difficult	Somewhat difficult	Very difficult	Extremely difficult
1. Starting a conversation with one person	1	2	3	4	5
2. Narrating for 2–3 minutes	1	2	3	4	5
3. Introducing oneself to a group of people	1	2	3	4	5
4. Continuing a one-to-one conversation for 10–15 minutes	1	2	3	4	5
5. Continuing a conversation with a group of people for 10–15 minutes	1	2	3	4	5
6. Debating with one person	1	2	3	4	5
7. Participating in a group discussion or debate	1	2	3	4	5
8. Speaking over the telephone	1	2	3	4	5
9. Asking a stranger for directions	1	2	3	4	5
10. Speaking to a person in authority	1	2	3	4	5
11. Chatting with friends	1	2	3	4	5
12. Having a relaxed conversation with a neighbour	1	2	3	4	5
13. Speaking to a colleague/classmate	1	2	3	4	5
14. Speaking to family members	1	2	3	4	5
15. Speaking to someone they know who they have met after a long time	1	2	3	4	5
16. Speaking with members of the extended family	1	2	3	4	5
17. Forming a good impression on someone of the same age group but of the opposite sex	1	2	3	4	5
18. Ordering food in a restaurant	1	2	3	4	5

(Continued)

(Continued)

	Not at all difficult	Not very difficult	Somewhat difficult	Very difficult	Extremely difficult
19. Asking a bus conductor for a ticket	1	2	3	4	5
20. Making an inquiry over a counter	1	2	3	4	5
21. Telling a joke to a group of people	1	2	3	4	5
22. Talking to a child	1	2	3	4	5
23. Speaking to a large crowd over a microphone	1	2	3	4	5
24. Talking to the family doctor	1	2	3	4	5

How do you think the attitudes of the following people would be towards this person?

		Extremely positive	Very positive	Somewhat positive	Not very positive	Not at all positive
25.	Family members	1	2	3	4	5
26.	Relatives	1	2	3	4	5
27.	Friends	1	2	3	4	5
28.	Neighbours	1	2	3	4	5
29.	Colleagues/classmates	1	2	3	4	5
30.	Acquaintances	1	2	3	4	5
31.	Superiors	1	2	3	4	5
32.	Subordinates	1	2	3	4	5
33.	Strangers	1	2	3	4	5

How much would the attitudes of the following people matter to this person?

		Not at all	A little	Somewhat	A lot	Extremely
34.	Family members	1	2	3	4	5
35.	Relatives	1	2	3	4	5
36.	Friends	1	2	3	4	5
37.	Neighbours	1	2	3	4	5
38.	Colleagues/classmates	1	2	3	4	5
39.	Acquaintances	1	2	3	4	5
40.	Superiors	1	2	3	4	5
41.	Subordinates	1	2	3	4	5
42.	Strangers	1	2	3	4	5

Section IV (Participation/QoL)

How much do you think this person's speech is negatively affecting the following?

		Not at all	A little	Somewhat	A lot	Extremely
1.	Relationships with family members	1	2	3	4	5
2.	Relationships with extended family	1	2	3	4	5
3.	Relationships with friends	1	2	3	4	5
4.	Relationships with colleagues	1	2	3	4	5
5.	Relationships with superiors	1	2	3	4	5
6.	Relationships with neighbours	1	2	3	4	5
7.	Intimate relationships	1	2	3	4	5
8.	Forming new relationships	1	2	3	4	5
9.	School life	1	2	3	4	5
10.	College life	1	2	3	4	5
11.	Getting a suitable job	1	2	3	4	5
12.	Maintaining a job	1	2	3	4	5
13.	Professional relationships	1	2	3	4	5
14.	Advancing in a career	1	2	3	4	5
15.	Social life	1	2	3	4	5
16.	Feeling content with life	1	2	3	4	5
17.	Feeling confident about oneself	1	2	3	4	5
18.	Feeling in control of one's own life	1	2	3	4	5

Number of statements attempted:
Total score:

Index

Note: Pages numbers in **bold** denote tables and *italics* denote figures.